Clinical D␣
Making in Optometry

Clinical Decision Making in Optometry

Edited by

Ellen Richter Ettinger, O.D., M.S., F.A.A.O.

Associate Professor of Optometry, Department of Clinical Sciences, State University of New York State College of Optometry, New York

Michael W. Rouse, O.D., M.S.Ed., F.A.A.O.

Professor of Optometry and Chief, Vision Therapy Service, Southern California College of Optometry, Fullerton

With a Foreword by

Richard L. Hopping, O.D., D.O.S. (Hon.), D.Sc. (Hon.)

President, Southern California College of Optometry, Fullerton

Butterworth–Heinemann

Boston   Oxford   Johannesburg   Melbourne   New Delhi   Singapore

Library of Congress Cataloging-in-Publication Data
Clinical decision making in optometry / edited by Ellen Richter
Ettinger, Michael W. Rouse ; with a foreword by Richard Hopping.
p.   cm.
Includes bibliographical references and index.
ISBN 0-7506-9571-4 (alk. paper)
1. Optometry—Decision making.   2. Optometry—Case studies.
I. Ettinger, Ellen Richter.   II. Rouse, Michael W.
[DNLM: 1. Optometry—methods.   2. Vision Disorders—diagnosis.
3. Vision Disorders—rehabilitation.   4. Decision Making.   WW 704
C6405   1996]
RE952.C57   1996
617.7'5—dc20
DNLM/DLC   96-30120
for Library of Congress   CIP

British Library Cataloguing-in-Publication Data
A catalogue record for this book is available from the British Library.

The publisher offers special discounts on bulk orders of this book.

For information, please contact:
Manager of Special Sales
Butterworth–Heinemann
313 Washington Street
Newton, MA 02158-1626
Tel: 617-928-2500
Fax: 617-928-2620

For information on all medical publications available, contact our World Wide Web
home page at: http://www.bh.com/med

10 9 8 7 6 5 4 3 2 1

Printed in the United States of America

To Henry, Lori, my parents, my sister, and my family for their love and support

E.R.E.

To Janet, Kayla, and my parents for their love and support

M.W.R.

Give a man a fish and you have fed him a meal. Teach a man to fish and you have taught him to survive.

Anonymous

Teach a student to handle one case and you have helped with one patient. Teach a student to think and you have prepared him or her for a career of life-long thinking and helping patients.

Ettinger and Rouse

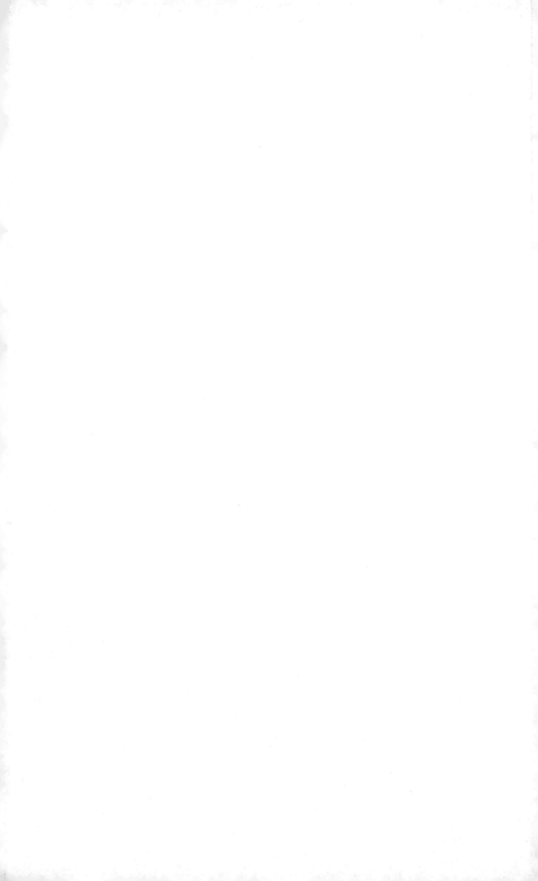

Contents

Contributing Authors

Eric Borsting, O.D., M.S., F.A.A.O.
Assistant Professor of Clinical Science, Southern California College of Optometry, Fullerton

Jerry D. Cavallerano, O.D., Ph.D., F.A.A.O.
Associate Professor of Optometry, The New England College of Optometry, Boston; Staff Optometrist, Beetham Eye Institute, Joslin Diabetes Center, Boston

Michael H. Cho, O.D., F.A.A.O.
Assistant Professor of Optometry, and Director of Optical Service, University of Alabama at Birmingham School of Optometry, Birmingham

Susan A. Cotter, O.D., F.A.A.O.
Associate Professor of Clinical Education, Illinois College of Optometry, Chicago

Timothy B. Edrington, O.D., M.S., F.A.A.O.
Professor and Chief, Cornea and Contact Lens Service, Southern California College of Optometry, Fullerton

Kia B. Eldred, O.D., F.A.A.O.
Visiting Assistant Professor of Optometry, University of Houston College of Optometry, Houston; Consultant, Head Injury Unit, The Institute for Rehabilitation and Research, Houston

Ellen Richter Ettinger, O.D., M.S., F.A.A.O.
Associate Professor of Optometry, Department of Clinical Sciences, State University of New York State College of Optometry, New York

Robin B. Fogel, M.L.S.
Assistant Librarian, Harold Kohn Vision Science Library, State University of New York State College of Optometry, New York

John B. Gelvin, O.D., F.A.A.O.
Adjunct Assistant Professor of Optometry, Indiana University School of Optometry, Bloomington; Medical Director, Faust-Gelvin Eye Center, Fort Wayne, Indiana

Elizabeth Hoppe, O.D., M.P.H., F.A.A.O.
Assistant Professor of Optometry, Southern California College of Optometry, Fullerton; Consultant, Foothill Center for the Partially Sighted, Foothill Presbyterian Hospital, Glendora, California

Alan G. Kabat, O.D.
Assistant Professor of Optometry and Attending Optometric Physician, University Eye Center, NOVA Southeastern University, North Miami Beach, Florida

Daniel Kurtz, O.D., Ph.D., F.A.A.O.
Professor of Optometry, Department of Clinical Skills and Practice, The New England College of Optometry, Boston

Gerald E. Lowther, O.D., Ph.D., F.A.A.O.
Professor of Optometry, Indiana University School of Optometry, Bloomington

Claudia A. Perry, M.L.S., Ph.D.
Head Librarian, Harold Kohn Vision Science Library, State University of New York State College of Optometry, New York

Michael W. Rouse, O.D., M.S.Ed., F.A.A.O.
Professor of Optometry and Chief, Vision Therapy Service, Southern California College of Optometry, Fullerton

Mitchell M. Scheiman, O.D., F.A.A.O.
Professor of Optometry and Chief, Pediatric/Binocular Vision Service, Pennsylvania College of Optometry, Philadelphia

Cristina M. Schnider, O.D., M.Sc., F.A.A.O.
Associate Professor of Optometry, The Pacific University College of Optometry, Forest Grove, Oregon

Dennis W. Siemsen, O.D., M.H.P.E., F.A.A.O.
Assistant Dean for Patient Care, Department of Clinical Education, Illinois College of Optometry, Chicago

Joel A. Silbert, O.D., F.A.A.O.
Associate Professor of Optometry and Director, Cornea and Specialty Contact Lens Service, The Eye Institute, Pennsylvania College of Optometry, Philadelphia

Dennis L. Smith, O.D., M.S.
Associate Professor of Optometry, The Pacific University College of Optometry, Forest Grove, Oregon

Joseph Sowka, O.D., F.A.A.O.
Associate Professor of Optometry and Attending Optometric Physician, University Eye Center, NOVA Southeastern University, North Miami Beach, Florida

Carole A. Timpone, O.D., F.A.A.O.
Associate Clinical Professor of Optometry, The Pacific University College of Optometry, Forest Grove, Oregon; Director of Clinic, Pacific University Family Vision Center, and Chief of Ocular Disease and Special Testing Service, The Eye Surgery Center at Pacific University, Portland, Oregon

Foreword

The clinician's ability to properly diagnose, treat, and manage conditions within the scope of his or her practice is critical to the successful delivery of ethical, high-quality care to every patient.

The optometric profession is in a state of ongoing transformation as a result of changes to the educational curriculum, new research, improved technology, and the numerous legislative and administrative changes at the state and federal levels. The identification of the optometrist as a primary care provider has also increased the profession's fundamental responsibilities.

Every practitioner in a primary care profession must be able to take care of most of the problems presented by most of the people most of the time. If a particular patient's problems are not within the practitioner's scope of practice, it is the practitioner's responsibility to refer the patient to another clinician.

With the ever-increasing scope of optometric practice, new graduates, as well as established optometrists, are expected to do everything in their power to properly and efficiently diagnose, treat, and manage the varied eye and vision conditions presented by their patients. This requires the collection of meaningful data and proper clinical decision making as we combine old knowledge with the new knowledge obtained through education, optometric research, and the literature.

Ellen Richter Ettinger and Michael Rouse are to be commended for their pioneering efforts and leadership in developing a text that will be of invaluable assistance to both the student and practitioner in enhancing their clinical decision-making skills. They have made a significant contribution to the optometric literature. Included in the text are various models of clinical decision making (algorithmic reasoning, pattern recognition, and hypothetico-deductive method) that emphasize that clinical decision making must be an active process.

The authors have included a section on the various stages of diagnostic reasoning and highlighted a number of common errors in clinical decision making, with examples to illustrate their point. Clinical testing should assist the practitioner in diagnosis, monitoring of patient management and therapy, and the establishment of a database of information on the patient. A number of helpful maxims, which can be used as guidelines to ensure effective clinical decision making, are included. The authors effectively address the issue of clinical uncertainty and provide techniques and strategies for addressing that uncertainty.

The practical discussion of epidemiology demonstrates how the process of clinical decision making can be improved through the practitioner's application of the principles of epidemiology. A number of examples are presented to prove this point. A practical approach to the problem of information access and management in the clinical setting directs the clinician to the appropriate information-management skills essential to the delivery of high-quality patient care.

It is appropriate and encouraging to find that the authors have also included a chapter on ethical decision making. In addition to the four principles of biomedical ethics, a set of guideline statements pertaining to the ethical delivery of clinical care is provided.

One of the unique and positive features of this text is that the largest portion of the book consists of a significant number of practical case scenarios prepared by an array of distinguished clinical optometrists. This approach exposes the reader to the thought processes—from start to finish of each case—of the author. For the student or practitioner who has not yet learned a structured approach to clinical decision making, the text, accompanied by helpful flow charts, is available for future review, study, analysis, and debate to assist the clinician in the development of his or her decision-making skills.

Richard L. Hopping

Preface

How do optometrists make clinical decisions? Patients enter the doctor's office with symptoms, referred to as presenting problems. Through a process that is still not understood completely, the astute practitioner evaluates the patient's symptoms, conducts an examination, arrives at a diagnosis, and develops a patient management plan. How does the optometric student learn to accomplish this task?

Students initially receive academic training that concentrates on the visual biology and pathophysiology of clinical conditions. Preclinical training then prepares the student for the hands-on skill to administer examination techniques necessary for making clinical observations and collecting clinical data. It is assumed that the student will integrate these preclinical skills and knowledge (often by osmosis) and enter clinical care functioning as an effective diagnostician. Unfortunately, patients' presenting complaints are often abstract and vague. In addition, patients with the same clinical condition frequently present with different descriptions of their problems and may not always present with the classic syndrome of clinical findings. The clinical uncertainty surrounding patient care complicates the decision-making process, expecially for the new and inexperienced clinician.

The goal of this book is to examine the process of clinical decision making in vision care, in an effort to help students and optometrists develop and refine their decision-making skills. We acknowledge that learning to make clinical decisions is an active process in which clinical examples are essential.

In Part I, the principles used in clinical decision making are explored. The chapters in this section investigate models of clinical decision making, dealing with clinical uncertainty, using epidemiology in making clinical decisions, accessing the biomedical literature, and making ethical clinical decisions. Brief clinical examples are used to illustrate underlying issues and concepts.

In Part II, clinical decision making is viewed within the context of expert clinicians solving the underlying cause of a series of entering patient complaints. These clinical scenarios use 18 common clinical conditions to illustrate the decision-making process. Each clinician presents an entering clinical scenario, develops a working hypotheses list, and discusses the thinking that leads to selecting problem-specific data to rule in or out each hypothesis and why certain other data is needed for database or baseline evaluation. The clinical decision-making process is then summarized in a flow chart.

The chapters for Part II are listed in the table of contents as case scenario numbers, not by topic or diagnosis, so we do not give the patient's diagnostic identity away. This will allow the reader to experience the thought processes of the author of each scenario as he or she investigates the patient's problem. A full list of the case scenarios, with the final diagnosis, is available in the Appendix, for those who wish to reread and reference specific cases. (For educational purposes, this may be especially useful for clinical faculty members and students.) In addition, the cases are not grouped or ordered by diagnostic categories (e.g., binocular problems, ocular pathology) in order to simulate actual clinical encounters, which are variable.

It is hoped that the information presented in this book will help take some of the mystery out of decision making and introduce some practical and useful strategies that can be used to provide care to patients.

E.R.E.
M.W.R.

Acknowledgments

We express our appreciation to Barbara Murphy and Karen Oberheim of Butterworth–Heinemann for their support and dedication to this project. Appreciation is also extended to Patricia T. Carlson for her assistance with book references, and to Wayne Grofik for his help with some figures in Part I.

E.R.E.
M.W.R.

I

Principles

1

Clinical Decision-Making Skills

Ellen Richter Ettinger

In order to help patients, good clinical reasoning skills are essential. Through rigorous training, clinicians learn to perform tests and use clinical equipment. This is the technical component of clinical care. It is what the clinician *does* with this information that is usually more complex.

The diagnostic thinking process has been compared to juggling while climbing a ladder.[1] The clinician keeps juggling background knowledge, observation skills, and reasoning abilities as he or she climbs steps on a ladder. As more information is obtained through case history and examination, additional steps are taken up the ladder, until a diagnosis is reached.

Albert and colleagues[2] considered the image of the clinician as a detective, carefully gathering and evaluating evidence suggestive of diseases. They point out, however, that conclusive evidence may be obtained in some cases only by autopsy or life-threatening procedures—too high a price to pay for a definite diagnosis. They also look at the diagnostician as an artist, having a special talent for doing the right thing at the right time, making subtle observations, asking the right questions, and pursuing lines of inquiry while remaining open to new possibilities.

Although none of these images alone may be sufficient to explain the clinical decision-making process, each contributes to an appreciation of the complex responsibilities and skills involved in this process. This chapter examines models of clinical decision making, steps involved in the decision-making process, common errors in diagnostic reasoning, factors that contribute to a doctor's diagnostic skills, and clinical "pearls" used in decision making. The goal is to assist the reader in becoming better at decision making in the clinical environment.

MODELS OF CLINICAL DECISION MAKING

What process do doctors use in making clinical diagnoses? Three models of clinical decision making have been described: algorithmic reasoning, pattern recognition (template matching), and hypothetico-deductive reasoning.[3–7]

Algorithmic Reasoning

The thinking process involved in algorithmic reasoning is usually demonstrated by a diagram or table that shows a sequence of questions with a number of possible paths. The answer to each question determines the pathway to follow. It is as if the doctor follows an internal flow sheet with decision points and subsequent steps that lead to a diagnosis. Figure 1.1 illustrates a series of questions appropriate for investigating the cause in a patient who presents with complaints of a red eye. These questions are concerned with the location of the redness (e.g., subconjunctival, conjunctival, or scleral-episcleral; eyelids), the presence of pain, the presence and type of discharge, recent history of upper respiratory infection (URI), history of allergies, presence of inflamed preauricular nodes, and presence of itching.

A strength of the algorithmic reasoning model is that it reflects a logical method in which the characteristics and associated factors of a clinical problem are considered carefully in determining a diagnosis. A shortcoming of this model is that it suggests that a *specific* sequence is followed in determining the diagnosis for a particular problem. For example, Figure 1.1 indicates that, in making a diagnosis of bacterial conjunctivitis, a sequence of questions about location of redness, pain, and discharge is pursued. In actual clinical practice, not every patient fits into the algorithm as illustrated, and the sequence of questions for investigating the problem may differ depending on the patient's presenting symptoms. If the patient comes in with a chief complaint of a sticky, yellow discharge, the characteristic of discharge is handled before an inquiry about pain. However, the model is helpful as a didactic tool to illustrate examples of reasoning sequences that can be used, as well as to demonstrate that clinical decision making is a logical, sequential (albeit variable) process.

Pattern Recognition

In pattern recognition, a diagnosis is made instantaneously as a doctor realizes that the patient's presentation conforms to a previously learned picture (or pattern) of disease.[3] The point of recognition when the

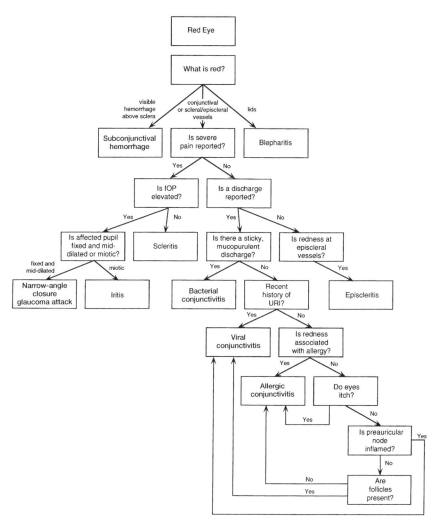

Figure 1.1 Algorithm for diagnosing the problem when the complaint is a red eye. (IOP = intraocular pressure; URI = upper respiratory infection.)

match is identified has been described as a sudden "a-ha" experience.[4] Pattern recognition generally occurs when a clinical diagnosis has a very recognizable pattern that is easily differentiated from other presenting patterns.

Examples of pattern recognition that occur in the eye care environment include cases of subconjunctival hemorrhage, Graves' disease, and albinism (tyrosine-negative). The visibility of blood above the sclera and below the conjunctiva in the case of the subconjunctival hemorrhage, the bilateral exophthalmos observed in the patient with Graves' disease, and the lack of pigment in the albino patient's skin and hair make these cases easily recognizable. Sackett and colleagues[3] also consider cafe au lait spots in neurofibromatosis, skin signs of psoriasis, and lesions in herpes zoster as readily recognizable patterns: That is, the observation of the patient is easily matched to a template in the clinician's memory.

Pattern recognition usually involves visual cues, although it may also involve auditory or tactile cues, as in cases of speech disorder or prominent tumors, respectively. Tables are sometimes used to identify the prominent features of clinical problems (Table 1.1). The salient features—for example, the obvious visible blood of the subconjunctival hemorrhage—are usually the ones that are immediately obvious to the doctor and lead to the quick "a-ha" or "I know what it is" response. The sticky, yellow discharge of bacterial conjunctivitis stands out as an identifying feature of that disorder. Viral conjunctivitis, however, has features that are much less prominent and much less likely to be recognized instantaneously.

Although pattern recognition may be effective in identifying diseases that are easily recognizable and distinguishable from other disease entities, it is not the most efficacious process in diagnosing conditions with less distinctive features.

Hypothetico-Deductive Method

The hypothetico-deductive method involves generating (early in the clinical encounter) a list of possible diagnoses (or working hypotheses) that correspond with a patient's presenting symptoms, and collecting data during the examination sequence to test these hypotheses. As data are gathered, some hypotheses are reinforced, some are rejected, and other new ones are generated. A cyclic, reiterative process of continuing data collection and testing hypotheses occurs until a final diagnosis is made. This is the process of *differential diagnosis*.

Studies in which physicians were asked to describe their thinking process in making a diagnosis suggest that the hypothetico-deductive strategy is the process used by most clinicians.[3] Studies of internists found that the first hypothesis was generated an average of 28 seconds after the chief complaint was heard and the correct hypothesis was generated from 1 to 7 minutes into the examination, with some variation across different clinical cases.[8] Another study provided insights into the point at which clinicians-in-training start to use the hypothetico-deductive method. Neufeld and colleagues[9] found that even students in their first year of medical school started generating hypotheses within approximately 30 seconds of hearing the patient's chief complaint and that, like

Table 1.1
Differential diagnosis of red eye.

	Visual Acuity	Discharge	Pertinent History, Description of Pain	Distinctive Clinical Findings	Pupil	Cornea
Subconjunctival hemorrhage	Normal	—	Hx of Valsalva maneuver common	Visible hemorrhage	Normal	Normal
Conjunctivitis						
Bacterial	Normal	Purulent	Irritated, matting of lids on awakening	Yellow, purulent discharge	Normal	Normal
Viral	Normal	Watery (thick)	Recent upper respiratory infection common	Follicles on lids, preauricular nodes	Normal	Normal
Allergic	Normal	Watery (thinner)	Itching, may have Hx of allergy, usually bilateral	Redness; thin, watery discharge	Normal	Normal
Acute iritis	Decreased	—	Severe pain, photophobia	Cells and flare in anterior chamber; variable IOP (high or normal), ciliary flush	Pupils small (miotic) and fixed	Sometimes cloudy
Acute angle-closure glaucoma	Decreased	—	Severe pain, photophobia, vomiting	Elevated IOP, steamy cornea, ciliary flush	Pupils large (mid-dilated) and fixed	Steamy

Table 1.1
(continued)

	Visual Acuity	Discharge	Pertinent History, Description of Pain	Distinctive Clinical Findings	Pupil	Cornea
Blepharitis	Normal	—	Itching	Lids red and irritated	Normal	Normal
Episcleritis	Normal	—	Mild pain	Sector redness (usually) of bulbar Conjunctiva and underlying epi-scleral tissue (but can be diffuse)	Normal	Normal
Scleritis	Variable	—	Deep pain, frequently associated with systemic connective tissue disorders	Diffuse redness and swelling of sclera	Normal or small	Normal
Contact dermatitis	Normal	—	Lid itching, Hx of contact with allergic substance (e.g., new eye cosmetics, skin moisturizers, nail polish)	Redness and dryness around lids	Normal	Normal

Hx = history; IOP = intraocular pressure.

the experienced doctors, they generated approximately five or six hypotheses during the clinical encounter. Notable differences were that experienced clinicians were more likely than early medical students to generate the correct hypothesis, to generate it earlier in the examination, to generate more specific hypotheses, and to consider other alternative hypotheses during the examination that were probably more related to the patient's problem.[9]

The hypothetico-deductive method does *not* involve an exhaustive listing of potential hypotheses that may be present but a list of *likely* hypotheses based on the patient's signs and symptoms. The number of hypotheses considered during the examination varies as some are rejected, reinforced, and added. For each clinical sign or symptom, extensive lists of all potential diagnoses can be considered,[10] but it is believed that the clinician considers the most likely set of possibilities based on the patient's entering symptoms and the available clinical profile at any point in the examination. It also is believed that clinicians consider only three to five hypotheses at a time because more than that is too many to store in short-term memory.[6, 7]

Although the hypothetico-deductive process is considered the strategy used most by clinicians, pattern recognition may help elicit hypotheses in cases of highly recognizable conditions.[3] It is reasonable to expect, however, that the clinician would continue to test and obtain data to confirm the likely hypothesis.

A modified type of pattern recognition sometimes occurs when a match is made to a template in the clinician's memory after some case history and clinical testing have taken place. A number of hypotheses may be considered, and case history information and data are gathered by the clinician. At some point, a match is found between the pattern of symptoms and clinical findings of a patient and a template of a particular etiology. Although instantaneous recognition at the *onset* of the clinical encounter may not occur, the point of recognition (the "a-ha" moment) is still significant.

Tables sometimes are used to display the significant features of diagnostic categories that have some similar features (e.g., red eye; see Table 1.1). Part of the diagnostic process is choosing which of the diagnoses in these tables is most likely and then comparing the characteristics of the patient's condition with the special features of the most-likely group. An initial symptom—for example, red eye—may elicit a category of diagnostic classifications. For example, in Case Scenario 4 in Part II, the patient presents with symptoms of ocular irritation and a red eye, and the doctor's initial hypothesis is conjunctivitis. (If the patient had complained of severe pain, the initial hypotheses would more likely have included a narrow-angle glaucoma attack, iritis, or

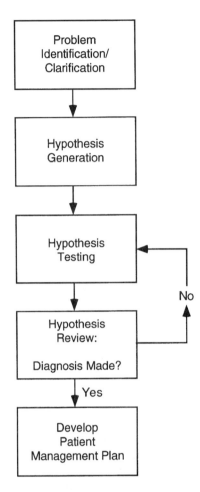

Figure 1.2 Five steps of diagnostic reasoning.

scleritis.) The doctor then proceeds to differentiate the problem by asking about the significant features of the three types of conjunctivitis. A sticky yellow discharge would strongly suggest the presence of a bacterial conjunctivitis. Recent occurrence of a URI would increase the likelihood of a viral conjunctivitis. A history or knowledge of an allergy would increase the probability of an allergic conjunctivitis. Clinical testing is performed to confirm the doctor's working hypothesis. (The final diagnosis can be determined by reading Case Scenario 4.)

DIAGNOSTIC REASONING

Diagnostic reasoning usually involves five stages (Figure 1.2).

Stage 1: Problem Identification and Clarification

The clinician's first opportunity to identify that the patient has a problem is at the onset of the examination, during the case history. The patient's chief (or entering) complaint may contribute much to the clinician's knowledge of the problem, or the major problem may be elicited further into the case history. In many patient encounters, first mention of a problem is nonspecific (e.g., eyes hurt, blurred vision). At this point, the doctor must ask additional questions to define the problem more clearly. It is the clinician's improved understanding of the patient's problem during the case history that allows him or her to start generating relevant hypotheses. For example, a patient may first express that his or her eyes hurt (nonspecific complaint). By discussing the complaint further with the patient during the case history, the doctor more clearly identifies and clarifies the patient's problem. The doctor may determine that the patient's complaint (e.g., eyes hurt) is eye fatigue, a foreign-body sensation, or actual eye pain. The clinician's improved articulation of the problem during the case history, and before beginning the clinical examination, enables him or her to consider effectively the etiology of the problem.

Many student clinicians move on to the examination sequence before understanding the patient's problems and symptoms clearly, which is counterproductive with regard to efficient diagnostic reasoning. Skilled diagnosticians usually obtain a high-level understanding of the patient's problem early in the patient encounter, before the case history ends. This first step in effective diagnostic reasoning prepares them for identifying the most probable hypotheses. Good case history and interviewing skills are essential to this task.[11]

Stage 2: Hypothesis Generation

Once the doctor understands the patient's problem, he or she can generate a list of possible working hypotheses. The hypotheses are based on the patient's complaints, the patient profile (age, gender, racial or ethnic background, occupation, environmental factors), and the doctor's knowledge of disease and epidemiology.

Stage 3: Hypothesis Testing

Through further inquiry in the case history and testing in the clinical examination sequence, the doctor gathers information that enables him or her to test the various hypotheses being considered. Some hypotheses are kept on the list, some are ruled out, and others are added as new data are collected.

Stage 4: Hypothesis Review—Diagnosis Made?

When an adequate level of certainty is reached, given the clinical information obtained, a diagnosis is made. Until this point, the doctor continues to gather information to make a proper diagnosis. Information obtained after this point is usually for the purpose of gathering a more extensive database on the patient's ocular status (e.g., refractive status, ocular health, binocular status) or monitoring a patient's progress over time.

Stage 5: Developing a Patient Management Plan

Once a diagnosis is made, the doctor can determine an appropriate patient management plan. This will depend on the diagnosis, the patient's particular condition level (e.g., early versus late diagnosis of glaucoma), the possible treatment or management options available, and other unique factors of the patient such as age, family history, medical history, and occupational requirements.

DIFFERENTIAL DIAGNOSIS

The term *differential diagnosis* has several meanings. As a noun, it refers to the doctor's list of likely hypotheses that may be attributed to the patient's presenting signs and symptoms.[4] For example, for the patient presenting with a red eye in Case Scenario 4, the differential diagnosis is conjunctivitis, iritis, and narrow-angle glaucoma attack. These are the clinical conditions most likely present, given the patient's symptoms.

Used as a verb, *performing a differential diagnosis* refers to the process of gathering clinical information to test the working hypotheses that have been identified, and finally determining the actual diagnosis. This is the cyclic process of hypothesis generation, data collection, and hypothesis testing illustrated in Figure 1.2. It is believed that clinicians usually consider four to six hypotheses at a time; more than that is too much to keep in short-term memory.[6, 7] Therefore, a clinician would not be expected to generate an exhaustive list of possible hypotheses, but to come up with a short list of the most likely hypotheses. The number of hypotheses generated during a clinical encounter is usually five to seven.[6–9]

In some cases, a general category is considered and, as more information is obtained, the clinician narrows the search and considers more specific classifications. For example, for a patient with the initial symptom of a red eye, the initial hypothesis is conjunctivitis. With more specific data, the clinician can consider and assess more specific categories such as bacterial conjunctivitis, allergic conjunctivitis, and viral conjunctivitis.

HYPOTHESIS GENERATION AND TESTING

Hypothesis generation and testing has been discussed and described by several sources.[2-9, 12] A diagram of the five-stage diagnostic process just described is presented in Figure 1.3. As shown, an initial list of possible hypotheses is generated early in the clinical encounter to correspond with the patient's presenting signs and symptoms. During the clinical testing sequence, as hypotheses are tested, some are reinforced and continue through the decision-making process as likely categories. Some are rejected and crossed out. In some cases, initial categories that are broad can become more specific as testing continues (e.g., H2 in Figure 1.3, which becomes H2A and H2B). In addition to the generation of more specific categories from initial ones, other totally new hypotheses are identified to address new clinical information (e.g., H5 and H6 in Figure 1.3).

Figure 1.4 illustrates hypothesis generation and testing for a clinical case involving a patient with a red eye. The clinical diagnoses considered are shown as they are generated, confirmed, eliminated, and determined as final. Similar flow charts will be provided with the cases in Part II of this book to illustrate how hypotheses are generated, eliminated (ruled out), and confirmed (ruled in).

COMMON ERRORS OF CLINICAL DECISION MAKING

In addition to discussing models of decision making and the steps involved, it has been suggested that demonstrating common errors of decision making is a useful didactic tool.[13, 14] By understanding common barriers to good decision making, students can become conscious of avoiding these types of problems. A number of common error patterns are discussed in this section (Table 1.2).

Premature Closure (Freezing)

Premature closure occurs when the clinician draws conclusions before adequate information is available to settle on a diagnosis. Early in the clinical encounter, the clinician observes some clinical symptom or sign

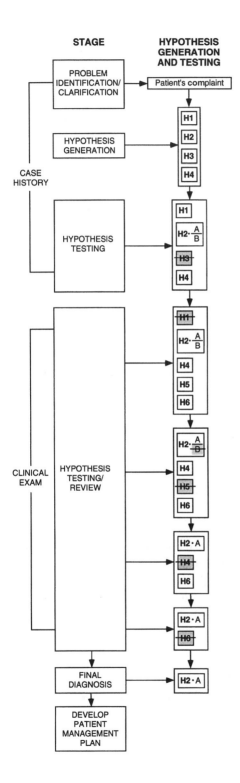

Figure 1.3 Hypotheses are reinforced (ruled in), eliminated (ruled out), and confirmed (final diagnosis) during hypothesis testing and generation.

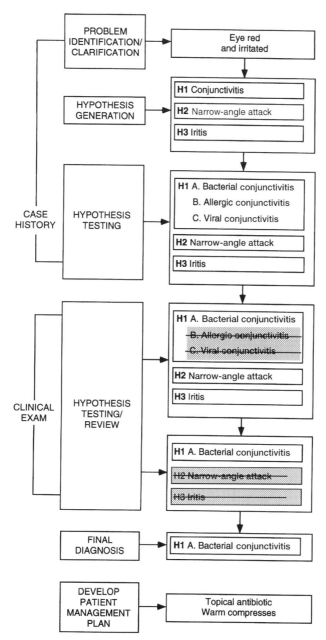

Figure 1.4 An example of hypothesis generation and testing for a case of a patient presenting with a red eye.

Table 1.2
Common errors of clinical decision making.

Premature closure (freezing)	Conclusions about hypotheses are made before adequate information is available, and the search is stopped.
Anchoring	Conclusions about hypotheses are made before adequate information is available, and additional relevant information is ignored.
Pseudodiagnosticity	There is active data collection, but the data do not result in a diagnosis.
Inadequate synthesis	Information is not put together fully, and conclusions that could be made from the data are not made.
Incorrect synthesis	Information is put together incorrectly, and an erroneous conclusion is drawn.
Technical nonsynthesis	Extensive, painstaking collection of data occurs; diagnostic decision making begins after all data are collected.
Patient unfamiliarity	Relevant information about the patient is not considered.
Representative heuristic	The clinician fails to make a proper diagnosis because the patient's sign and symptom complex does not correspond with the clinician's internal representation of the condition.
Availability heuristic	A doctor's atypical experience in seeing patients with a condition erroneously affects the estimate of probability used in future patients who may (or may not) have that particular problem.
Anchoring and adjustment heuristic	A doctor's initial probability estimate (based on early evidence from the anchor) is not adjusted sufficiently to formulate a revised probability, in spite of new information that becomes available later in the examination.

that suggests a particular diagnosis. *Freezing* is said to occur if he or she settles on this diagnosis before adequate data are available to support (or disconfirm) it.

Example
A 63-year-old man presents with complaints of blurred vision. He has been a diabetic for 7 years and reports that he recently has forgotten to take his medication for the diabetes on several occasions. Premature closure occurs if the clinician surmises that the patient has diabetic retinopathy, ignoring other possibilities including cataracts, macular

degeneration, a regular (non–diabetes-induced) change in refractive error, and other potential problems resulting in blurred vision.

Anchoring

Anchoring occurs when the clinician holds onto an early piece of information that leads to a diagnosis associated with that detail, ignoring other useful and relevant facts. This prevents the clinician from making an appropriate diagnosis. Like premature closure, anchoring involves retaining an early hypothesis and making a decision on the basis of inadequate data. However, in anchoring, the clinician continues to gather data but ignores relevant data that does not confirm his or her presumed diagnosis, whereas in premature closure the doctor stops gathering information because he or she believes that the appropriate diagnosis has already been identified correctly. Anchoring is an example of the phenomenon that we tend to see what we look for and ignore what we do not want (or expect) to see.

Example
A 69-year-old man presents for an eye examination complaining of blurred vision at distance and near. His last eye examination was 4 years ago, and his glasses are 5 years old. The clinician, who is focused on the fact that this presbyope has not had a change in glasses in 5 years, concludes that this person's problem is a change in refractive error. During the examination, the doctor finds that an updated refraction improves the patient's distance and near vision in the left eye from 20/40 to 20/30, but ignores the fact that pigmentary changes in the patient's maculas suggest that macular degenerative changes have resulted in reduced visual acuity. This clinician has anchored.

Pseudodiagnosticity

Pseudodiagnosticity occurs when the clinician continues to seek data that are not helpful in making a diagnosis.[13, 15] Data gathering may make the clinician feel that he or she is involved in decision making, but the active data collection is not contributing to a diagnostic decision.

As discussed, a useful strategy in clinical decision making involves identifying a set of working hypotheses early in the clinical encounter and testing the working hypotheses by continuing to gather *relevant* data to help differentiate which condition is present. In pseudodiagnosticity, there is a tendency to continue choosing tests that provide information about only one of the possible diagnoses being considered but to ignore other alternatives. An exhaustive search of findings related to the first hypothesis and a lack of information about other hypotheses does not enable the doctor to rule in or rule out the alternative hypotheses. Pseudodiagnosticity, therefore, is a nonoptimal strategy of data selection that results in inadequate analysis of a patient's status.

Example
A patient presents with symptoms of ocular discomfort at the end of the day. She uses a computer approximately 4–5 hours per day and reports that her eyes feel very irritated at the end of the day. The clinician initially thinks that these symptoms may be the result of a binocular or accommodative problem that results in asthenopia at the end of the day or, alternatively, a dry-eye problem that becomes manifest at the end of a long working day, especially after many hours at the computer. The clinician investigates the categories of binocular and accommodative problems exhaustively. She finds that the patient has 10Δ esophoria, with a reduced negative fusional convergence at near. These findings indicate a convergence excess. She also finds a reduced accommodative amplitude using the push-up method and then repeats the test using minus lenses. An accommodative infacility was diagnosed using ±1.50 lenses; the test was then repeated using ±2.00 lenses. The clinician continues to probe the visual functional system, performing additional tests that investigate the initial diagnostic classification but ignoring the second alternative of dry eye. Red lens, Worth four-dot, Wirt circles, and fixation disparity testing and Keystone visual skills are performed. The doctor checks near retinoscopy with two different methods—the Monocular Estimation Method (MEM) and book retinoscopy.

Observing that the patient shows reduced and abnormal findings on vergence and accommodative testing, the doctor diagnoses that the patient has a convergence excess and accommodative infacility. Though these findings are true, the doctor has forgotten to explore the possibility of a dry eye, which may also be present and may be contributing to the patient's discomfort. The nonoptimal strategy of gathering exhaustive data in a particular area while ignoring data relevant to another possible hypothesis results in a misleading evaluation. In this case, the patient had a binocular and accommodative problem in addition to a dry eye. Had the clinician tested, she would have found that the patient had a tear breakup time of 1 second in both eyes, representing an almost immediate breakup of the tear film. Staining with fluorescein dye would have shown a superficial punctate keratitis in both eyes, especially inferiorly. Recommending artificial tears as therapy for dry eyes would have been an important aspect of the management plan to reduce the symptoms in this patient.

Inadequate Synthesis

Inadequate synthesis occurs when conclusions that could be support-ed by available data are not made.

Example
A patient presents complaining of headaches at work. During the exam-ination, normal ocular health, pupillary responses, and visual fields are found. Binocular testing reveals orthophoria at distance and 15Δ exopho-ria at near, with base-out vergence findings (positive fusional conver-gence) at near of 6/10/2. The patient's near point of convergence is 10 cm break/13 cm recovery, with diplopia reported. Inadequate synthesis occurs if the doctor fails to recognize that the patient's complaint of headaches is related to the fact that he has a convergence insufficiency.

Incorrect Synthesis

Incorrect synthesis occurs when available clinical data contradict a doc-tor's conclusion. Fortunately, this type of error is rare in clinical prac-tice,[16] although it may occur more with students who are still learning to identify the clinical findings associated with specific clinical conditions. For example, if a clinician makes a diagnosis of convergence excess when the patient has high exophoria at near, instead of esophoria, incorrect synthesis is said to have occurred. This type of error is rare in practice because well-trained clinicians are not likely to make incorrect diagnoses based on the evidence. The types of errors discussed previously are more common because they occur even among individuals who are well-trained and knowledgeable about clinical problems and conditions.

Example
The same case used for inadequate synthesis can be used to illustrate this type of error. The patient presents complaining of headaches at work. The clinician finds all ocular health tests to be normal and binoc-ular test results are as described earlier. Incorrect synthesis occurs when the doctor concludes that this patient has a divergence insufficiency. This is an incorrect diagnosis: The patient is orthophoric at distance, and there is no divergence problem. The problem, instead, is at near and, based on the clinical findings of a high exophoria at near, a reduced positive fusional convergence, and a receded near point of convergence, is a convergence insufficency.

Technical Nonsynthesis

Technical nonsynthesis is the type of error encountered frequently among novice clinicians, who are preoccupied with collecting data

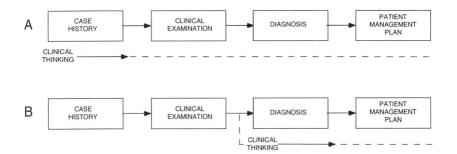

Figure 1.5 Clinical thinking during the examination. A. Clinical thinking occurs throughout the examination from the onset of the patient encounter. B. The clinician starts thinking and analyzing the case *after* all data have been collected. Model B is an inefficient method of decision making because the clinician may miss many cues and signs (e.g., head tilt; patient anxiety, fatigue, or discomfort) that are readily available to the clinician in Model A. Model A is by far the preferred method of clinical testing and decision making.

rather than generating and evaluating hypotheses. The quantity of the data is impressive, but the relevance and usefulness of the information collected is limited. Sackett and his colleagues[3] describe how such a clinician painstakingly collects data and, once all the data are collected, *then* searches through the data to make a diagnosis. Ideally, clinical thinking should occur *throughout* the examination, from the onset of the patient encounter, as illustrated in Figure 1.5A. Technical nonsynthesis is illustrated in Figure 1.5B; the clinician's evaluation begins *after* all the clinical data have been collected.

Technical nonsynthesis is an inefficient method of collecting data and making diagnoses because unnecessary tests may be performed merely to fill in the blanks on the examination forms. Likewise, tests that may generate useful information during the examination sequence may be left out. A medical study in which patients arriving for hospital admissions underwent a battery of 50 routinely performed tests showed that the exhaustive strategy did not produce any improvements in mortality, morbidity, or disability; in fact, the cost of care rose, and patient satisfaction was lowered.[17] To avoid technical nonsynthesis, the clinician should remember that every test should be performed for a reason, not randomly or aimlessly.

Like pseudodiagnosticity, technical nonsynthesis is a nonoptimal method of gathering data. However, in the case of pseudodiagnosticity, the clinician has at least worked on generating hypotheses and selecting tests that address a hypothesis (although only one hypothesis is investigated), whereas in the case of technical nonsynthesis, clinical tests are performed independent of working hypotheses, solely in the interest of generating data.

Example

A patient comes in complaining of headaches. The clinician conducts a full examination, concentrating essentially on performing tests and obtaining clinical data. More and more data are collected, independent of the patient's presenting complaint. The clinician's goal in this strategy is generating data. After all of the information is collected, the doctor starts to consider the possible diagnosis. With this type of strategy, the doctor may miss important cues that assist diagnosis (e.g., the patient may vocalize discomfort during binocular testing, which may lend support to the presence of a binocular problem if the appropriate clinical data are found).

Patient Unfamiliarity

The error of patient unfamiliarity does not occur as a result of failing to collect appropriate data or to synthesize clinical results adequately. In fact, this type of error is not at all dependent on the quality or quantity of clinical data. Rather, it reflects a failure of the clinician to become familiar enough with the patient to make a proper diagnosis. This occurs most frequently when an incomplete case history is taken or the clinician fails to obtain relevant information about the patient's status. It can occur also when a patient presents without any symptoms and the clinician, after a problem is found in clinical testing, fails to investigate further the existence of symptoms. For example, in a patient who presents without symptoms but who demonstrates binocular problems during clinical testing, the conclusion that a patient is asymptomatic at near would be incorrect if based merely on the fact that she does not complain about it at the onset of the examination. Some patients hesitate to complain about problems because they consider the symptoms unimportant or unrelated or because they are embarrassed. Some have temporarily forgotten about certain symptoms because they have developed ways of avoiding them. For instance, a patient may not complain of near problems because he or she currently does not do much near work, or the patient may have developed a habit of avoiding near work to avoid the problem. If the patient suddenly is required to perform increased near work, as with a change in job responsibilities, he or she may become symptomatic. Some patients do not complain because they fail to recognize their symptoms as anything abnormal. Children, for example, often do not report symptoms because they are unaware that not everyone functions as they do; they fail to recognize symptoms as symptoms (e.g., "Doesn't everyone see double?").

Getting to know patients, and paying attention to psychological and sociologic influences, is an important aspect of clinical care.[11] It is also an important factor in identifying management plans with which patients are likely to comply. The error of patient unfamiliarity may have an even greater impact on selecting the proper management plan for patients than on making a proper diagnosis.

Example
A patient presents for an eye examination with a chief complaint of a black eye. The doctor observes periorbital ecchymosis and conjunctival injection. The optometrist dilates the patient's eyes and finds the retinas are healthy, with no sign of internal trauma or pathology. The doctor informs the patient that no sign of ocular pathology was found and that the bruises around the eye will improve over the next 2 weeks. He recommends routine eye care in 1 year but provides no additional recommendations or intervention. The doctor in this example failed to ask the patient how she acquired the bruises around her eye. If he had asked the patient about the incident that resulted in the bruised eye, he might have elicited that she is a victim of domestic violence and that her husband had caused the injuries. He also might have found out that she went to a clinic 1 month ago with ocular and facial injuries caused by another abusive incident at home.

Battering is the single major cause of injury to women in the United States (more common than automobile accidents, muggings, and rapes combined), and more than 40% of injuries to adult domestic violence victims involve the face, neck, or head.[18] The doctor in this situation treated the superficial clinical sign—in this case, a black eye—but failed to address the underlying cause of the problem, domestic abuse. Had this doctor used facilitative interviewing techniques,[11] he might have educated the patient about local resources and community services (counseling agencies, battered women's shelters, domestic violence hotlines) but, because he did not take the opportunity to get to know the patient well enough, he did not help the patient optimally.

ERRORS CAUSED BY HEURISTICS

The previous seven types of errors are examples of poor decision-making processes that are consistently ineffective. Heuristics, in contrast, are general rules or strategies that usually support and assist *good* decision making. Nonetheless, they may result in errors at times.[19–22] Because heuristics often are used by clinicians intuitively and unconsciously in making judgments on the likelihood of clinical problems, it is important to understand how heuristics can impede proper decision making.

Representative Heuristic

Pattern recognition is an example of the representative heuristic. In pattern recognition, the clinician recognizes that a patient's sign/symptom complex is very similar to the sign/symptom complex of a disease or condition with which he or she is familiar. The diagnostic reasoning that occurs with this heuristic is as follows: Because this patient's sign/symptom complex matches my internal representation (sign/symptom complex) of disease X, there is a high probability that this patient has disease X. This rule of thumb works very well in most cases and is usually a very efficient and economical method of handling the complicated job of identifying a patient's problem. However, a clinician's internal representation of a disease often is based on his or her own experience of seeing patients with the disease. Although this image may differ from the classic textbook characteristics seen in most patients with the given disease, clinicians often still hold their own representation as the standard for the disease.

Errors in clinical decision making may occur if clinicians incorrectly match patients to their own potentially deviating image (representation) of a disease or if they fail to match patients to the more common, characteristic portrait of the clinical problem. Even if a clinician's representation of the disease matches the usual picture, errors still may occur if the patient's own presentation of the condition does not match the typical pattern seen in most patients.

Example
A patient with a rare presentation of retinitis pigmentosa (RP) is seen for an examination. The patient's symptoms and clinical signs do not match the doctor's internal representation of RP. In the representative heuristic, the doctor fails to make a diagnosis of RP because she does not match the patient's sign/symptom complex with her characteristic image of RP.

Availability Heuristic

The availability heuristic is a reflection of the fact that things that happen more frequently in our personal experience affect our estimates of probability. For example, if a clinician happens to have seen 10 cases of a rare disease recently, that diagnosis may come to mind more readily, despite the fact that this frequency is out of line with epidemiologic statistics. For a patient coming in with the same presenting complaint as previous patients who have a rare disease, the doctor may place strong emphasis on the hypothesis that this patient also has the rare disease, despite its rarity and the greater prevalence of other conditions with similar features. The availability heuristic is an example that what one sees in practice is what is likely to come to mind. However, an individual patient's condition may not be consistent with a particular doctor's recent exposure to clinical disease and pathology. The availability heuristic may be misleading if a clinician has seen a very vivid and memorable presentation of a rare case or has experienced multiple random repetitions of cases that are usually rare. A clinician must remain open-minded beyond his or her own sphere of clinical experiences when making clinical judgments.

Example
A doctor has recently seen a patient with strabismus, who is diagnosed with a brain tumor. He sees a new patient with strabismus, and consequently makes an initial diagnosis of a brain tumor.

Anchoring and Adjustment Heuristic

When clinicians estimate the probabilities of patients having clinical diagnoses, they usually consider an initial probability when an initial characteristic or so-called anchor brings the diagnosis to mind; this probability is adjusted as more clinical features and test results become known during the examination. A potential error can occur if the clinician sets the initial probability estimate (based on the anchor) too high.

Experiments have shown that initial probability estimates tend to be extreme—either very close to 0 (no probability) or 1.00 (absolute certainty).[3] Extreme initial estimates mean that very significant information must be obtained during the examination to produce prominent changes in probability. Another potential error can occur if clinicians do not adjust their probability estimates sufficiently when new information becomes available.[3]

Example
A 20-year-old woman presents for an eye examination with complaints of blurred vision in one eye. The patient has no history of ocular disease or injury. The clinician initially assigns a very high probability to an uncorrected refractive error; a very low probability is assigned to keratoconus, since it is a much rarer condition. Despite a typical "scissors" reflex on retinoscopy and distorted mires on keratometry, the

clinician fails to revise significantly the estimate of the probability of keratoconus in this patient. Had the doctor attended to the evidence that became available, a correct diagnosis of keratoconus would have been made. This clinician has fallen prey to an error in the anchoring and adjustment heuristic.

DECISION RULES

Decision rules bear some similarities to heuristics, as they both help to direct decision making. However, decision rules are much more explicit directions that guide clinical care and decision making. Following are some decision rules used in optometry:

- In patients with symptoms of flashes of light, the patient's pupils must be dilated and retinal detachment should be considered.
- Patients with intraocular pressures (IOPs) in excess of 22 mm Hg are suspects for glaucoma and must have visual field testing (in addition to tonometry and ophthalmoscopic evaluation).
- Patients with cup-to-disc ratios of 0.50 or higher are suspects for glaucoma and must have visual field testing (in addition to tonometry and IOP measurements).

Students and clinicians often learn about clinical care in textbooks, journals, lectures, and other sources. They must act on this knowledge by articulating decision rules for themselves based on this information (e.g., making a diagnosis or performing a new clinical procedure, under certain clinical conditions).

As they attend to their instructors and preceptors in clinics, students learn to adopt their own set of decision rules by observing those used by their instructors. Practicing clinicians must constantly review and modify their decision rules as new information becomes available. An important aspect of clinical care, one that requires a willingness to be a lifelong learner, is that the clinician must maintain updated decision rules that reflect the current understanding of clinical problems and treatment.

Not all practitioners use the same decision rules, and a clinician's decision rules may reflect how conservative or receptive he or she is to certain types of testing or treatment. A clinician must ensure, however, that his or her decision rules accurately reflect the state of scientific and clinical knowledge, and that they are tailored adequately to the needs of individual patients.

Sets of clinical decision rules have been discussed and developed in the form of clinical guidelines by professional groups and associations.[23–47]

These are usually recommendations for the diagnosis, management, and treatment of patients with specific types of clinical problems. They generally are based on modern scientific knowledge and clinical research, and expert clinical opinions are used to develop such recommendations. These guidelines help educate practitioners about important recommendations in the interest of patient care. They may also be of interest to government organizations, public health agencies, other health care professionals, insurance companies, managed care providers, and others who affect health care delivery. It is important to remember, however, that these are *recommendations* and *general guidelines* only; the individual practitioner who knows the patient's needs and concerns is best prepared to determine the care that is optimal for each patient.

REASONS TO PERFORM CLINICAL TESTS

Pseudodiagnosticity and technical nonsynthesis, described previously, should remind the doctor that extensive, unguided, or random collections of data do not contribute efficiently to diagnostic reasoning. The clinical examination should not be an exercise in filling in the blanks on an examination form. There should always be a purpose for performing a test. Reasons to perform clinical tests include the following:

1. *To assist in diagnosis.* Choosing tests appropriately helps identify the correct diagnosis. Clinical tests are selected to rule in and rule out hypotheses considered during the examination.
2. *To assist in monitoring patient management and therapy.* It is often helpful to use clinical tests to evaluate therapeutic interventions over time. Comparing IOPs before and after the initiation of drug treatment for glaucoma, for example, is essential. Uncertainty regarding the effects of treatment exists, with variability across individuals and within individuals over time. Monitoring therapy helps to reduce this uncertainty.
3. *To establish a database of information about the patient.* Obtaining a database of information in a comprehensive examination enables the doctor to identify problems of which a patient may be unaware or may fail to mention. Some problems, such as chronic open-angle glaucoma, are asymptomatic in the early stages. Patients may have other problems in addition to their chief complaint but may forget to mention them or may think they are unimportant.

To reduce the likelihood of missing other problems unrelated to a patient's presenting complaints and to ensure that the differential diagnosis includes all the likely conditions, it is important to obtain a database of information from the patient. A comprehensive general examination should include testing in each of the following areas: refraction and visual acuity; binocular vision, accommodation, and sensory assessment; ocular health testing; and screening for neurologic and systemic conditions.

An example of guidelines for the comprehensive adult eye examination, developed by the American Optometric Association, is provided in Table 1.3.[23] These recommendations are an example, but each practitioner should consider his or her own guidelines for a database for the comprehensive examination. It should be understood that modifications may be necessary depending on the cooperation and comprehension of the patient, the symptoms and problems of the patient, and the judgment of the doctor. In addition to the tests in the general database, problem-specific tests should be performed to address particular problems. For example, patients with complaints of diplopia or near-point asthenopia should have additional binocular testing and investigation; contact lens wearers should have appropriate evaluation of lens fit, lens condition (presence of deposits), and corneal health; and patients with ocular pathology should have additional problem-specific testing.

In Part II of this book, each patient presents for an eye examination, some for a general examination and some with specific complaints. Each patient undergoes a comprehensive eye examination, with appropriate additional problem-specific tests. Not all data obtained relate to the patient's presenting complaints or to ruling in or out diagnostic hypotheses drawn from these symptoms; additional data are obtained to compile a database that enables the optometrist to rule out other problems.

FACTORS CONTRIBUTING TO A DOCTOR'S CLINICAL DECISION-MAKING SKILLS

Clinicians make many decisions in the course of caring for patients. Choosing the proper questions to ask during the case history, selecting the tests to perform during the examination, identifying the likely diagnoses, and determining an optimal management plan all rely on the doctor's decision-making skills.

Factors that contribute to a doctor's clinical decision-making skills (Figure 1.6) include the doctor's knowledge base, analytic and diagnostic reasoning skills, clinical experience, and professional style. The doctor's knowledge base (including clinical training, books, jour-

Table 1.3
Comprehensive adult eye examination.

A. Patient history
    1. Nature of presenting problem, including chief complaint
    2. Visual and ocular history
    3. General health history, which may include social history and review of systems
    4. Medication usage and medication allergies
    5. Family eye and medical histories
    6. Vocational and avocational visual requirements
B. Visual acuity
    1. Distance visual acuity testing
    2. Near visual acuity testing
C. Preliminary testing
    1. General observation of patient
    2. Observation of external ocular and facial areas
    3. Pupillary responses
    4. Versions and ductions
    5. Near point of convergence
    6. Cover test
    7. Accommodative amplitude
    8. Stereopsis
    9. Color vision
D. Refraction
    1. Measurement of patient's most recent optical correction
    2. Measurement of anterior corneal curvature
    3. Objective measurement of refractive status
    4. Subjective measurement of monocular and binocular refractive status at distance and near
E. Ocular motility, binocular vision, and accommodation
    1. Evaluation of ocular motility and alignment
    2. Evaluation of vergence amplitude and facility
    3. Assessment of accommodative amplitude and facility
    4. Assessment of suppression
    5. Measurement of fixation disparity and associated phoria
F. Ocular health assessment and systemic health screening
    1. Evaluation of the anterior ocular segment and adnexa
    2. Measurement of intraocular pressure
    3. Evaluation of the ocular media
    4. Evaluation of the posterior ocular segment
    5. Visual field screening (confrontation)
    6. Systemic health screening tests

Source: Reprinted with permission from the American Optometric Association. Comprehensive Adult Eye and Vision Examination (Clinical Practice Guideline). St. Louis: AOA, 1994.

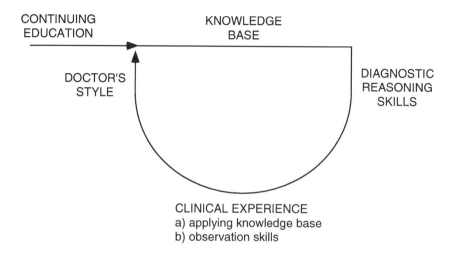

Figure 1.6 Factors that contribute to a doctor's decision-making skills. The factors include the doctor's (1) knowledge base, including clinical training programs, books, journals, study groups, continuing education; (2) analytic and diagnostic reasoning skills, including the ability to clarify a patient's problems, generate likely hypotheses, select appropriate testing that leads to final diagnoses, and design appropriate patient management plans; (3) clinical experience, including patient encounters with experiences in applying the knowledge base and developing observation skills, and refining clinical reasoning skills; and (4) professional style, including the doctor's attitudes, beliefs, biases, preferences for treatments, and demeanor with patients.

nals, and continuing education) is the foundation for clinical care. Video and computer learning programs are two more recent sources that can contribute to a doctor's knowledge base. An appropriate knowledge base must exist for a doctor's analytic and diagnostic reasoning skills to be fully realized. The doctor's experience in applying that knowledge base and making good clinical observations is also essential.

Clinicians who are training or who have graduated within the past few years probably are facing many new types of clinical experiences that they have not handled previously. Students-in-training are developing and honing their observational skills. Over time in a clinical setting, doctors learn to apply their knowledge base to clinical problems. They learn to refine their ability to make astute clinical observations. They also gain experience in refining the analytic reasoning skills used in the clinical setting.

Clinicians must be aware of their attitudes and beliefs and must be sure that they do not let any biases affect their delivery of care. They must also remember that their demeanor and manner with patients affects their ability to obtain clinical information and, therefore, their ability to make a correct diagnosis. It is important for doctors to remain open-minded and to willingly obtain and consider new clinical data.

It is very likely that clinicians who have been practicing for many years are facing clinical problems and treatment options that they did not learn about in optometry school. For example, many practicing clinicians have had to learn about the human immunodeficiency virus and treatment of the acquired immunodeficiency syndrome through continuing education. Similarly, clinicians must continue the educational process throughout their career to stay up-to-date on new ocular diagnostic techniques and therapeutic drugs. To maintain a current knowledge base, clinicians in practice must be motivated to pursue continuing education. Figure 1.6 should remind practitioners that clinical excellence is a lifelong pursuit.

COGNITIVE PROCESSES IN DECISION MAKING

Researchers have investigated the cognitive processes used by novice and expert clinical decision makers. Understanding how doctors think and make decisions effectively can help student clinicians learn to model behaviors to improve their own diagnostic and decision-making abilities.

One model of the cognitive processes used by expert clinicians suggests that relevant knowledge is organized and stored in memory in the form of *illness scripts*, within a database of previously observed patients.[48] Illness scripts are composed of three pieces of information: enabling conditions, faults, and consequences. Enabling conditions are predisposing factors (e.g., age, gender, genetic factors, smoking and drug or alcohol use, environmental factors) that put a patient at risk for disease. Faults are the causes or *labels* of the problem, in the form of either a diagnosis or a brief description of a pathophysiologic mechanism (e.g., vitamin deficiency). Consequences include signs, symptoms, and complaints that result from the diagnosed condition. Illness scripts thus are stored memories of previous patients that link the three components (enabling factors, faults, and consequences).

Over time and with increasing clinical experience, clinicians store illness scripts of patients with different pathologic processes. Expert clinicians are able to retrieve these illness scripts as needed. Characteristics of new patients evoke memories of previous patients with similar features. Experience affords the clinician vast opportunities to store and make linkages among enabling conditions, signs and symptoms, and their associated diagnoses. Illness scripts are patient-centered, sign and symptom–oriented representations of disease rather than typical dictionary or textbook definitions. In contrast, inexperienced clinicians and doctors who have not been exposed to a particular type of problem tend to resort to a more pathophysiologic, textbook analysis of a given problem when the patient database is not available.[48]

Another difference in the cognitive processes of expert and novice clinicians is that expert clinicians appear to translate the enabling conditions and consequences (signs and symptoms)[49] more effectively into categoric concepts referred to as *semantic axes*.[50] *Semantic*, defined as *meaning*, is used in this term because it helps the clinician capture the meaning (or context) associated with signs and symptoms: the diagnosis, or the underlying problem. The term *axes* demonstrates that characteristics are observed along opposite ends of a continuum. Examples of semantic axes that relate to clinical care include, among others, unilateral-bilateral, constant-intermittent, recent-longstanding, acute-chronic, severe-mild, local-diffuse, and young-old. Clinicians learn to translate the patient's enabling conditions and symptoms within semantic axes, which helps them recognize patterns as they relate to specific clinical problems.[49, 50] Dr. David Corliss[49] provides an example in optometry: The statement by a 45-year-old man ("I suddenly started having this sharp pain in my right eye 3 days ago that comes and goes and seems to be getting worse") is abstracted by the clinician as "a sharp, unilateral, peripheral, acute, intermittent, and progressive pain of recent onset in a middle-aged man."

Researchers who observed novice and expert clinicians found that successful diagnosticians had the most diverse set of semantic relationships and were able to obtain the broadest, deepest representation of a patient's problem.[50] Diagnostic abilities were not tied only to knowledge base but specifically to the ability to understand the patient's problem. This task is underscored as stage 1 in Figure 1.2 and is repeated again here to remind the reader of the importance of this step. It is believed that a deep understanding of the patient's problem helps to generate the proper hypotheses and to rule out the incompatible ones.

CLINICAL "PEARLS" FOR DECISION MAKING

A number of maxims have been used as guidelines to promote effective clinical decision making.[5, 22, 51] Ten of these are highlighted here.

1.   *When you hear hoofbeats, think of horses, not zebras.*[5, 22, 51] This aphorism reminds the clinician that common diseases are far more likely to be seen than rare diseases. Students often are eager to look for rare, esoteric diagnoses that they read about in textbooks, but they must remember to consider these etiologies as likely hypotheses only when the possibility of such conditions is realistic. In other words, one should think of the obvious before looking for the obscure.

2.   *Uncommon manifestations of common diseases are more common than common manifestations of rare diseases.*[5, 22, 51] This aphorism reminds us that a clinical sign or symptom is more likely to come from a common etiology than a rare one, even if it occurs more frequently in the rare condition.

3.   *We tend to see what we are looking for; similarly, we tend not to see what we don't want (or expect) to see.*[22] By this aphorism we are reminded that the clinician is not always an objective observer, processing information like a neutral, nonthinking, indifferent machine. If the doctor has settled on an initial diagnosis, he or she may tend to see the clinical signs that confirm that hypothesis and to ignore signs that do not correspond to that line of clinical thinking.

4.   *Remain open-minded; avoid making hasty decisions.* Hasty decisions can lead to premature closure and anchoring. These errors not only are ineffective methods of data collection and decision making but also may be dangerous because of the clinician's confidence that a diagnostic decision has already been reached. If premature closure ensues, important data may never be collected. It has been said that "premature closure in effect represents closure."[16] Similarly, important data may be collected but ignored in the case of anchoring. Both of these errors may lead to incorrect treatment decisions because the doctor has a false sense of confidence in the diagnosis that is held.[16]

Researchers have found that experienced clinicians may be more prone to anchoring and premature closure errors than students and residents, who are more willing to reject their earlier hypotheses in the presence of conflicting data.[51, 52] *All* clinicians—not just those in training—must remember to keep an open mind. An important exercise in remaining open minded is to be conscious of considering alternatives in diagnostic decision making: If you find yourself settling on a diagnosis early in your examination of a patient, force yourself to come up with at least one other plausible alternative and be sure to analyze why your original hypothesis is better.

5.   *Remember to look for diseases and conditions that you cannot afford to miss.*[5] This aphorism reminds the doctor that it is important to consider the presence of dangerous clinical problems, especially those that are potentially serious if untreated or not managed within a certain

period of time. This clinical principle is the reason that optometrists habitually measure IOPs in patients, even in the absence of symptoms or a positive glaucoma history. Glaucoma tends to be asymptomatic in the early stages (except in the presence of narrow-angle attacks), and patients may not know that they have glaucoma. The potential outcomes of this condition, including severe visual defects, blindness, and diminished quality of life,[53] underscore the importance of investigating the possibility of glaucoma in patients presenting for routine eye examinations, even in the absence of symptoms or a previous personal or family history of glaucoma.

6.   *Remember the law of parsimony: The simplest explanation that fits the clinical description is likely to be the best.*[5] This aphorism reminds the clinician to look for simple explanations before considering more complex, esoteric factors. The law of parsimony is really a reminder of the law of probability and the understanding that high-prevalence problems are more likely to be seen than are low-prevalence problems. A symptom or sign is more likely caused by a common disease than an uncommon one.

The exception to this rule is to consider rarer diseases when the clinical profile suggests that a less common problem may be present. As Riegelman[21] reminds us, "It is important to look for a zebra when the pattern suggests something unusual."

An important clinical application of the law of parsimony is to consider whether several problems may be contributing to the same presenting complaint: That is, if a patient comes in with a particular complaint, and the clinician conducts a differential diagnosis looking for the one correct diagnosis, might the doctor be ruling out the possibility that two or more conditions may be present simultaneously and contributing to the same problem? The answer, based on laws of probability (and, consequently, the law of parsimony), is that, except in rare cases, the patient's complaint is attributable to one problem. Sox and coworkers[5] explain that the probability of two unrelated diseases occurring at the same time is the probability of one disease multiplied by the probability of the other. The product of the probabilities of the two diseases is much lower (indicating a lower likelihood) than the probability of either disease occurring alone. An exception to this reasoning, as pointed out in the explanation, is that the probability of two common diseases occurring simultaneously is greater than the probability of one rare disease. Another exception is that in patients with chronic disease, new symptoms are not always the result of the initial condition and may indicate the presence of additional problems. In patients with cataracts, for example, additional vision loss is not always the result of progressive cataracts, and the doctor must be certain to rule out new contributing factors, such as age-related macular degeneration or other ocular problems.

7.   *To make a good diagnosis, you must understand the patient's problem clearly.* Expert diagnosticians take time to identify and define the patient's problem, asking appropriate questions during the case history and throughout the examination. During investigation of the case history, *and before the testing sequence begins*, the doctor begins to generate clinical hypotheses and to rule in or rule out possibilities as information is gathered. The perceptive diagnostician picks up cues of hidden agendas,[54] in which the patient does not mention his or her chief concerns until well into the examination and often toward the end. Without identifying the patient's concern, the doctor may be unsuccessful in making an appropriate diagnosis and solving the patient's problem.

8.   *Understand how heuristics can help you but do not allow them to mislead you.* Heuristics are general rules that help the clinician make decisions on a regular basis. The availability, representative, and anchoring and adjustment heuristics demonstrate that these rules must be used properly, or they can result in errors.

9.   *Avoid relying on personal and anecdotal evidence; instead, rely on good epidemiologic and probabilistic reasoning.* Relying on anecdotal evidence results in clinical thinking and decision making based on one's personal experience rather than on the collective experience across populations of patients. Personal experience is essential in making observations and in practicing analytic reasoning, but decision making should be based on sound epidemiologic reasoning. (See Chapter 3 for more on the use of epidemiology in clinical decision making.)

10.   *Decision making must be individualized to a patient's unique set of needs, desires, goals, and concerns.* Different patients describe illness differently and may have varying psychological experiences and responses. Although we stress that decision making is carried out based on epidemiologic and probabilistic principles, clinical care must be tailored to the individual patient. Remember, "No disease is rare to the person who has it."[51] It is the ability to make sound clinical and scientific decisions while tailoring care to the individual patient that exemplifies clinical excellence. In applying principles of good decision making, know that the most important factor in pursuit of clinical excellence is remembering that *each patient is a person*.

REFERENCES

1. Barresi BJ. Ocular Assessment: The Manual of Diagnosis for Office Practice. Boston: Butterworths, 1984.

2. Albert DA, Munson R, Resnik MD. Reasoning in Medicine: An Introduction to Clinical Inference. Baltimore: Johns Hopkins University, 1988.
3. Sackett DL, Haynes RB, Guyatt GH, et al. Clinical Epidemiology: A Basic Science for Clinical Medicine (2nd ed). Boston: Little, Brown, 1991.
4. Kurtz D. Teaching clinical reasoning. J Optom Educ 1990;15:119–122.
5. Sox HC Jr, Blatt MA, Higgins MC, et al. Medical Decision Making. Boston: Butterworths, 1988.
6. Bradley GW. Disease, Diagnosis and Decisions. New York: Wiley, 1993.
7. Elstein AS, Shulman LS, Sprafka SA. Medical Problem Solving: An Analysis of Clinical Reasoning. Cambridge, MA: Harvard University Press, 1978.
8. Barrows HS, Norman GR, Neufeld VR, et al. The clinical reasoning of randomly selected physicians in general medical practice. Clin Invest Med 1982;5:49–55.
9. Neufeld VR, Norman GR, Feightner JW, et al. Clinical problem-solving by medical students: a cross-sectional and longitudinal analysis. Med Educ 1981;15:315–322.
10. Roy FH. Ocular Differential Diagnosis (5th ed). Philadelphia: Lea & Febiger, 1993.
11. Ettinger ER. Professional Communications in Eye Care. Boston: Butterworth-Heinemann, 1994.
12. Werner DL. Teaching clinical thinking. Optom Vis Sci 1989;66:788–792.
13. Kern L, Doherty ME. "Pseudodiagnosticity" in an idealized medical problem-solving environment. J Med Educ 1982;57:100–104.
14. Kassirer JP. Teaching problem-solving: how are we doing? N Engl J Med 1995;332:1507–1509.
15. Wolf FM, Gruppen LD, Billi JE. Use of the competing-hypotheses heuristic to reduce "pseudodiagnosticity." J Med Educ 1988;63:548–554.
16. Voytovich AE, Rippey RM, Suffredini A. Premature conclusions in diagnostic reasoning. J Med Educ 1985;60:302–307.
17. Durbridge TC, Edwards F, Edwards RG, et al. An evaluation of multiphasic screening on admission to hospital. Precis of a report to the National Health and Medical Research Council. Med J Aust 1976;1:703–705.
18. New York State Office for the Prevention of Domestic Violence. Domestic Violence Data Sheet. Troy, NY: New York State Office for the Prevention of Domestic Violence, 1990.
19. Detmer DE, Fryback DG, Gassner K. Heuristics and biases in medical decision-making. J Med Educ 1978;53:682–683.
20. Tversky A, Kahneman D. Judgment under uncertainty: heuristics and biases. Science 1974;185:1124–1131.
21. Riegelman RK. Minimizing Medical Mistakes: The Art of Medical Decision Making. Boston: Little, Brown, 1991.
22. Carroll JS, Johnson EJ. Decision Research: A Field Guide. Newbury Park, CA: Sage Publications, 1990.
23. American Optometric Association. Comprehensive Adult Eye and Vision Examination (Optometric Clinical Practice Guidelines). St. Louis: AOA, 1994.
24. American Optometric Association. Pediatric Eye and Vision Examination (Optometric Clinical Practice Guidelines). St. Louis: AOA, 1994.
25. American Optometric Association. Care of the Patient with Diabetes Mellitus (Optometric Clinical Practice Guidelines). St. Louis: AOA, 1994.
26. American Optometric Association. Care of the Patient with Amblyopia (Optometric Clinical Practice Guidelines). St. Louis: AOA, 1994.

27. American Optometric Association. Care of the Patient with Primary Angle Closure Glaucoma (Optometric Clinical Practice Guidelines). St. Louis: AOA, 1994.

28. American Optometric Association. Care of the Patient with Age-Related Macular Degeneration (Optometric Clinical Practice Guidelines). St. Louis: AOA, 1994.

29. American Optometric Association. Care of the Patient with Anterior Uveitis (Optometric Clinical Practice Guidelines). St. Louis: AOA, 1994.

30. Cataract in adults: management of functional impairment. Clinical practice guideline; no. 4. [AHCPR Pub. No. 93-0543.] Rockville, MD: US Department of Health and Human Services, Public Health Service, Agency for Health Care Policy and Research, Feb. 1993.

31. American Academy of Ophthalmology. Quality of Ophthalmic Care (Preferred Practice Patterns). San Francisco: AAO, 1988.

32. American Academy of Ophthalmology. Glaucoma Suspect (Preferred Practice Patterns). San Francisco: AAO, 1989.

33. American Academy of Ophthalmology. Cataract in the Otherwise Healthy Adult Eye (Preferred Practice Patterns). San Francisco: AAO, 1989.

34. American Academy of Ophthalmology. Retinal Detachment (Preferred Practice Patterns). San Francisco: AAO, 1990.

35. American Academy of Ophthalmology. Low to Moderate Refractive Errors (Preferred Practice Patterns). San Francisco: AAO, 1991.

36. American Academy of Ophthalmology. Conjunctivitis (Preferred Practice Patterns). San Francisco: AAO, 1991.

37. American Academy of Ophthalmology. Blepharitis and the Dry Eye in the Adult (Preferred Practice Patterns). San Francisco: AAO, 1991.

38. American Academy of Ophthalmology. Primary Open-Angle Glaucoma (Preferred Practice Patterns). San Francisco: AAO, 1992.

39. American Academy of Ophthalmology. Primary Angle-Closure Glaucoma (Preferred Practice Patterns). San Francisco: AAO, 1992.

40. American Academy of Opthalmology. Esotropia (Preferred Practice Patterns). San Francisco: AAO, 1992.

41. American Academy of Ophthalmology. Comprehensive Adult Eye Evaluation (Preferred Practice Patterns). San Francisco: AAO, 1992.

42. American Academy of Ophthalmology. Comprehensive Pediatric Eye Evaluation (Preferred Practice Patterns). San Francisco: AAO, 1992.

43. American Academy of Ophthalmology. Amblyopia (Preferred Practice Patterns). San Francisco: AAO, 1992.

44. American Academy of Ophthalmology. Diabetic Retinopathy (Preferred Practice Patterns). San Francisco: AAO, 1993.

45. American Academy of Ophthalmology. Age-Related Macular Degeneration (Preferred Practice Patterns). San Francisco: AAO, 1994.

46. American Academy of Ophthalmology. Precursors of Rhegmatogenous Retinal Detachment in Adults (Preferred Practice Patterns). San Francisco: AAO, 1994.

47. American Academy of Ophthalmology. Rehabilitation: Management of Patients with Low Vision (Preferred Practice Patterns). San Francisco: AAO, 1992.

48. Schmidt HG, Norman GR, Boshuizen HP. A cognitive perspective on medical expertise: theory and implication. Acad Med 1990;65:611–621.

49. Corliss DA. A comprehensive model of clinical decision making. J Am Optom Assoc 1995;66:362–371.
50. Bordage G, Lemieux M. Semantic structures and diagnostic thinking of experts and novices. Acad Med 1991;66:S70–S72.
51. Judge RD, Zuidema GD, Fitzgerald FT. Clinical Diagnosis: A Physiological Approach. Boston: Little, Brown, 1989.
52. Friedlander ML, Phillips SD. Preventing anchoring errors in clinical judgment. J Consult Clin Psychol 1984;52:366–371.
53. Prevent Blindness America. Vision Problems in the U.S. Schaumburg, IL: Prevent Blindness America, 1994.
54. Barsky AJ. Hidden reasons some patients visit doctors. Ann Intern Med 1981;94:492–498.

2

Dealing with Clinical Uncertainty

Ellen Richter Ettinger

Dealing effectively with uncertainty is the hallmark of an excellent clinician. Patients rarely come in with every classic textbook sign and symptom of a disease or condition. In reality, they usually come in with *some* of the signs and symptoms of a condition. The doctor performs additional testing until *enough* information is available to identify the clinical problem and to choose the appropriate management plan.

Clinical certainty can be expressed and illustrated (Figure 2.1) in terms of percentages (0–100%) or probability (0–1.0). Both extremes represent certainty; an event with a probability of 1.0 (or 100%) is *certain* to occur, whereas one with a probability of 0 (or 0%) is certain *not* to occur. Clinical certainty rarely reaches a 100% confidence level because of limited available information.[1-4] Most situations fall somewhere in between, making clinical diagnosis more complicated. The goal of the clinician-in-training should not be to avoid uncertainty, because clinical uncertainty is inescapable; rather, the goal should be to understand how to approach uncertainty in a manner that optimizes what is known about the patient.

The goal of this chapter is to examine the sources of uncertainty and to present strategies to help clinicians deal more effectively with ambiguity or doubt. Chapter 1 described the basic thinking processes used by practitioners to make decisions; this chapter presents additional techniques that are useful when the degree of uncertainty is still high. Discussed are techniques and tools that can be used to reduce uncertainty, including closed-loop decision making, decision trees, and computer-assisted diagnostic support systems.

SOURCES OF UNCERTAINTY

Uncertainty occurs as a result of a number of factors.

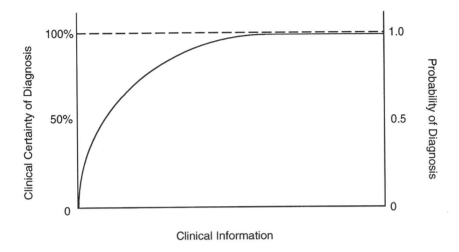

Figure 2.1 Quantifying clinical certainty. Clinical certainty can be expressed in terms of percentages (0–100%) or probability (0–1.0). Clinical certainty rarely reaches a 100% level of confidence because of the sources of uncertainty discussed.

Limited Availability of Clinical Information

It may be difficult to obtain data from some patients.[1] This is especially true for children and patients from special populations in which data often are limited because of the patient's ability to respond to testing. In other cases, data may not be available because conducting certain tests (especially invasive procedures) may pose a risk outweighing the benefits. In each of these cases, the ability to gather data is limited.

Limited Quality of Information

Limits on the quality of information occur in patients who responsd to clinical testing but whose responses are ambiguous or unreliable.[1] Such limits also occur frequently in young children and patients from special populations.

Limited Ability to Gather Definitive Information

If a clinician wanted to know whether a patient had a brain tumor, the most direct way of testing this hypothesis would be to operate and examine the patient's brain for a tumor. Clearly, this is too risky a procedure to use for diagnosis in patients (with *and* without tumors) and would have too many complications and detrimental effects.

As a result of the types of problems that could occur if clinicians insisted on seeking conclusive, definitive evidence (as in the previous example), we use clinical tests and procedures to indicate the presence of disease when we are not able to inspect an internal part of the body directly.[2] The state of technology and modern instrumentation has made it easier to gain insights into such problems as those previously listed, which make it difficult or impossible to inspect the suspected part of the body directly. Radiologic imaging tests, for example, have been very helpful; still, there are times when current instrumentation does not provide definite answers to clinical questions.

Advances in technology, such as computerized visual-field testing, have made diagnosis of many pathologies, including glaucoma, easier in many cases. Because it would be physically impossible to inspect the optic nerve head manually to assess whether any damage is present, clinicians use other methods and make inferences in the absence of autopsy or other risky vision-threatening procedures. We analyze cup-to-disc ratios visually, evaluate visual-field findings, and measure intraocular pressures (IOPs) as indicators of whether glaucomatous conditions are present. Computer-driven digitized analyses of optic nerve heads also have made it easier to assess early signs of optic nerve changes and damage. Still, there are times when a clinician is limited in assessing whether optic nerve damage is present, given the current state of technology.

Limited Ability or Ambiguity in Interpreting Clinical Data

Does an IOP of 23 mm Hg mean the patient has glaucoma? Does 24? Does 25? Even when good, reliable clinical data are available, they are often subject to interpretation.[3] In addition to analyzing individual test results, the art and science of correlating appropriate tests with related tests further affects the interpretation of data.

Uncertainty in Patients' Responses to Treatment

Different patients frequently react differently to the same therapeutic modality, whether it is a drug, a vision therapy procedure, a low-vision device, or other form of intervention.[3] Even the same individual may respond differently to a particular treatment at a different time of day or a different period in a lifetime. Patient management plans must be monitored carefully as a result of this uncertainty.

Examiner Uncertainty

An additional source of uncertainty is the clinician's own confidence in his or her clinical findings and activities. A clinician's doubts in generating working hypotheses, gathering and analyzing adequate data, determining the final diagnoses, and choosing optimal patient treatment plans contribute to uncertainty in a clinical encounter. Students frequently doubt the quality of their clinical results or their interpretations, an aspect of a clinician's uncertainty often reduced by experience.

Even experienced clinicians, however, encounter uncertainty in making decisions. Different doctors with the same set of clinical data may express different levels of certainty with respect to their diagnostic and therapeutic decisions. One clinician may look at Figure 2.1 and state an 80% certainty regarding a decision; another with the same clinical information may claim a 60% certainty.

Clinicians often build confidence in their decisions by monitoring successful cases over time, obtaining feedback from clinical experts through consultations and referrals, and expanding their knowledge base through additional training and continuing education.

Whereas the previous categories emphasize the components of uncertainty that arise from a patient's ability to respond and from technology's capacity to test, this category emphasizes that clinicians themselves contribute their own component of uncertainty to the decision-making process.

STRATEGIES FOR ADDRESSING SOURCES OF UNCERTAINTY

Strategies for reducing each category discussed in the previous section are addressed here.

1.   *Limited availability of information.* When it is difficult to collect data, as with many pediatric patients or individuals from special populations, consider using one of several strategies. Be familiar with special testing procedures to help gather data in populations that are difficult to test. For example, picture charts, the Broken-Wheel test, and Allen picture cards are preferable for many patients when traditional procedures using Snellen acuity charts are not helpful. Alternatively, when the clinician is unable to obtain subjective responses from a patient, he or she must rely more heavily on objective test results. For example, if a patient does not provide reliable results during subjective testing for refractive error, the doctor must rely more

heavily on objective findings (such as retinoscopy) that provide information on refraction.

2.   *Limited quality of information.* When the quality of information obtained from patients is questionable, following certain other strategies may be valuable. Ensure that the patient understands instructional sets; repeat or clarify the directions, if necessary. Ensure that the patient is not distracted or fatigued; if such is the case, try to regain the patient's attention or reschedule. Alternatively, if the patient does not respond well to a test, try to obtain the information using other tests that provide comparable information. For example, if the patient does not respond well to binocular testing behind the phoropter, try to assess the patient's binocularity with open-space testing such as a cover test, prism bar vergence testing, stereopsis testing, or other out-of-phoropter procedures that reflect a patient's binocular function.

3.   *Limited ability to gather definitive information.* Staying up-to-date in the latest standards of care and using modern instrumentation and procedures in clinical practice are essential in minimizing the uncertainty in this category. Sometimes the high costs of modern technology, however, may necessitate patient referrals for certain types of testing rather than acquiring all specialized equipment in one's office. For example, as corneal topography has developed, some clinicians have chosen to refer patients for topographic analysis rather than to obtain the instrumentation themselves; others have found it valuable to have the corneal topographer in their own offices. Some clinicians have their own ultrasound equipment, whereas others refer patients for this type of testing. Many clinicians do not perform laboratory testing, magnetic resonance imaging, or computed tomography scans in their offices.

Several strategies can help minimize limitations that arise in this category. One strategy is to remain knowledgable in the latest methods of clinical testing and use the highest standards of clinical care. Alternatively, if access to various specialized equipment or testing procedures is not immediately available, use appropriate referrals, consultations, and laboratory test orders to obtain the information needed.

4.   *Limited ability or ambiguity in interpreting data.* Certain strategies apply here as well. For instance, if the patient's responses in a test do not provide a clear or likely interpretation, consider bringing the patient back to repeat the test. If, for example, the patient's IOP is 22 or 23 mm Hg, reschedule the patient to recheck the pressures for further elevation. If the responses in one test are inconclusive, consider conducting other tests that provide similar information. For example, if the IOPs are borderline, assess whether the optic nerve heads and visual fields suggest that the patient has glaucoma.

5. *Uncertainty in patient's responses to treatment.* The primary strategy for addressing this source of uncertainty is to monitor a patient's response to treatment over time. Reschedule a patient on a regular basis to assess whether the management plan is working effectively. Educate patients thoroughly about side effects that result from drug therapy or other therapeutic intervention and encourage them to contact you if they have any questions or problems. Warn them about any important signs that require an immediate phone call to the doctor or a return to the doctor's office before the next scheduled appointment.

6. *Uncertainty on the part of the examiner.* Clinicians have to address the sources of their own uncertainties to minimize the effects in this category.

Increase your confidence by monitoring successful cases in your experience. Then again, increase your confidence and reinforce your knowledge base by additional training, reading, study groups, and continuing education. When you are unsure of what to do for a patient, use consultations and referrals to obtain feedback from clinical experts. Over time, outside feedback can help the clinician develop his or her expertise and confidence in making many of these decisions independently. Remember that the clinician does not have to be 100% certain to be confident of a decision; uncertainty is a basic component of clinical decision making.

STUDENTS' UNCERTAINTY IN DECISION MAKING

Students frequently doubt the quality of their clinical results or their interpretations. They frequently express concern and have difficulty in the decision-making process. Many of the problems about which students complain (e.g., inability to get clinical results from a patient, not knowing how to interpret results, or not knowing how to put everything together) are related to the sources of uncertainty discussed in the categories in the preceding section. Students' complaints often are similar to those in the left-hand column of Table 2.1. Strategies to help solve each of these problems are provided in the column on the right.

Another common strategy used by students when they are uncertain about what to do is to try to gather more information. Some students attempt an extensive, random collection of data similar to the pseudodiagnosticity or technical nonsynthesis modes of decision making described in Chapter 1. Students should remember that additional tests should always be done with a purpose, not aimlessly. In considering

Table 2.1
Uncertainties in clinical encounters.

Problem	Suggested Strategies
Unable to generate initial working hypotheses	Review your case history information and ensure that you have a clear concept of the patient's problem(s). Go back and ask more case history information to help you generate possible diagnostic hypotheses. Think of broad categories, rather than forcing yourself to generate very specific diagnostic categories.
Unable to obtain clinical results from patient (limited quantity or quality of information)	Ensure that your instructions to the patient are clear. If you are unsuccessful in obtaining data for a particular test (e.g., von Graefe phorias), try to use other tests that provide the same or similar types of information (e.g., cover test). If the subjective data are questionable or unattainable, rely more on objective testing. Ensure that the patient is not distracted or fatigued. If your patient's results are questionable but the patient appears to be responding properly, ensure that your equipment is calibrated properly and is in proper working order. Consider whether the patient may be malingering.
Uncertain how to interpret the results of a clinical test (ambiguous data)	If a patient's results are ambiguous, consider repeating the test to obtain a new set of results. Consider using other tests that provide similar information. Check the clinical literature and the manufacturer's guide for any information regarding how to interpret rare or unusual responses.
Unable to integrate clinical findings, unsure how to put the results together (limited analytic ability, limited diagnostic ability)	Look for patterns in the data: (1) Compare the results of tests that generate abnormal findings; (2) compare the results of tests that evaluate the same (or similar) information; (3) relate clinical findings to the information obtained in the case history.

Table 2.1
(continued)

Problem	Suggested Strategies
	Eliminate working hypotheses not supported by the data collected; re-evaluate the remaining likely hypotheses based on the data collected. If still unsure, consider whether new and more appropriate hypotheses must be generated (on the basis of patterns in the data.
	Consider whether other clinical tests would be useful in allowing you to put the results together and make a final diagnosis.
Uncertain that treatment plan will be successful (limited treatment predictability)	Reschedule the patient for monitoring progress; modify the treatment plan, if necessary.
	Warn the patient of any side effects or signs that warrant calling the doctor or returning to the office.

additional tests, it is important to think about whether a particular test is likely to contribute to one's ability to make a clinical decision. If the test is only an exercise in data gathering, it is not a useful test.

Another consideration is the degree of certainty required to make a decision. Is 80% sufficient? Is 90%, or 100%? If the doctor is 90% certain of a diagnosis, is it worthwhile to bring the patient back to do additional tests? For example, it would not be an efficient use of time to require a patient with no risk factors for glaucoma (and a history of normal IOPs, cup-to-disc ratios, and visual fields) to return for repeated daily IOP measurements for an extended period (e.g., a month). Similarly, it would not be an efficient use of time to repeat automated visual-field tests daily for an extended period in a patient who provides reliable data. Students should remember that clinical decisions rarely are made with 100% confidence. In trying to decide whether additional tests should be done, clinicians must consider the risks of performing the tests and the benefits or usefulness of the tests in contributing to diagnostic decisions (e.g., false-positive and false-negative results; see Table 3.19 and Chapter 3 for a discussion of using *new* tests).

As illustrated in Figure 2.1, as clinicians gather more relevant clinical information, their level of certainty can increase. Beyond a point, however, additional clinical information does not yield a significant increase in a doctor's level of confidence (as with the previously mentioned case in which daily measurements of IOP in a patient with no glaucoma risk factors would not be useful). Clinicians should consider both the probabilities at which they would want to perform additional testing before making a confident diagnosis and the levels of certainty at which they would be confident in initiating treatment for a diagnosis. (The clinician should ask him- or herself at what level of certainty would he or she feel comfortable enough to stop testing and make a confident diagnosis, or at what level of certainty would he or she feel confident in starting treatment for a diagnosis—say, glaucoma—without performing additional tests.) In the presence of high probabilities, a clinician may feel certain of a diagnosis and be ready to start treatment without additional testing; at low probabilities, further testing may be required to help increase the level of certainty.

Testing thresholds and test-treatment thresholds are *quantitative* assessments of probability values that help determine when it is useful to perform additional specific tests.[4] They are calculated with information about the risks of a test and the risks and benefits of treating patients with a particular disease. (Below a testing threshold probability, with a low probability of disease, the outcome of the test would not affect a decision that no treatment is required; thus, the test would not be considered necessary. Above a test-treatment threshold, the probability of disease is high enough that the test result would not affect the management decision to treat; thus, the test would not be deemed necessary.) Similarly, the term *therapeutic threshold* can be computed from data related to the benefits and risks of a specific treatment.[4] (Below a therapeutic threshold probability, the clinician would want to gather more clinical information through additional testing to reach an adequate level of certainty with regard to proper treatment.)

Although quantitative measures from the clinical literature are not always readily accessible to a doctor actively engaged in seeing patients, many clinicians consider these types of assessments intuitively,[5] and it is useful to consider the issues mentioned with regard to the potential risks and benefits of clinical tests and therapies. Clinicians also should remember the Chapter 1 guidelines for searching for additional information: Additional tests are considered useful if they are problem-specific and assist in making a diagnosis, if they provide information useful for monitoring therapy over time, or if they help to establish a database of information on the patient. Clearly, these concepts hold true when the potential benefits of the tests outweigh the potential risks. A highly risky procedure that would not alter the diagnostic or therapeutic decision would not be indicated.

SPECIAL TECHNIQUES FOR MANAGING UNCERTAINTY

Besides the previously discussed strategies for strengthening a clinician's decision making, the following tools and techniques are also helpful. Closed-loop decision making, decision trees, and computer-assisted diagnostic support systems can reduce uncertainty and enhance doctors' confidence in their decisions.

Open-Loop Versus Closed-Loop Decision Making

Using the proper technique at the right time can reduce clinical uncertainty.[1] A model of open-loop decision making is presented in Figure 2.2A. In this model, the doctor evaluates the patient's status, considers the available alternatives, then makes a decision. When a simple decision is being considered and the doctor is highly confident of the decision, this model is adequate. An example is found in considering a minor refractive change. A myopic patient complains of slightly blurred vision at a distance and, on examination, shows a small increase in myopia corresponding to the decrease in acuity. The doctor is confident that providing this change in prescription to the patient will eliminate the symptoms of blurred vision.

A modification to this model is possible. In Figure 2.2B, the initial steps are the same but, instead of the process ending after the third step (determining the patient management plan), the activity continues with feedback that leads to a re-evaluation. For example, a doctor performs a subjective examination with visual acuities, and trial frames the change found. The patient experiences discomfort with the large change in prescription, and prefers the old prescription. This feedback gives the doctor an opportunity to evaluate decisions made. In Figure 2.2A, the decision itself is the end point, and there is no feedback. In Figure 2.2B, a closed-loop system exists, and the clinician evaluates the consequences of decisions made. This gives the doctor an opportunity to take any necessary corrective steps to optimize the outcome of the decision-making process.

An example of the use of a closed-loop system is found in the fitting of a patient with contact lenses. Soon after dispensing the lenses, the doctor brings the patient back to evaluate the patient's status. This involves taking visual acuities and evaluating the fit and comfort of the lens. When problems are identified, the doctor considers possible alternatives: modifying the lens (e.g., changing the peripheral curves, blending the transition zones, changing the diameter of the lens or optic zone), changing the lens care system or schedule (e.g., using dif-

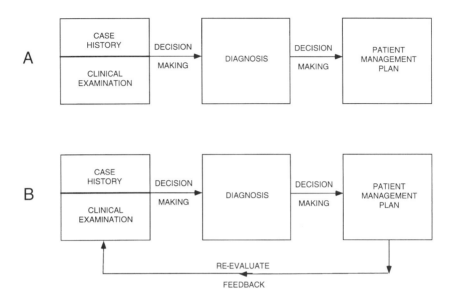

Figure 2.2 Open-loop and closed-loop decision making. A. The steps involved in an open-loop model of decision making. B. The same steps, illustrating that a closed-loop system provides a mechanism to obtain feedback after patient management plans have been determined.

ferent solutions, modifying the wearing schedule), or changing to a different lens (e.g., a different material or lens design). By considering the alternatives in relation to the data obtained from the current and previous examination, the doctor makes a decision about what to do. Once again, the doctor can reschedule the patient to determine the effects of the new corrective action.

The more confident a doctor is of a decision, the more likely open-loop decision making will be sufficient. However, sometimes the doctor does not have enough information at one point to predict how a patient will respond to a given action. Uncertainty calls for closed-loop decision making. Knowing that they will have the opportunity to evaluate their actions can increase doctors' confidence in their ability to maximize their decisions in the long run.

Decision Trees

Decision trees are visual representations of decisions and are used in decision analysis. Although decision analysis is not unique to medicine, it has been used to assist decision making in clinical care. This analysis is an explicit, quantitative method of separating a complex problem into its component parts, identifying available courses of action, evaluating the probabilities of each potential outcome, and making a choice based on the calculations found. By laying out all the options and outcomes, decision analysis provides a systematic approach for making a choice. Formal decision analysis is not meant to be a simulation of the actual process of decision making,[2, 3] but it can help the clinician to make decisions under conditions of uncertainty.

A decision is represented on a decision tree by a square and is referred to as a *decision node*. A common decision in clinical care involves whether to recommend surgery or prescribe drug treatment for a problem. The two decision alternatives are listed in Figure 2.3 as surgery or medical treatment.

Next, the clinician outlines each immediate outcome for each decision alternative. These are written after chance nodes, which are represented on the decision tree by circles. Chance nodes are points on the tree at which chance dictates the outcome. In Figure 2.3, if surgery is done, disease may or may not be present; similarly, following medical treatment, disease may or may not be present. Additional decision nodes and chance nodes are added to the decision tree to illustrate the sequence of events that can occur within the context of the clinical situation considered. If the surgeon chooses a radical procedure and attempts a cure, as in this scenario (very top branch of Figure 2.3), the patient may survive or die an operative death. Alternatively, the surgeon may choose a less risky, palliative procedure having a much lower risk of operative death.

The final outcomes for each decision alternative, the fruit of the tree, are located at the very end of the branches. The final outcomes for the surgical alternative are that the patient will either survive and be cured, will survive without a cure and die of the disease, or will die from the operation. The final outcome for the decision alternative of medical therapy for the patient is that the patient will either survive cured or will die of the disease.

After the decision nodes and possible outcomes are laid out, probabilities are assigned to each event that is controlled by chance, and the decision tree is labeled with these probabilities. The probabilities usually come from statistics available in the clinical literature. In cases in which published probabilities are not known or available, clinicians sometimes substitute their own estimate based on their knowledge and experience. Because probabilities are based on a total likelihood of 1.00 (100%), the sum of the probabilities at each chance node must equal 1.[5] The number of immediate outcomes at a particuar chance node is unlimited, but the outcomes must be mutually exclusive and the sum of their probabilities must equal 1.[5]

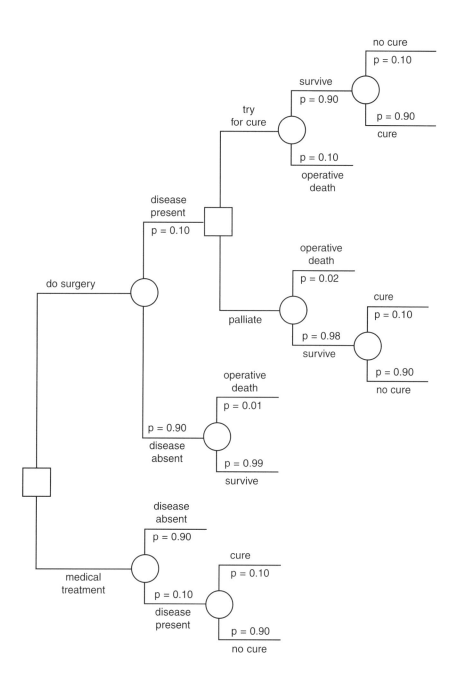

Figure 2.3 A decision tree for comparing medical and surgical treatments of a hypothetical disease. (Reprinted with permission from HC Sox Jr, MA Blatt, MC Higgin, et al. Medical Decision Making. Boston: Butterworths, 1988;156.)

After the probabilities are inserted, the *expected value* of each decision alternative is determined by a calculation known as *folding back the decision tree*. The term *folding back* is used because the mathematic calculation starts at the tips of the branches of the tree (far right) and proceeds back to the root of the tree (far left). Expected value can be calculated for life expectancy adjusted for the quality of life, cost-effectiveness, utility, or other outcome variables. The outcome variable is selected by the person performing the analysis. (Life expectancy is adjusted to take quality of life into account because length of life itself is not an accurate measure of outcome. Cost analysis requires an adjustment with respect to potential outcomes, because pure cost of treatment does not reflect the possible results; cheaper treatments may produce worse outcomes. *Cost-effectiveness* is defined as "the cheapest treatment for an equal or better health care outcome."[6] Utility analysis is a quantitative measure of the strength of a patient's preference for an outcome.) The complex calculations involved in folding back are beyond the scope of the discussion here but are described in further detail in various sources.[2, 5-7]

Forming a decision tree for a clinical problem can be an insightful experience because it forces the clinician to define the problem clearly, to identify all the decision alternatives, to list the possible outcomes for each alternative, to consider the probability for each outcome, and to analyze the situation logically.

Critics of formal decision analysis argue that it is time-consuming, too rigorous, and that it dehumanizes decision making and reduces the caring role of the doctor by focusing the decision on numbers, probabilities, and computations.[2, 6] Supporters of decision analysis respond that the systematic analysis provided with this technique is preferable to basing decisions on unrealistic or improbable hopes of doctors or patients and that it is possible to incorporate the preferences of patients with an analysis of utility.

One of the major advantages of decision analysis is that it forces the decision maker to lay out *all* the alternatives and to consider all the outcomes in a logical way. Decision analysis helps the clinician address uncertainty by providing a system for looking at the component parts of a decision (alternatives and options) analytically. Even if exact probabilities are not known or available, it forces the clinician to analyze the alternatives and outcomes comparatively. In many cases, just sketching out a decision tree with all the alternatives and possible outcomes helps suggest the preferred option, even without numbers.[3]

Patient management decisions in eye care usually involve a subset of the following options: corrective lenses, vision therapy, prisms, surgery, drug therapy, low-vision devices, environmental recommendations, and patient education recommendations.[1] For example, a clinician may work to determine whether surgery or drug therapy will provide an optimal outcome for a patient with an ocular pathology. For a patient with binocular problems, a clinician may try to decide among corrective lenses, vision therapy, prisms, and surgical intervention. When a clinician is unsure of how to manage a particular patient, it may be helpful first to draw a decision tree and list *all* the decision alternatives for that situation, listing each potential outcome for each decision alternative, and then to consider probabilities. Although probabilities may not be available for all the options, the clinician may be able to incorporate personal estimates or a ranking of high to low among the choices. Finally, even without considering any numbers, just going through the process of considering *all* the management options and their potential outcomes (advantages and risks) may enable the clinician to come to a final decision.

Computer-Assisted Diagnosis and Support Systems

Many clinicians are interested in how computers can aid in diagnosis. Computers are very helpful in storing information regarding statistical probabilities and in maintaining detailed information about diseases and therapies. These characteristics have been used to develop computed systems that affect decision making. Four approaches to computer-assisted diagnosis are discussed here: expert systems, computer-assisted testing and evaluation equipment, simulation models, and external computer-assisted support systems.

Expert Systems

Artificial intelligence is concerned with building systems that simulate human intelligence.[8] *Expert systems* in clinical care are computer programs that simulate the decision making ability of clinicians. Such systems can be developed by having expert clinicians (referred to as *domain experts*) work with computer engineers (referred to as *knowledge engineers*).[8] The clinicians describe the rules they use for making decisions. The computer experts then translate the expertise of the clinicians into machine-usable programs.[9] Combining many rules generates computer systems that have the capacity to make decisions for complicated cases. Such systems are referred to as *rule-based* because they are built on and developed after the rules of the clinical experts.

An alternative method for developing an expert system is to provide a sufficient number of clinical cases along with the decisions reached by the clinical experts. The expert system then generates its own rules on the basis of the cases provided. Such a system is referred to as *example-based*.

One problem in the development of computed expert systems has been that one of the strengths of computers—holding a lot of information and expanding on information—would make it easier for computed systems to create an explosion of possible hypotheses,[6] rather than to narrow down the hypotheses to several most likely choices, as in the hypothetico-deductive process of clinicians. In expert systems, it has been difficult to simulate the narrowing down of possible hypotheses to those that are the most likely.[6]

A common criticism of expert diagnostic systems is that, at this point, computed systems are not able to detect in patients' responses such subtle nuances as tonal quality; speed of response; and body posture suggestive of nervousness, pain, discomfort, or doubt.[9] Psychosocial information necessary for proper clinical decision making may not be processed.

Another obstacle has been the high cost and time needed to develop these systems. Questions have been raised about the cost-effectiveness of developing expert systems for functions generally handled easily by clinicians.[9, 10] It appears more likely that expert systems developed in eye care will address the more complex, unusual, or specialized cases and will be used by clinicians as consultants for very difficult patient problems.[6, 11]

Expert systems build on the strengths of computers but do not have to serve as a substitute for doctors; instead, they can complement a doctor's ability to make judgments by contributing the computer's memory, reliability, and processing capacities to the decision-making situation.[8]

Computer-Assisted Testing and Evaluation

Computer-assisted instrumentation and equipment that assist in testing and evaluating patients have had a significant impact on the information used by clinicians to make diagnoses. Automated perimeters, computed assessment of corneal topography, and digitized photographic analyses of optic nerve heads used in glaucoma management are just three examples of the improved level of clinical data possible as a result of computerized equipment.

Computerized testing equipment offers high speed and efficiency not always attainable with the human examiner. The computer uses a consistent testing procedure across the spectrum of patients and over time; it eliminates examiner bias and error. As has been said, the "computer never becomes bored, tired, or ill."[12]

If computerized instrumentation results in better testing procedures and, consequently, better clinical data, it can facilitate better decision making. The instrumentation described in this category is not designed to replace or serve as a substitute for the doctor, but to *support* the doctor's decision-making process. These instruments help address sources of uncertainty encountered in some previously described clinical situations (see Table 2.1).

Simulation Models

Computer simulations and computer-assisted instructional techniques have been used to develop diagnostic skills.[13, 14] Frequently, models of realistic patient encounters are used for students or practitioners in interactive tutorial sessions.

Simulations are especially useful for allowing students to learn and practice skills that require expensive equipment, difficult or risky procedures, or very limited resources. In this way, learning is accomplished in a "forgiving" environment.[13] Learning to make diagnoses of unusual patient problems not widely accessible to students or to perform risky surgical techniques would be useful patient simulations both for students and for practicing clinicians. The goal of these techniques is not to intervene directly during an actual patient encounter but to prepare the clinician better to handle the uncertainty that would otherwise occur in the absence of these training opportunities.

External Computer-Assisted Support Systems

The final category of computer-assisted support systems includes performing computed biomedical literature searches (see Chapter 4), communicating with expert clinicians through e-mail, and contacting expert clinicians through telemedicine. Although the resources in these examples may not be available directly at the clinical site, each of them can help reduce uncertainty and enhance decision making.

Will computers replace clinicians? One challenge in developing expert computerized diagnostic systems has been in the ability to program the complexities of clinical problem solving.[15] Although computers can perform impressively when handling statistical and numeric analyses related to clinical problems, there are still limits to a computer's ability to simulate a clinician's thinking. A computer can do only what it is programmed to do,[2] and at present it has been difficult to program the more abstract components of clinical analysis. How do clinicians make observations of patients? Can a computer recognize whether a patient is depressed? A fundamental problem with the con-

cept of computed diagnosis involves programming the more imagina-
tive aspects of human thinking into a computer.[6] Those concerned that
computers may replace doctors may be reassured by remembering that,
at this point, computers lack the "intuition, inspiration and insight
which the [human] brain uses in coming to decisions."[6] Although the
computer may be able to handle admirably some aspects of the science
of clinical care, it has much more difficulty with the art. The computer's observational skills and ability to get to know the patient as an individual are limited. Is the patient experiencing mild discomfort or severe
pain? Is the patient afraid or calm? Is the patient compliant? How do
the patient's beliefs and attitudes interact with his or her clinical care?
Such questions should help reassure the concerned human clinician
that computers may be helpful in *assisting* in diagnosis but are not likely to *replace* the human clinician in the near future. Doctors may find
it helpful to use computers as an adjunct to clinical problem solving
but not as a substitute for the human doctor.

WHERE TO BEGIN

Although computers and decision trees can assist in diagnostic and
therapeutic decision making, clinicians often find that the hardest step
is getting started. Sometimes clinicians find it difficult to start generating diagnostic hypotheses. In complicated cases, trying to make a specific diagnosis early in the encounter can make the clinician feel lost.
When you are puzzled and perplexed at the beginning, how do you
get started?

In cases of uncertainty, when you do not know what disease or condition the patient has and you are not sure how to proceed, think in
terms of broader categories rather than of very specific conditions (e.g.,
conjunctivitis rather than viral conjunctivitis; retinal disorder rather
than central serous retinopathy). Often, identifying a broad category
and investigating with further testing can bring you to a more specific
diagnosis.

One strategy in considering broad classifications for ocular problems
is to consider a front-to-back approach.[16] Visual problems may start as
anteriorly as the lids and may extend as far back as the visual cortex.
If you are not certain of the cause of a visual problem, consider the
part(s) of the eye affected (Table 2.2). Is it more likely the lids or the
lashes? Is it the conjunctiva, the sclera, the cornea, the iris, the lens,
the vitreous, or the retina? Is it the optic nerve or visual pathway
involvement? After you identify a broad category, you are more prepared to narrow your diagnosis to a more specific cause. Think corneal,

Table 2.2
Front-to-back approach.

Source	Examples of Pathologies
Lids and lashes	Blepharitis, entropion, ectropion, trichiasis
Conjunctiva	Conjunctivitis, subconjunctival hemorrhage
Cornea	Abrasions, opacities, keratoconjunctivitis sicca
Anterior chamber	Glaucoma
Iris	Iritis
Lens	Accommodative dysfunctions, cataracts, sub-luxated lens
Vitreous	Opacities, vitreal hemorrhages
Retina	Hemorrhages; exudates; cotton-wool spots; artery and vein occlusions; retinal, disc, or macular edema
Neurologic involvement	Optic neuritis, cranial nerve palsies

retinal, and neurologic rather than keratoconus versus central serous retinopathy versus sixth nerve palsy when you do not have enough information to consider actual diagnoses.

The technique described above can be very useful for diagnosing anatomically based problems such as corneal and retinal problems. When using this model, remember to include functional problems, such as accommodative dysfunctions, in your thinking.

When the problem is not centered at the eye, it may be helpful to consider a set of broad etiologies grouped together in the mnemonic device VITAMINES (vitamins, plus E; Table 2.3).[17] This system provides 18 broad classifications that may help bring to mind the types of possible causes of a patient's problems.

In cases in which you are still unsure of the patient's problem and how to proceed, consider these suggestions.

1.   *Get a clearer understanding of the patient's problem by returning to the case history.* In many cases in which the patient's problem is hard to define, it is because the clinician has not obtained a full understanding of the problem. By returning to the case history and asking the patient more questions, the doctor is better able to frame the problem and to comprehend what the patient is experiencing. This is stage 1 of the diagnostic reasoning process (see Chapter 1), a critical step that is the antecedent to hypothesis generation.

2.   *Perform problem-specific tests and reassess your level of certainty after these tests.* In many cases, performing additional tests can reduce uncer-

Table 2.3
Clinical diagnostic categories.

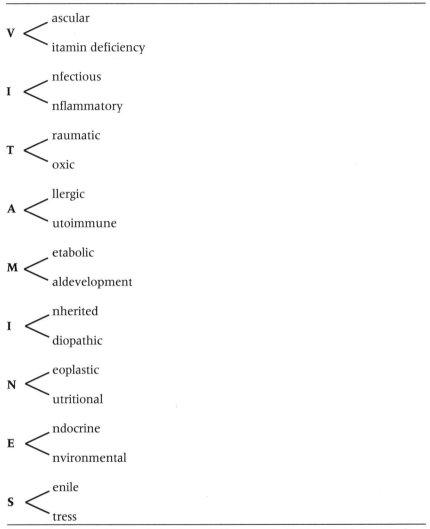

V	ascular / itamin deficiency
I	nfectious / nflammatory
T	raumatic / oxic
A	llergic / utoimmune
M	etabolic / aldevelopment
I	nherited / diopathic
N	eoplastic / utritional
E	ndocrine / nvironmental
S	enile / tress

Source: Reprinted with permission from JS Sherman. A clinician's guide to special testing. Optom Manage 1992;27:62.

tainty. Select tests that are appropriate, given your understanding of the patient's problem; once problem-specific tests are done, *re-evaluate* your level of understanding. Sometimes the dedication under uncertainty is aimed so strongly at collecting new information that analysis takes a back seat. This can lead to technical nonsynthesis (see Chapter 1) in which excessive testing interferes with data evaluation and assessment. Continuing to think about information provided by new tests keeps the doctor on track with regard to diagnosis and evaluation.

3.   *Think normal versus abnormal.* Under conditions of uncertainty, when you are unsure how to proceed, think about what is normal and what is abnormal in the patient's clinical data. What findings fall outside the expected ranges? Identifying abnormalities can help generate diagnostic hypotheses that can direct further investigation.

4.   *Look for relationships between clinical findings you have obtained.* Look for patterns in the data and try to correlate and integrate the results of related tests (e.g., IOPs, optic nerve head assessments, visual fields; or near cover test, convergence near point, von Graefe phoria at near, positive fusional convergence at near). Relate the patient's chief complaint and case history to the data.

5.   *Under conditions of uncertainty, when you are really not sure what is occurring, consider your* highest *level of understanding of the patient's problem (Figure 2.4) and work to increase your level of understanding.* A diagnosis is the highest level of understanding. If all you have is the patient's description of the problem but no clinical data or observations, this is the lowest level. Consider what clinical tests you can perform to provide information related to the patient's symptoms. If you have clinical data or you have made observations related to the patient's sympoms, determine what additional tests you must perform to reach a diagnosis. When you do not have a diagnosis, you should work toward a higher level of understanding of the patient's problem through further testing, until you reach a diagnosis.

6.   *Under uncertain conditions, when there is inadequate information to make a conclusive assessment, do not close your mind and settle on a diagnosis too early.* Keep an open mind to new data and continue to collect data that can contribute to good decision making. This can help prevent errors of premature closure and anchoring (see Chapter 1).

7.   *Under conditions of uncertainty, consider using a closed-loop process of decision making.* Sometimes it is helpful to bring the patient back for further testing or to determine whether your initial management plan is effective. By looking for feedback and re-evaluating decisions, the doctor can take advantage of opportunities to fine-tune management strategies.

8.   *Remember that good record keeping is an adjunct to effective problem solving.* Under conditions of uncertainty, it is *especially* important to keep clear records, which helps to follow the patient's status and the doctor's management plans.

The problem-oriented medical record was developed by Dr. Lawrence Weed to improve record keeping in medicine.[18, 19] This system has also been used in optometry. It consists of four parts: the database, the prob-

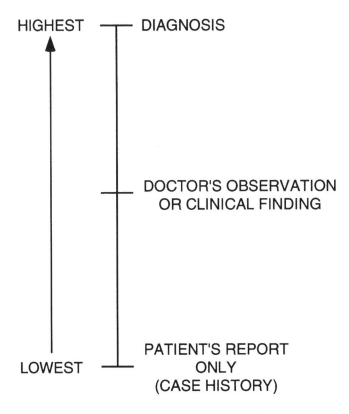

Figure 2.4 A doctor's level of understanding of a patient's problem. Clinicians should work to increase their level of understanding of a patient's problem from the lowest level (patient's report) to the highest level (a final diagnosis).

lem list, the plan, and progress notes. The database is composed of two parts, the minimum database collected on all patients and problem-specific data that address a particular patient's individual concerns and problems.

Two types of problem lists are used. A working problem list, found at the end of each examination, provides a list of all the patient's problems at that visit. A master problem list, generally found at the front of the patient's record, provides the doctor with an overview of the patient's cumulative problems and has been referred to as a *table of contents* of the record.[20]

Progress notes are composed of four parts, often referred to by the acronym SOAP: subjective, objective, assessment, and plan. *Subjective* notes consist of information provided by the patient about symptoms, problems, and concerns. *Objective* notes include the doctor's clinical examination results. *Assessment* is the doctor's evaluation of the patient's problems and status. The *plan* presents the doctor's management strategy for the patient.

Good record keeping can help organize the collection of clinical data and, therefore, assist in the clinical decision-making process. It is especially helpful in assessing the patient's progress over time.

9.   *Don't be overwhelmed by the complexities of a case.* Remember that patients may present with a variety of symptoms and several diagnoses that exist simultaneously. To wade through the complexities of clinical diagnosis, it is important to adopt a systematic method of problem solving. A *comprehensive* evaluation of the patient's ocular status (suggested in the example in Table 1.3) can help determine each of the patient's problems. For example, a patient with an uncorrected refractive error, convergence insufficiency, and dry eye may present for an examination. Detecting any of the problems without the others means that the patient may remain symptomatic. A comprehensive approach to eye care will help the doctor detect and address the full set of a patient's ocular and vision-related problems.

In cases in which extensive problem-specific tests are required or a problem requiring immediate attention is identified (e.g., corneal abrasion), it may be preferable to defer some tests from the general database until the patient's primary problem is handled. In such cases, remember to address the remaining database at appropriate follow-up visits.

When several diagnoses are identified, it may be necessary to prioritize the plan, depending on the immediacy of care required. Pathologic problems, such as a retinal detachment, iritis, or corneal abrasion, require rapid action. These examples illustrate that, in addition to making decisions regarding diagnosis and management plan, doctors must also make assessments regarding the time course of care provided.

When cases are complex and alternative modes of therapy have to be compared for a particular problem, decision trees can provide a system for evaluating and comparing the alternatives.

10.   *Seek other expert opinions.* When you are still uncertain about the diagnosis or appropriate treatment, seek expert opinions through consultations and referrals. Consultations occur when a doctor sends a patient to another professional for (1) a specific test, (2) a set of tests, or (3) an expert opinion. Referral generally indicates a transfer of responsibility in the care of the patient that is expected to continue over an extended period.[21] Making your intentions clear to both the patient and the other doctor makes it easier for appropriate diagnosis, management, and follow-up to occur. Computer-assisted expert opinions are becoming increasingly available and provide another source of information for decision making.

SUMMARY

Uncertainty is an unavoidable aspect of clinical care. The wise clinician learns to manage uncertainty optimally by understanding the sources of uncertainty and the strategies for addressing them. Knowing how to use decision trees, closed-loop decision making, and computer-assisted diagnosis and support systems can improve decision making and reduce a clinician's uncertainty.

REFERENCES

1. Ettinger ER. Clinical Decision Making in Special Populations: Dealing With Incomplete Data. In DM Maino, RL London (eds), Diagnosis and Management of Special Populations. St. Louis: Mosby–Year Book, 1995;207–226.
2. Albert DA, Munson R, Resnik MD. Reasoning in Medicine: An Introduction to Clinical Inference. Baltimore: Johns Hopkins University, 1988.
3. Weinstein MC, Fineberg HV. Clinical Decision Analysis. Philadelphia: Saunders, 1980.
4. Pauker SG, Kassirer JP. The threshold approach to clinical decision making. N Engl J Med 1980;302:1109–1117.
5. Sox HC Jr, Blatt MA, Higgin MC, et al. Medical Decision Making. Boston: Butterworth-Heinemann, 1988.
6. Bradley GW. Disease, Diagnosis and Decisions. New York: Wiley, 1993;96.
7. Sackett DL, Haynes RB, Guyatt GH, et al. Clinical Epidemiology: A Basic Science for Clinical Medicine. Boston: Little, Brown, 1991.
8. Reggia JA, Tuhrim S (eds). Computer-Assisted Medical Decision Making. New York: Springer-Verlag, 1985.
9. Madsen EM, Reinke AR, Fehrs MH, et al. Applications of expert computer systems. J Am Optom Assoc 1991;62:116–122.
10. Madsen EM, Reinke AR, Fehrs MH, et al. Exploring the optometric application of expert computer systems: refractive error correction. J Am Optom Assoc 1991;62:621–629.
11. Madsen EM, Kaminski MS, Yolton RL. Automated decision making: the role of expert computer systems in the future of optometry. J Am Optom Assoc 1993;64:479–489.
12. Maino JH, Maino DM, Davidson DW (eds). Computer Applications in Optometry. Boston: Butterworths, 1989.
13. Leroy A, Zeitner D, Smith DL, et al. The optometry game: enhancing test selection and lens prescribing skills by use of computer simulations. J Am Optom Assoc 1994;65:221–229.
14. Baro JA, Lehmkuhle S, Sesma MA. InSight: a series of interactive experiments and demonstrations in vision science for the Macintosh computer. J Optom Educ 1991;16:82–87.
15. Judge RD, Zuidema GD, Fitzergald FT (eds). Clinical Diagnosis: A Physiologic Approach (5th ed). Boston: Little, Brown, 1989.

16. Ettinger ER. Managing patients with lupus erythematosus. N Engl J Optom 1994;46:126–132.
17. Sherman JS. A clinician's guide to special testing. Optom Manage 1992; 27(7):58–62.
18. Weed LL. Medical records that guide and teach. N Engl J Med 1968;278:593–600, 652–657.
19. Weed LL. Medical Records, Medical Education, and Patient Care. Cleveland: Press of Case Western Reserve University, 1969.
20. Barresi BJ. Ocular Assessment: The Manual of Diagnosis for Office Practice. Boston: Butterworths, 1984.
21. Ettinger ER. Professional Communications in Eye Care. Boston: Butterworth-Heinemann, 1994.

3

Use of Epidemiology in Clinical Decision Making

Elizabeth Hoppe

REASONS FOR USING EPIDEMIOLOGY

Every time clinicians see patients, they are required to make a series of decisions. What is the probability of ocular or systemic disease? What is the likelihood that this patient has a visual disorder? Which diagnostic tests will best determine the cause of the patient's symptoms? How accurate are the results of the test? Are the results normal? If disease or disorder is found, what are the expected consequences? How will reduction of a patient's risk factors reduce the risk of disease?

In most clinical situations, the diagnosis, prognosis, treatment options, and best course of management have a level of uncertainty. For any given patient, an eye care provider does not know, in advance of the diagnosis, how this patient's condition will progress, or how the patient will respond to the recommended therapy or treatment regimen. With technology ever expanding, the number, variety, and reliability of tests available to the doctor of optometry is increasing dramatically. Knowledge of disease distribution, the ability to assess the information obtained in clinical testing, and the measurement of treatment effectiveness can be improved through application of the principles of epidemiology.[1–4]

Historically, principles of epidemiology have been used by eye care professionals to make major breakthroughs in the understanding of human disease patterns. In 1941, congenital cataracts and characteristic retinal signs were used to identify an outbreak of congenital rubella. In the 1970s, bilateral optic atrophy in a 3-year-old boy helped to identify the toxicity of diiodohydroxyquin, a drug used to treat colitis. Clinical

Table 3.1
The six *E*s.

	Areas of Health Care and Health-Care Decision Making
Etiology	Identifying and quantifying causal factors, risk factors, or risk indicators
Efficacy	Establishing the degree to which clinical or public health practices are either beneficial, useless, or harmful
Effectiveness	Measuring the degree to which an efficacious practice actually benefits a defined population
Efficiency	Measuring the effectiveness of a given expenditure of resources
Evaluation	Assessing the extent to which a stated goal, objective, or standard actually is reached as the result of specific health practices
Education	Introducing clinicians, public health practitioners, administrators, and policy makers to the epidemiologic perspective and to the value of applying quantitative science to clinical and public health problems

Source: Reprinted with permission from RD Newcomb, EC Marshall. Public Health and Community Optometry (2nd ed). Boston: Butterworth-Heinemann, 1990;73.

findings of aniridia helped to identify Wilms' tumor, and the association between amblyopia and the incidence of foreign bodies in the better-seeing eye made a strong case for the use of safety eye wear.[5] As we look ahead to the scope and mode of the expanding practice of optometry, epidemiologic principles may be applied to health care program planning, human resources needs assessment, and quality assurance programs. An understanding of basic methods used in epidemiology will enhance any doctor's clinical practice. Table 3.1 lists the Six *E*s, six areas in which epidemiology may be useful in health care and health care decision making.[6]

DEFINITION

Simply put, *epidemiology* has been defined as the study of disease occurrence and its relation to various characteristics of individuals or their environment. Epidemiology and clinical diagnosis use similar processes. The main difference between them is that clinical diagnosis focuses on the patient, whereas epidemiology traditionally focuses on some aspect of a population, community, or neighborhood. A blend of the two results

Table 3.2
Definition of incidence and prevalence.

Incidence	Number of new cases of a condition that occur in a given period of time, usually a year	New cases/population at risk
Prevalence	Number of existing cases of a condition at a given time	Existing cases/ total population

in a hybrid known as *clinical epidemiology*. It is concerned with studying groups of people to gather evidence to help make clinical decisions in patient care; it is the study of variation in the outcome of illness and of the reasons for that variation. Clinical epidemiology may also be thought of as the study of determinants and effects of clinical decisions.

Epidemiology, and therefore clinical epidemiology, relies on the basic assumptions that human disease does not occur at random and that human disease has both causal and preventive factors that may be identified through a systematic investigative process. The tools used in epidemiology rely heavily on the measurement of disease frequency, the distribution of disease, and the determinants of disease. Both the theory of probability and various mathematic concepts are used to make calculations that can be applied in a clinical setting. This chapter serves as a basic introduction to these concepts and illustrates ways to integrate epidemiology into the clinical decision-making process.

RATES OF DISEASES AND DISORDERS

Because diagnosis, treatment, and management of diseases and disorders have their basis in prior experience with patients, an understanding of the distribution and rates of disease in a population is essential. In epidemiology, the rates of disease are expressed in terms of *incidence* and *prevalence* (Table 3.2).

Incidence Rates

Incidence rates measure the probability that healthy people will develop a disease over a specified period of time. In other words, incidence measures the rate at which a new disease occurs in a group of people who are disease-free. To determine accurately the incidence rate of a disease, it is necessary to follow a specific group of people, or a population, forward in time and to measure the rate at which new cases of a disease appear. This process is often difficult for many reasons. First, it assumes that there is an adequate ability to determine the health status of the people being followed. Usually this is done by direct examination or by auditing medical records. Second, the time of onset must be determined. For an acute condition (e.g., bacterial conjunctivitis or uveitis), this may be relatively easy to determine. For a chronic condition (e.g., glaucoma or diabetic retinopathy), the time of onset is more difficult to ascertain. Third, an incidence rate requires specification of the numerator. The definition of incidence in Table 3.2 indicates that the numerator is the number of new cases. Often, this is specified as the number of people who develop the disease, but in optometric and ophthalmologic literature, it also may be the number of *eyes* with the disease or condition. The denominator then must be specified to match the numerator—either *people at risk* or *eyes at risk*. In specifying incidence rates, the denominator should not include those who already have the disease or those who are not susceptible to the disease. For example, people who are not susceptible to the disease may have had the disease already and acquired immunity, as in the case of chickenpox, or they may be immunized against the disease. Incidence rates of prostate cancer should include only men in the denominator, and the denominator of incidence rates of uterine cancer should include only women who have not undergone hysterectomies. Most often, the denominator is given in a standardized form. For example, incidence rates may be expressed in percentage form (that is, cases per 100 people at risk), cases per 1,000, or cases per 100,000. A general rule of thumb is that the numerator should be expressed as a whole number. For example, the incidence of ocular cancer is better expressed as 1/100,000 per year instead of 0.1/10,000 per year.

Finally, in measuring an incidence rate, the period of observation must be specified. This is usually 1 year but may be any specified period. In the case of an extremely rare disease, it may take more than 1 year to identify enough cases to measure the incidence. In the case of a very common disease, 6 months or even 1 month may be a more appropriate period.

There are a number of examples of studies that have followed populations over time to determine incidence rates. The Framingham study[7] was begun in 1948 by enrolling 5,209 subjects. Subjects have been examined every 2 years since. Originally, the Framingham study was designed to study heart disease, but additional measures, including incidence of ocular conditions, have been included. The Baltimore Longitudinal Study on Aging[8] is a prospective study being conducted by the National Institute on Aging. It began in 1958 by enrolling a representative sample of adults aged 21 and older. Complete medical examinations are conducted periodically to collect data on physical, mental, and social changes that occur with aging. Numerous reports of eye conditions found in this study are available in the literature. The Orinda Longitudinal Study of Myopia[9] is a community-based cohort study of school children aged 6–14 years. Data collection began in 1989, and the study is ongoing. It includes measures of refractive error, corneal curvature, crystalline lens power, and axial ocular dimensions.

Prevalence Rates

As shown in Table 3.2, prevalence rates measure the probability of people having a particular disease at a given time. Both the number of people who have had the disease in the past and the duration of their illness have an impact on prevalence. This effect is *additive* (i.e., even if the number of new cases of disease—incidence—is low, the prevalence may be high if the disease has a long duration). In the example of a chronic disease for which there is no cure (say, diabetes), prevalence is equal to all the previously diagnosed cases and any new cases. In the example of an acute condition that is self-limiting or effectively treated (say, corneal abrasions), prevalence (P) is related to the incidence (I) of disease by the following equation:

$$P = I \times d$$

where *d* is the duration of illness.

Prevalence may be expressed either as a point prevalence or a period prevalence. *Point prevalence* attempts to measure the number of cases of a disease at one point (i.e., on one day). *Period prevalence* consists of prevalence at a point, plus new cases, and recurrences within a given period, most often 1 year. In the case of a disease such as AIDS, the duration of which effectively lasts until the death of the patient, the period prevalence for 1 year might be calculated as the sum of the monthly incidence rates less the number of people who die from AIDS divided by the total population at midyear.

Because of the relationship between prevalence and the duration of a disease, prevalence rates tend to favor chronic conditions over acute conditions. This tendency will give falsely high rates for chronic disease and falsely low rates for acute disease. Generally, for an acute or infectious disease, the incidence rate will be most helpful, whereas for a chronic condition, prevalence rates will provide the most useful information.

Often, prevalence rates are obtained by survey. A typical survey might ask the question, "In the last 2 weeks, have you been sick with a cold?" In 1956, the National Health Interview Survey was established to provide information on disease rates across the United States.[8] The health examination survey includes both a questionnaire and a physical examination, and the health records survey samples institutional health records, with a supplemental survey of patients and practitioners. All three instruments provide excellent resources of epidemiologic data. In addition, information about both incidence and prevalence rates may be found in optometric and medical literature, local databases (e.g., a state-based blindness registry), or your own experience in your own clinical setting.

When using these rates in clinical practice, it is important to assess the "generalizability" or external validity of the information. Is the population studied in the literature the same as the population you are seeing clinically? For example, the National Health Interview survey represents the civilian noninstitutionalized population. If you are practicing in a military setting, you might expect your patients to be generally younger and healthier than the population at large. The fact that they were inducted implies a certain level of health. This is an example of the phenomenon known as the *healthy worker effect*.[10] If you practice in an institutional setting (a nursing home or long-term care facility), you might expect your patients generally to be older and sicker. Rates can vary widely on the basis of ethnicity as well. For example, optometrists practicing within the Indian Health Service might expect to see rates of diabetes much higher in the Native American population than in overall U.S. rates. The prevalence of diabetes among Navajo Indians aged 45–64 is almost four times higher than among the general U.S. population.[11] Optometrists who have a patient base consisting mainly of blacks may find that their patients are at high risk for glaucoma. Studies have shown that glaucoma is five times more likely to occur in blacks than in whites, and glaucoma is approximately four times more likely to cause blindness in blacks than in whites.[12]

USING DISEASE RATES IN CLINICAL PRACTICE

As described earlier in this chapter, clinical decision making involves dealing with uncertainty. Using incidence and prevalence rates can help diminish the level of uncertainty by allowing you to determine the likelihood of a particular diagnosis. As will be seen later in this chapter, incidence and prevalence play an important role in screening and in the selection of appropriate clinical tests.

In the work of a health care administrator, incidence and prevalence are important for program planning and allocation of funds. Both incidence and prevalence can also be expressed for specific population groups and can be subdivided by age, gender, or ethnicity. This information may be helpful when planning services for a Native American health service facility, an urban clinic that serves a primarily black population, or a school-based screening program. In each of these situations, eye care needs may vary tremendously, resulting in varying requirements for the type and frequency of testing or for eye care professional staffing levels.

Incidence and prevalence rates may also serve as a quality assurance check. If the prevalence of a specific condition in the general population is known, it can be compared with the number of cases actually detected. Barresi[13] suggests that if it is expected that approximately 8% of the male population demonstrates some type of color deficiency, and a clinical facility is documenting less than that number in the charts of its male patients, you may wish to assess whether patients are being screened properly for color deficiency.

To illustrate some of the incidence and prevalence rates important to an optometrist, Tables 3.3 through 3.8 have been compiled from several different sources.[14-23] (Rates are for the general U.S. population unless otherwise specified.) For ease of comparison across conditions, all the rates are shown per 100,000 population.

RISK FACTORS FOR DISEASE

In addition to knowing the rates of disease for a population, often it is helpful to be able to determine the risk factors for a specific disease for an individual patient. Risk factors for disease are calculated by studies of precursors, or exposure to some factor, and the subsequent clinical events. Most of what we know about risk factors comes from either cohort or case-control population-based epidemiologic studies.

The word *cohort* originally described a division of an ancient Roman legion or a band of warriors.[24] Since then, it has come to mean a group of individuals having a statistical factor (such as age, socioeconomic status, or exposure status) in common in a demographic or epidemiologic study. Cohort studies may be done either prospectively (e.g., following an identified group of people ahead in time) or retrospectively (e.g., reviewing medical records). The cohort is evaluated to determine differences in the rate at which disease develops and the exposure to a specific environmental factor or the possession of a specific characteristic. A cohort study allows us to calculate the *relative risk* of a disease, given a certain exposure or characteristic. The relative risk may be expressed as an increased likelihood of disease.

Table 3.3
Chronic ocular disease rates.

Condition	Rate	
Glaucoma	Incidence:	81.68/100,000
	Prevalence:	500/100,000
	Prevalence over the age of 40:	2,000/100,000
	Prevalence by age:	
	52–64	1,400/100,000
	65–74	5,100/100,000
	75–85	7,200/100,000
Cataract	Incidence:	449.18/100,000
	Prevalence range:	200–20,000/100,000
	Prevalence by age:	
	52–64	4,600/100,000
	65–74	18,000/100,000
	75–85	46,000/100,000
Macular degeneration	Prevalence:	9,000/100,000
	Prevalence by age:	
	52–64	2,000/100,000
	65–74	11,000/100,000
	75–85	28,000/100,000
Diabetic retinopathy	Incidence:	22.65/100,000
	Prevalence among diabetics by age:	
	65–74	3,000/100,000
	75–85	7,000/100,000

Table 3.4
Acute ocular condition rates.

Condition	Rate	
Allergic disorders	Incidence	98.50/100,000
Abrasion of cornea and eye	Incidence	219.66/100,000
Uveitis	Incidence	15/100,000

Table 3.9 illustrates this concept using an epidemiologist's "2 × 2" table (later, this table will be important conceptually). Cell A represents persons who have the disease and have been exposed to the risk factor of concern. Cell D represents members of the cohort who do not

Table 3.5
Systemic condition rates.

Condition	Rate	
Diabetes	Prevalence overall:	2,300/100,000
	Prevalence age <45:	500/100,000
	Prevalence age >65:	8,000/100,000
Hypertension	Prevalence readings above:	
	160/95 mm Hg	20,000/100,000
	140/90 mm Hg	45,000/100,000
Sickle cell anemia	Prevalence among U.S. blacks:	
	trait	8,000/100,000
	disease	400/100,000
Familial hypercho-lesterolemia	Prevalence:	200/100,000

Table 3.6
Refractive error rates.

Condition	Rate	
Myopia	Prevalence by age:	
	5 years	1,000/100,000
	10 years	8,000/100,000
	15 years	15,000/100,000
	12–54 years	25,000/100,000
Hyperopia (>+1.25 D)	Prevalence ages 5–50 years:	4–7,000/100,000
	Prevalence among adult rural population:	2,450/100,000
Astigmatism	Prevalence:	
	any amount	70,000/100,000
	≥1.25 D	3,000/100,000

develop the disease and who have not been exposed to the risk factor. Cells B and C represent mixed exposure and disease outcomes.

Relative risk (RR) of disease is expressed as the incidence among the exposed divided by the incidence among the unexposed:

$$RR = [A/(A + B)] \div [C/(C + D)]$$

Case-control studies compare people in whom a disease has been diagnosed (cases) to similar people who do not have the disease (controls). The purpose of this comparison is to determine whether the two groups

Table 3.7
Binocular conditions.

Condition	Rate	
Exophoria >9Δ	Prevalence:	670/100,000
Esophoria >7Δ	Prevalence:	670/100,000
Any strabismus	Incidence:	198.48/100,000
	Prevalence:	3,000–5,000/100,000
Exotropia	Prevalence:	170/100,000
Esotropia	Prevalence:	670/100,000
Convergence insufficiency	Prevalence among elementary school children (Canada):	2,250/100,000
Amblyopia	Prevalence:	1,700/100,000

Table 3.8
Other conditions.

Condition	Rate	
Keratoconus	Incidence:	1.5/100,000
	Prevalence:	30/100,000
Color deficiency	Prevalence in males:	8,000–10,000/100,000
Legal blindness (all causes)	Incidence:	15/100,000
	Prevalence:	160/100,000
Congenital toxoplasmosis	Incidence:	3.48/100,000
Retinoblastoma	Incidence:	5/100,000
All ocular cancers	Incidence:	1/100,000
	Prevalence:	12/100,000

differ in the proportion of persons who had been exposed to a specific factor or who posses a certain characteristic. To analyze a case-control study, epidemiologists use the same 2 × 2 table shown in Table 3.9. By definition, all the cases *have* the disease and would be entered either in cell A or cell C, depending on their exposure status. All the controls do not have the disease and would be entered in cell B or cell D.

Case-control studies use an odds ratio (OR) to describe the relationship between exposure and disease. The OR can be considered the odds in favor of having a disease with the risk factor present. Another definition of odds is the ratio of the likelihood of the event occurring over the likelihood of the event not occurring. ORs for a case-control

Table 3.9
Cohort study.

	Disease Present	Disease Absent	Total
Exposed to risk factor	Cell A	Cell B	A + B
Not exposed to risk factor	Cell C	Cell D	C + D
Total	A + C	B + D	A + B + C + D

study are calculated as the odds of disease with the risk factor divided by the odds of having the disease without the risk factor:

$$OR = (A \times D) \div (B \times C)$$

Cohort studies and case-control studies have unique strengths and weaknesses. Generally, a cohort study takes more time because it is necessary to wait for the disease to develop. Case-control studies are faster because the disease status already is known. Case-control studies are better for rare diseases and are usually less expensive to conduct.[1, 6, 25]

Though population-based epidemiologic studies do not predict accurately the likelihood of disease for an individual patient in your examination chair, they do give you some idea of the strength of association between specific diseases and specific risk factors. This approximation can give you a ballpark estimate of what can be expected for an individual patient, given a certain set of circumstances. The best source of risk factors and ORs is the current professional literature. It is not unusual to find different numbers quoted for the same risk factors, depending on the study design; thus, a review of more than one published article is recommended. Table 3.10 gives examples of ORs and relative risks for various ocular conditions and associated risk factors.[26–33] It should be noted that these risk factors come from only one study; other studies may report different risk factors. To read this table, it is helpful to remember the phrase, "A patient with risk factor x has y times greater odds of developing disease z." For example, shown in the first row, "A patient with fair skin has 5.4 times greater odds of developing ocular surface epithelial dysplasia."

PRINCIPLES OF SCREENING

Optometric practice uses the principles of screening in several areas. School-based vision screenings have been found critical in the identi-

Table 3.10
Relative risk and odds ratios.

Condition	Risk Factor	
Ocular surface epithelial dysplasia	Fair skin	odds ratio 5.4
	Propensity to sunburn	odds ratio 3.8
Graves' disease	Smoking	odds ratio 1.6
Graves' ophthalmopathy	Smoking	odds ratio 7.7
Postoperative endophthalmitis	Intraocular lens with Prolene haptics	odds ratio 4.5
Acute contact lens–related disorders	Extended-wear soft contact lenses	relative risk 2.7
Esotropia	Maternal smoking through pregnancy	odds ratio 1.8
	Low birth weight (<2,500 g)	odds ratio 8.2
Retinal vein occlusion	Systemic hypertension	odds ratio 3.86
	Open-angle glaucoma	odds ratio 2.89
	Male gender	odds ratio 2.61
Posterior subcapsular cataract	History of cortisone use	odds ratio 8.39
Death from secondary primary tumors	Bilateral retinoblastoma	relative risk 60.0

fication of undetected refractive error, ocular pathology, and binocular vision problems that may diminish a child's ability to learn. Vision screening has become an integral part of licensure for driving, and many service organizations work to provide cataract and glaucoma screenings. In addition to screening groups of people, many of the tests performed as part of a comprehensive eye examination may actually be considered screening tests. For example, performing the Amsler chart test may serve as a screening for macular degeneration, tonometry may be thought of as a screening for glaucoma, and glucometry is a screening test for diabetes.

A *screening test* is one that can be performed efficiently and cost-effectively. It does *not* provide a definitive diagnosis of disease but indicates an increased likelihood of disease or the need for further testing. A positive screening test is followed by a *diagnostic* test to determine whether the disease state truly exists. For example, in screening for glaucoma by tonometry, a definitive diagnosis of glaucoma cannot be made without evaluation of the optic nerve and the visual field. Screening for macular degeneration with the Amsler chart might include fluorescein angiography as a follow-up diagnostic test.

Table 3.11
Screening test.

Results	Disease Present	Disease Absent
Positive	True positive Cell A	False positive Cell B
Negative	False negative Cell C	True negative Cell D

   Screening tests always are compared to the true disease state. Although determining the true disease state often is difficult, in evaluating a screening test, it is assumed that a "gold standard" exists by which the true state of disease might be determined. Table 3.11 shows the possible relationships between the true disease state and the results of the screening test.

   As shown in this table, if the disease is present but the screening test fails to detect the disease, a false-negative registers (shown in cell C). If the disease is absent and the screening test is positive, a false-positive appears (shown in cell B). Cells A and D occur when the screening test accurately predicts the disease state, yielding a true positive or a true negative. An ideal screening test will result in few false responses.

   To quantify the rate of false-positive and false-negative results of a screening test, two measures are used: sensitivity and specificity. *Sensitivity* is defined as the proportion of people who have the disease and have a positive test for the disease. Another way to think of sensitivity is to consider how many people the screening test will detect of all those who have the disease. The calculation to determine a screening test's sensitivity is:

$$\text{Sensitivity} = A \div (A + C)$$

Specificity is defined as the proportion of people who do not have the disease and have a negative screening test. Alternatively, of all those who do *not* have the disease, how many people will screen negative? The calculation to determine a screening test's specificity is shown in the following equation:

$$\text{Specificity} = D \div (D + B)$$

   Sensitivity and specificity are related inversely. To ensure that sensitivity is 100% (i.e., *no one* with the disease would test negative), a large number of false-positive results would be produced. This result has an impact on cell B and, in turn, would result in lowering the specificity of the screening test. To balance the trade-off between speci-

Table 3.12
Sensitivity and specificity.

Blood Sugar Level 2 hrs After Eating (mg/dl)	Sensitivity (%)	Specificity (%)
70	98.6	8.8
80	97.1	25.5
90	94.3	47.6
100	88.6	69.8
110	85.7	84.1
120	71.4	92.5
130	64.3	96.9
140	57.1	99.4
150	50.0	99.6
160	47.1	99.8
170	42.9	100.0
180	38.6	100.0
190	34.3	100.0
200	27.1	100.0

Source: Reprinted with permission from Diabetes Program Guide, Public Health Service pub. no. 506, 1960.

ficity and sensitivity, it is important to pick a *cutoff point* for the screening test. This cutoff point is a somewhat arbitrary division between normal results and abnormal results requiring a diagnostic test. For example, in screening for glaucoma, you might select a cutoff point of 21 mm Hg.

Table 3.12 illustrates the trade-off between sensitivity and specificity for blood glucose measurement as a screening test for diabetes. Fletcher et al. describe the relationship as follows:

> If we require that a blood sugar taken 2 hours after eating be greater than 180 mg/dl to diagnose diabetes, all of the people diagnosed as diabetic surely would have the disease, but many other people with diabetes would be missed. This test would be very specific at the expense of sensitivity. At the other extreme, if anyone with a blood sugar of greater than 70 mg/dl were diagnosed as diabetic, very few people with the disease would be missed, but most normal people would be falsely labeled as having diabetes. The test would then be very sensitive but nonspecific. There is no way, using a single blood sugar determination under standard conditions, one can improve both the sensitivity and specificity of the test at the same time.[34]

Table 3.13

Hypothetical screening test for glaucoma with intraocular
pressure cutoff of 21 mm Hg.

Results	Disease Present	Disease Absent
Positive	40 Cell A	460 Cell B
Negative	10 Cell C	9,490 Cell D

Generally, a blood glucose measurement of 140 mg/dl is used as a cut-off point for diabetes screening. This cutoff point corresponds to a sensitivity level of 57.1% and a specificity level of 99.4%. Therefore, there would be few false-positive results using this cutoff point.

Another important measurement used in screening is the predictive value. The *predictive value* is defined as the probability of disease, given the results of the screening test. Positive predictive value is the probability of disease in a patient with a positive screening test result. In other words, the positive predictive value tells us how many of all the people who test positive for a condition actually have it. This value is important in evaluating the results of a screening test. Not all those who test positive in the screening will actually have the disease; therefore, not all the people who undergo further diagnostic testing will have positive diagnostic test results. The equation given here shows the calculation for positive predictive value (PPV), using the screening cells from Table 3.11:

$$PPV = A \div (A + B)$$

Table 3.13 shows the hypothetical results of a screening for glaucoma. Ten thousand people were screened, using applanation tonometry; then they were evaluated for glaucoma through a complete battery of optometric testing. The cutoff point for the screening was set at 21 mm Hg. The prevalence of glaucoma in this population matches that of the general population: 500/100,000.

Sensitivity is calculated as $A/(A + C)$ or 40/40 + 10 = 80%. Specificity is calculated as $D/(D + B)$ or 9,490/9,490 + 460 = 95.4%. Positive predictive value is calculated as $A/(A + B)$ or 40/40 + 460 = 8%. That is, of all of the people who test positive and are subsequently given a complete evaluation, only 8% actually will have the disease. Each of these calculations will change if any of the underlying conditions of the screening are changed. For example, if the cutoff point were set high-

Table 3.14
Hypothetical screening test for glaucoma with intraocular
pressure cutoff of 18 mm Hg.

	Disease Present	*Disease Absent*
Positive	49	601
	Cell A	Cell B
Negative	1	9,349
	Cell C	Cell D

Table 3.15
Change in intraocular pressure cutoff point.

	Cutoff at 21 mm Hg	*Cutoff at 18 mm Hg*
Sensitivity	80.0%	98.0%
Specificity	95.4%	94.0%
Predictive value	8.0%	7.5%

er or lower or if the population being screened were at a higher or lower risk for glaucoma, these values would change.

Table 3.14 shows what might happen to the values if the cutoff point were set at 18 mm Hg instead of at 21 mm Hg. This assumes the same prevalence of glaucoma in the population. Now, instead of 500 people testing positive in the screening, 650 people might test positive. Table 3.15 shows the difference in sensitivity, specificity, and predictive value when the cutoff point is changed. Sensitivity increases to 98%, specificity is decreased to 94%, and the predictive value is slightly decreased to 7.5%. This change in the cutoff point results in nine more people being identified correctly, but it also increases by 150 the number who are required to undergo full diagnostic testing. There is a trade-off between increasing the number who are identified correctly and promoting worry, stress, and additional costs among the additional 150 who register as false-positives.

If the screening were performed on a population older than 75, the prevalence of glaucoma would increase to 7,200/100,000. Using the same cutoff point of 21 mm Hg and the same specificity of 95.4%, the screening results may be calculated as shown in Table 3.16. Table 3.17 shows the difference in screening results when the prevalence is changed. The change in the sensitivity shows a better identification of the true positives. The large change in predictive value shows the bigger pay-off achieved by screening a high-risk population.

Table 3.16
Hypothetical screening test for glaucoma with intraocular pressure
cutoff of 21 mm Hg, high prevalence.

Results	Glaucoma Present	Glaucoma Absent
Positive	680	427
	Cell A	Cell B
Negative	40	8,853
	Cell C	Cell D

Table 3.17
Change screening results with change in prevalence of glaucoma.

Prevalence in General Population: 500/100,000	Prevalence in Population >75: 7,200/100,000
Cutoff at 21 mm Hg	Cutoff at 21 mm Hg
Sensitivity 80%	Sensitivity 94.4%
Specificity 95.4%	Specificity 95.4%
Predictive value 8%	Predictive value 61.4%

It is readily apparent that the higher the prevalence of a condition, the higher the positive predictive value of the screening test. For further comparison, Table 3.18 shows the change in positive predictive value relative to the prevalence of disease. In this example, both the sensitivity and specificity of the screening test are held constant at 95%.

The concepts of sensitivity, specificity, predictive value, and prevalence are important in evaluating a screening program. Additionally, these concepts are used to evaluate diagnostic tests.

USING EPIDEMIOLOGY TO SELECT AND INTERPRET DIAGNOSTIC TESTS

Sackett et al.[35] list five reasons for performing a diagnostic test: (1) to determine the cause of illness or symptoms, (2) to determine the severity of the illness or condition, (3) to predict the subsequent clinical course and prognosis, (4) to possibly predict likely responsiveness to therapy in the future, and (5) to determine the actual response to therapy in the

Table 3.18
Positive predictive value versus prevalence.

Prevalence (%)	Predictive Value (%)
99	99.9
95	99.7
90	99.4
80	99
70	98
60	97
50	95
40	93
30	89
20	83
10	68
5	50
1	16
0.5	9
0.1	2

Source: Modified with permission from DL Sackett, RB Haynes, GH Guyatt, et al. Clinical Epidemiology (2nd ed). Boston: Little, Brown, 1991;90.

present. With all these possible uses, a clinician performs many routine diagnostic tests throughout the course of a comprehensive eye examination and may add special diagnostic testing when evaluating a specific ocular condition or disease. Which tests are the best? How should you decide which tests to perform, and how do you evaluate the test results? Principles of epidemiology can help guide you through the process.

If you are considering the purchase of new diagnostic testing equipment, determining whether to order special laboratory tests, or simply performing extra refractive testing in your office, eight guidelines for selecting a test have been proposed. Table 3.19 lists the questions to ask yourself, to research in the literature, or to ask the diagnostic equipment manufacturer.

In addition to these general guidelines, it is also important to evaluate the test's sensitivity, specificity, predictive value, and two previously unmentioned elements: validity and reliability. The *validity* of a test is the degree to which the results of a measurement match the true state of the phenomenon being measured (i.e., the accuracy of the test). *Reliability* of a test is the degree to which repeated measures of the same relatively stable phenomenon fall closely together. It is the reproducibility or the precision of a test. Unlike that between specificity and sensitivity, no implicit relationship exists between validity and reli-

Table 3.19
Guidelines for selecting a diagnostic test.

1. Has there been an independent blind comparison with a gold standard of diagnosis?
2. Has the diagnostic test been evaluated in a patient sample that included an appropriate spectrum of mild and severe, treated and untreated disease, plus individuals with different but commonly confused disorders?
3. Was the setting for this evaluation, as well as the mechanism for sampling patients, adequately described?
4. Has the reproducibility of the test result (precision) and its interpretation (observer variation) been determined?
5. Has the term normal been defined sensibly as it applies to this test?
6. If the test is advocated as a part of a cluster or sequence of tests, has its individual contribution to the overall validity of the cluster or sequence been determined?
7. Have the tactics for carrying out the test been described in sufficient detail to permit their exact replication?
8. Has the utility of the test been determined?

Source: Reprinted with permission from DL Sackett, RB Haynes, GH Guyatt, et al. Clinical Epidemiology (2nd ed). Boston: Little, Brown, 1991;52.

ability. A test may be both valid *and* reliable, neither valid *nor* reliable, or some combination of the two (Table 3.20).

The ideal test is both valid and reliable. As mentioned previously, though a test can be both valid and reliable, it may not be possible for one test to have both good sensitivity and good specificity because of their trade-offs. How do you decide which is more important—sensitivity or specificity?

A highly sensitive test should be used when there is an important consequence for missing a treatable but serious disease or condition. Sensitive tests are also helpful early in a diagnostic workup to rule out diseases or narrow your list of possible diagnoses. Sensitive tests are also useful when either the possibility or the prevalence of a disease is relatively low and the purpose of the test is to discover disease. For example, a sensitive test might be used on an asymptomatic patient who may have an underlying disease state.

Tests that are highly specific are useful to confirm, or rule in, a diagnosis that has been suggested by other clinical findings. Because highly specific tests have few false-positive results, they are helpful when a false-positive result can harm the patient physically, emotionally, or financially. Table 3.21 summarizes the advantages and uses of specific and sensitive tests.

Table 3.20
Validity and reliability example: tonometry.

True Value	Valid Test (But Not Reliable)	Reliable Test (But Not Valid)	Reliable and Valid Test	Not Reliable or Valid Test
16 mm Hg	16 mm Hg	18 mm Hg	16 mm Hg	20 mm Hg
16 mm Hg	18 mm Hg	18 mm Hg	16 mm Hg	14 mm Hg
16 mm Hg	14 mm Hg	18 mm Hg	17 mm Hg	14 mm Hg
16 mm Hg	20 mm Hg	18 mm Hg	16 mm Hg	22 mm Hg
16 mm Hg	12 mm Hg	19 mm Hg	16 mm Hg	24 mm Hg
avg = 16 mm Hg	avg = 16 mm Hg	avg = 18 mm Hg	avg = 16 mm Hg	avg = 19 mm Hg

Table 3.21
Comparison of specific and sensitive tests.

Sensitive Tests	Specific Tests
Few false-negatives	Few false-positives
For serious but treatable disease (e.g., tuberculosis, syphilis, glaucoma, brain tumor)	For disease with serious misdiagnosis consequences (e.g., dyslexia, human immunodeficiency virus, learning disability)
Use early to rule out disease	To rule in disease
Test people without complaints	To confirm a suspected diagnosis

Source: Data from RH Fletcher, SW Fletcher, EH Wagner. Clinical Epidemiology (2nd ed). Baltimore: Williams & Wilkins, 1988.

Earlier, we learned that the predictive value of a screening test is influenced by the prevalence of the condition being tested. The same is true of the predictive value of a diagnostic test. The predictive value of a diagnostic test is influenced by the sensitivity and specificity of the test and by the prevalence of the condition in the population being tested. Even a very specific test, when applied to a population with a low prevalence of disease, will yield mainly false-positive results. Conversely, when the probability of disease is very high (high prevalence), a negative test result does not rule out the disease, so the false-positive rate of a test becomes less important.

Table 3.22
Positive and negative likelihood ratios.

Positive likelihood ratio (LR+) =

$$\frac{\text{Probability that finding is present in diseased persons}}{\text{Probability that finding is present in nondiseased persons}}$$

$$\text{LR+} = \frac{\text{True-positive rate}}{\text{False-positive rate}}$$

Negative likelihood ratio (LR–) =

$$\frac{\text{Probability that finding is absent in diseased persons}}{\text{Probability that finding is absent in nondiseased persons}}$$

$$\text{LR–} = \frac{\text{False-negative rate}}{\text{True-negative rate}}$$

Another way to describe the performance of a diagnostic test is the likelihood ratio. A *likelihood ratio* compares the probability of that test result in the presence of disease to the probability of the same test result in people without the disease. Likelihood ratios can be calculated for both positive and negative test results. They answer the questions of how likely it is to find a positive test result for a person *with* the disease compared to a positive test result for a person *without* the disease and how likely it is to find a negative test result for a person *with* the disease compared to a negative test result for a person *without* the disease. The likelihood ratio is useful for diagnostic tests that do not have clear cutoff points. Table 3.22 defines these two likelihood ratios.

Table 3.23 illustrates known values for some diagnostic tests that an optometrist might use. To read the likelihood columns, for the example given for a computed tomography (CT) scan of the orbit, one might say that the likelihood of a positive CT scan in the presence of an orbital tumor compared to a positive CT scan in the absence of an orbital tumor is 29.7 to 1, or a positive test result is almost 30 times more likely in a patient with an orbital tumor.

Applying Bayes' Theorem

Given that no test is perfect in terms of validity, reliability, sensitivity, and specificity, how sure are you of your results? It is important

Table 3.23
Diagnostic tests.

Test	True-Positive Rate	False-Positive Rate	Likelihood Ratio Finding Present	Likelihood Ratio Finding Absent
Computed tomography scan of the orbit	0.89	0.03	29.7	0.11
VDRL test for syphilis (<30 d)	0.40	0.02–0.16	2.5–20.0	0.61–0.71
Erythrocyte sedimentation rate for temporal arteritis	0.99	0.04	24.8	0.01

to qualify the results you have obtained in terms of the certainty of results. *Bayes' theorem* is used for calculating the posterior probability or post-test odds of a disease or condition. That is, after your test has been performed and you have the results of the testing, what is the probability that the patient does or does not have the condition in question? This is known as *conditional probability*, because it is an estimate of the probability that one event is true, given the condition that we know another event to be true (e.g., the probability that a patient has a disease, given the clinical test result). To determine this conditional probability, three things are needed: prior probability of the disease, the probability of a test result conditional on the patient's *having* the disease, and the probability of the test result conditional on the patient *not having* the disease. Table 3.24 illustrates these three probabilities and their relationship to the concepts that already have been covered.

Though several methods for using Bayes' theorem in clinical decision making are available, the one that will be presented in this chapter uses likelihood ratios (see Table 3.22) and the odds of an event. The odds of an event are calculated as the probability that an event will occur divided by the probability that an event will not occur. Because odds total 100%, or 1.0, the probability that an event *will not* occur is equal to 1—the probability that an event *will* occur. This relationship is shown in the following equations:

$$\text{Odds} = \frac{\text{Probability that event will occur}}{\text{Probability that event will } not \text{ occur}}$$

Table 3.24
Conditional probabilities.

Conditional Probability	Related Concepts
Prior probability of disease—the probability of disease before new information is acquired	Prevalence, incidence, risk factor
Probability of a test result, conditional on the patient having the disease	Sensitivity, positive likelihood ratio, positive predictive value
Probability of the test result, conditional on the patient not having the disease	Specificity, negative likelihood ratio

$$\text{Odds} = \frac{\text{Probability that event will occur}}{1 - \text{Probability that event } will \text{ occur}}$$

To determine the odds, you may rely on published data (see Table 3.10), expert opinion, or your own clinical judgment. It is also possible to turn prevalence rates into pretest odds for calculation. In Table 3.3, prevalence rates were given for glaucoma specific to different age ranges. If a clinician wants to turn this into the pretest odds of a patient having glaucoma, a simple calculation may be made as shown in the calculations here. In the absence of reliable prevalence rates or expert opinion, pretest odds may be estimated as low, moderate, or high.

$$\text{Prevalence of glaucoma aged 52–64} = \frac{1,400}{100,000}$$

Odds of a patient aged 52–64 (with no other risk factors) having

$$\text{glaucoma} = \frac{1,400/100,000}{[1 - (1,400/100,000)]} = \frac{0.014}{(1 - 0.014)} \approx 0.014{:}1 \text{ or } 1.4\%$$

$$\text{Prevalence of glaucoma aged 75–85} = \frac{7,200}{100,000}$$

Odds of a patient aged 75–85 (with no other risk factors) having

$$\text{glaucoma} = \frac{7,200/100,000}{[1 - (7,200/100,000)]} = \frac{0.072}{(1 - 0.072)} \approx 0.072{:}1 \text{ or } 7.2\%$$

Using Bayes' theorem, the post-test odds then are calculated, using the following equation:

$$\text{Post-test odds} = \text{Pretest odds} \times \text{likelihood ratio}$$

In applying Bayes' theorem, an optometrist may interpret similar test results differently in different situations. For example, an intraocular pressure (IOP) reading of 22 mm Hg in a 12-year-old white male with C/D ratios of 0.2 will be interpreted differently from an IOP reading of 22 mm Hg in a 65-year-old black woman with C/D ratios of 0.7. This is because the pretest odds are assessed very differently for these two patients.

A formal application of these calculations may be difficult, owing to a paucity of information on likelihood ratios for standard optometric tests. Regardless, the general premise of Bayes' theorem may be applied consciously in the clinical decision-making process. As early in the examination as the case history, an optometrist must think consciously about the probability or pretest odds of ocular and visual conditions. The initial assessment of the pretest odds should be reconsidered each time new information is gained through the testing performed.

Rosenbaum and Wernick[36] demonstrated the use of Bayes' theorem in two different patient scenarios. In the first scenario, a patient with uveitis is worked up for toxoplasmosis by measuring an antibody titer to toxoplasmosis. The authors have determined that the pretest odds that a patient with uveitis will have toxoplasmosis is 5% or 0.05.[37] The probability that toxoplasmosis antibodies are present in patients with toxoplasmosis is 100% or 1.0.[38] In the United States, approximately one-half of the adult population has antibodies to toxoplasmosis.[39] Therefore, the probability that toxoplasmosis antibodies are present in patients without toxoplasmosis is 50% or 0.50. The positive likelihood ratio can be calculated as:

$$\frac{\text{Probability that finding is present in diseased persons}}{\text{Probability that finding is present in nondiseased persons}} = \frac{1.0}{0.5} = 2.0$$

The post-test odds that a patient with uveitis who has toxoplasmosis antibodies *actually has* toxoplasmosis is:

$$\text{Pretest odds} \times \text{positive likelihood ratio} = \text{Post-test odds}$$
$$0.05 \times 2.0 = 0.10 \text{ or } 10\%$$

Thus, even with a positive antibody titer, there is only a 10% chance that this patient has toxoplasmosis.

In the second scenario, a patient with chorioretinal inflammation is worked up for toxoplasmosis by using the same antibody titer test. The pretest odds that a patient with chorioretinal inflammation will have toxoplasmosis is somewhat higher at 20% or 0.20.[15] The positive likelihood ratio is still the same, 2.0. Therefore, the post-test odds are calculated as:

$$0.20 \times 2.0 = 0.40 \text{ or } 40\%$$

In these two examples, the positive antibody titer test result would be interpreted differently. A patient who has uveitis with antibodies present has only a 10% chance of actually having toxoplasmosis, whereas a patient who has chorioretinal inflammation with antibodies present has a 40% chance of having toxoplasmosis. Rosenbaum and Wernick[36] suggest that toxoplasmosis antibody titer is not a tremendously useful test for patients with uveitis and that even among patients with chorioretinitis, toxoplasmosis antibody titers should be reserved for patients whose lesions are suggestive of active toxoplasmosis.

Evaluating a Series of Tests

Often, an optometric evaluation may entail the performance of a battery of tests, rather than a single screening test or a single diagnostic test. When this is the case, it is important to consider the value of testing done either in serial or in parallel. How many tests are needed to make a good diagnosis? What number of tests is considered excessive?

Inexperienced clinicians sometimes use an exhaustive strategy of decision making (see Chapter 1). That is, they may conduct a painstaking search for all the medical facts about a patient, then search through all of the collected data that might possibly be pertinent to arrive at a tentative diagnosis. A study conducted at a hospital in Australia randomized 1,500 patients on admission. One-half the group underwent a battery of 50 tests as soon as they arrived, to provide clinicians with all the results. The other half underwent the usual testing ordered by the attending physician. The results showed that the exhaustive testing did not improve measures of mortality, morbidity, duration of monitoring, disability, patient progress, or length of stay in the hospital. It *did* result in an increase of 5% in total costs and decreased patient satisfaction.[40]

If more testing is not necessarily better, how can you concentrate on the most appropriate battery of tests? Although guidelines have been given for individual tests, different concerns arise in using more than one test together. In combining more than one test, the testing may be done either in serial or in parallel.

Serial testing occurs when testing is done consecutively, and each test is considered in light of the results of the previous test. Such testing commonly is done in comprehensive eye examinations, in office practices, and hospital clinics where ambulatory care is provided.

For example, during a comprehensive eye examination, a doctor of optometry might use serial testing to determine the frequency of an observed exotropia. The first test selected might be an assessment of stereopsis. The second test might be a unilateral cover test at 6 meters.

The cover test results would be interpreted in light of stereopsis results. If the patient demonstrated good stereopsis but movement on the unilateral cover test, the exotropia may be assessed as intermittent. If the patient demonstrated suppression or poor stereopsis and movement on the unilateral cover test, the exotropia may be assessed as constant.

Serial testing also may be used when some of the tests are expensive or risky. This type of testing strategy maximizes specificity and positive predictive value; thus, a clinician can be more confident that a positive test result truly indicates the presence of disease or ocular conditions. However, sensitivity may be lower, and there is potential that a disease or condition may be missed.

Parallel testing occurs when all the tests are performed at once, and a positive test result of any test is considered evidence of disease. During an comprehensive examination, a clinician may perform a threshold automated visual field test. The printout from the test will allow the clinician to evaluate simultaneously the visual field in terms of total deviation, pattern deviation, and the patient's sensitivity to the brightness of the target (decibel level). A positive result in any of these three areas can signify a clinical problem.

Other examples of parallel testing include blood work or other laboratory tests. Most frequently, this type of testing is done out of the office in a laboratory or diagnostic center. Multiple tests done in parallel increase the sensitivity of the testing above that expected for any individual test. Therefore, disease is less likely to be missed, but overdiagnosis (false-positives) may be more common. Parallel testing also may be helpful when a very sensitive test is needed (see Table 3.21) but the clinician only has available tests that are lower in sensitivity. The less sensitive tests may be combined in parallel to produce a more sensitive *final* analysis.

How does the outcome of one test influence another test? How should the results of the tests be interpreted? When all the tests are positive or all of the tests are negative, it is easy to interpret the results, but what must be done when the results are mixed? It is important to understand how new information affects the uncertainty of diagnosis to minimize the margin of error. Without knowing how new information has affected the probability of a diagnosis, the clinician may acquire too much or too little information and thereby overtest or undertest for what would be a wise clinical strategy.

Bayes' theorem and theories of conditional probability may be applied to serial groups of tests as well as to single tests. In applying Bayes' theorem to a group of tests, the post-test odds of the first test are used as the pretest odds for the next test done in the series. An example is shown in the following calculations:

Post-test odds test 1 = Pretest odds × likelihood ratio test 1

Post-test odds test 2 = Post-test odds test 1 × likelihood ratio test 2

Post-test odds test 3 = Post-test odds test 2 × likelihood ratio test 3

These equations show that the certainty of any test in the series is both influenced by the test preceding it and influences the test following it. The final post-test odds for the entire series is the post-test odds for the last test performed. This allows both positive and negative test results to be considered when making a final decision.

Use of Normative Data

After a clinician has selected the appropriate test and assessed the certainty of the results obtained, his or her next job is to make a determination whether the findings or groups of findings are normal. Rouse[41] suggests that case analysis systems such as graphic analysis, optometric extension program analysis, and clinical criteria help the doctor make decisions regarding binocular and accommodative anomalies. He adds that normative data also are a useful resource.

Normative data rely on large population-based studies to assess the distribution of a particular clinical finding. Statistical analysis of populations and the laws of probability show that physiologic phenomena, including measurements related to vision and ocular health, often follow a normal distribution. The statistical empiric rule states that within a normal distribution, 68% of the measurements will fall within ±1 standard deviations of the mean value, 95% of the measurements will fall within ±2 SD, and virtually all of the measurements will fall within ±3 SD of the mean (see Figure 3.1). How does the statistical concept of the normal distribution relate to *clinical* normality?

Morgan[42] relates that as a rule, statisticians accept as normal any measurement that falls in the range of the mean ±0.7 SD. Rouse[41] states that the values suggested for *normal* range from ±0.5 SD of the mean (in an attempt to avoid false-negative results) to ±2.0 SD (in an attempt to avoid false-positive results). He cautions clinicians to use normative data as a method to identify clinical data that are more extreme than those typically found in the general population but not necessarily *abnormal*.[21] Clinical data that are more extreme may be considered to place the patient at greater risk for an ocular or visual problem. When these extreme results are associated with visual symptoms or signs of physiologic changes, then they may be considered abnormal.

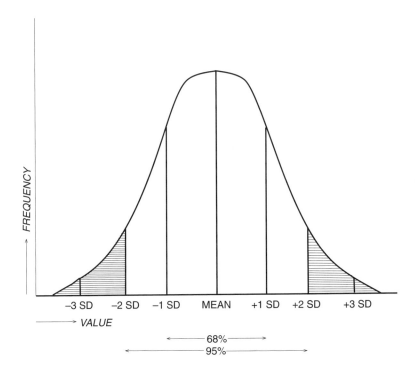

Figure 3.1 Normal distribution.

SUMMARY

In this chapter, we have discussed the relationship between epidemiology and clinical decision making; explained what epidemiology is and
some of the ways it can be applied in a clinical setting; identified what
incidence rates and prevalence rates are and some sources for information; identified what risk factors are in terms of relative risk and
ORs, how to calculate them, and where to find them in the literature;
described screening techniques and analysis of screening results; suggested ways to evaluate diagnostic tests and suggested the types of tests
best for certain types of conditions; discussed the application of Bayes'
theorem to clinical decision making; and discussed the differences
between a statistically normal distribution and clinical normality. In
reading the following chapters, you will want to test your understanding of these concepts and use some of these epidemiologic tools
to assist your clinical decision making. The following cases will apply
some of the principles covered in this chapter.

CLINICAL SCENARIOS

Case 1

Dr. A picks up the chart for her next patient. She pauses outside the examination room to scan the file quickly. The patient intake form contains the patient's name, age, and gender. Dr. A reads that Ms. K is 65 years old and makes a mental note of some ocular conditions that increase with age. She thinks about the prevalence rates of the following diseases among 65-year-olds: glaucoma, 5,100/100,000; cataract, 18,000/100,000; macular degeneration, 11,000/100,000; and diabetes, 8,000/100,000. From these prevalence rates, she lists the conditions in order, from most common to least common, and makes a preliminary estimation of the odds that Ms. K will have each of these conditions: cataract odds, high; macular degeneration odds, moderate; diabetes odds, moderate; and glaucoma odds, low.

After taking a minute or two to prepare mentally, Dr. A enters the examination room. When she meets Ms. K, she notes that Ms. K is black. Dr. A automatically readjusts the order of the four conditions and re-estimates the odds based on risk factors associated with ethnicity. Her new list reads: cataract odds, high; glaucoma odds, moderate; diabetes odds, moderate; and macular degeneration odds, low.

She also thinks about two more conditions based on risk factors associated with ethnicity and makes a mental note of their prevalence rates: sickle cell anemia trait, 8,000/100,000; and hypertension (140/90), 45,000/100,000.

During the case history, Dr. A learns that Ms. K's mother had glaucoma and that her sister has adult onset diabetes. Dr. A mentally increases the odds of glaucoma and diabetes from moderate to high. Now she adopts the position that these conditions will have to be ruled in because Ms. K has significant risk factors for each and Dr. A wants to confirm a suspicion.

During the course of the examination, what additional history questions should Dr. A ask Ms. K? What clinical tests will best help her to focus her examination on the basis of Ms. K's risk factors? Are sensitive tests or specific tests better? What additional findings will support or weaken Dr. A's primary concerns?

Discussion

Dr. A is concerned about Ms. K's high risk for glaucoma and diabetes. In the early stages, a person with open-angle glaucoma does not have any symptoms; thus, Dr. A cannot gain any more information by asking Ms. K about her eyes or vision. However, she might ask some additional history questions about the signs and symptoms of adult onset diabetes. Given Ms. K's risk, highly specific tests would be best because they have few false-positive outcomes. Dr. A will be paying special attention to the results of the IOP measurement, optic nerve assessment, visual-field analysis, and funduscopic findings.

Case 2

Mr. G is visibly upset as he tells Dr. B the reason for his visit. "They told me that I need to be checked for glaucoma. They think that I have it! That makes you go blind doesn't it?" Dr. B asks Mr. G a few more questions and discovers that Mr. G recently had participated in a community screening at the mall and that the club sponsoring the screening recommended that he have a complete workup for glaucoma. After reassuring Mr. G, Dr. B begins his examination.

He notes that Mr. G is Asian, aged 35, with no family history of glaucoma, no systemic conditions, and no medications. As Dr. B knows that Mr. G had no special risk factors, he thinks about the prevalence of glaucoma in the general population and the odds that Mr. G has it. He makes a mental note: glaucoma, 500/100,000; odds, low.

Dr. B believes that glaucoma will have to be ruled out (i.e., he is skeptical that Mr. G has glaucoma, because he considers Mr. G a patient without specific risk factors). What clinical tests will best help Dr. B to focus his examination on the basis of Mr. G's screening results? Are sensitive tests or specific tests better? What additional findings will support or weaken Dr. B's assessment of Mr. G's risk?

After the full examination, including a visual-field test and evaluation of the optic nerve head, Dr. B gives Mr. G a clean bill of health. He tells him that there is no sign of glaucoma. Over the next week, Dr. B sees 10 more patients, all with stories similar to Mr. G's: They have been to a screening at the mall, and the results indicated that they might have glaucoma. In 9 of the 10 cases, Dr. B determines that the patient does not have glaucoma. In the tenth patient, Dr. B finds early-stage open-angle glaucoma and initiates a therapeutic regimen.

Dr. B is concerned that the equipment being used in the screening might be broken or miscalibrated, because not all the patients who come to his office have glaucoma. He calls the club's president, who assures Dr. B that the equipment is in proper working order and that it is calibrated correctly. Should Dr. B be worried? On the basis of the patients coming to Dr. B's office, what is the predictive value of the screening?

Discussion

As Mr. G is considered to be at low risk for glaucoma, a sensitive test would be best. The predictive value can be calculated as:

$$PPV = A \div (A + B)$$

Without knowing the diagnostic results from *all* the patients who participated in the screening, the predictive value cannot be calculated accurately. However, on the basis of the patients Dr. B has seen, he can estimate the predictive value to be:

$$1 \div (1 + 10) = 9\%$$

The club may want to rethink the cutoff point for their screening if they are finding too many false-positive results. Raising the cutoff point will improve specificity but lower sensitivity.

Case 3

The county hospital calls Dr. C in for a consultation on a tough pediatric case. Baby T is 10 months old and appears to be delayed in her verbal and visual development. Baby T has not held still long enough for any of the pediatricians on staff to be able to assess her. She does not seem to be tracking objects, and her mother reports that at times one or the other eye seems to wander in. Dr. C immediately suspects esotropia, but she has a concern that retinoblastoma also must be ruled out. She thinks about the prevalence and incidence rates of each condition: esotropia prevalence, 670/100,000; retinoblastoma incidence, 5/100,000.

Dr. C knows that though esotropia is much more common, retinoblastoma poses a much greater concern. She asks Ms. T some history questions while observing Baby T at play. Ms. T reports that Baby T was born prematurely. Dr. C knows that premature birth is associated with low birth weight and that low birth weight has been associated with esotropia. She remembers reading a study[28] that concluded, "A patient with low birth weight less than 2,500 grams has 8.2 times greater odds of having esotropia."

Dr. C knows that Baby T's age and her inability to participate in testing will reduce the accuracy of her test results and render the conclusions less certain. She decides to do as many tests as she can as quickly as possible, to assess Baby T's visual functioning. After completing the series of tests, Dr. C determines that Baby T appears to have reduced acuity in one eye, signs of a tropia on cover test, and a suspicion of a slightly hazy pupil. She attempts to make sense of the test results. She develops the chart shown in Table 3.25, using Bayes' theorem and her prior experience with testing pediatric patients.

In comparing the odds for each condition, Dr. C feels that retinoblastoma cannot be ruled out totally, but she believes that esotropia is a much more likely diagnosis. She reassures Ms. T that an evaluation is precautionary but that the probability of finding a retinoblastoma is relatively low. She schedules Baby T for a dilated examination in her office, but, in the meantime, she prescribes patching of the dominant eye to initiate amblyopia therapy.

Table 3.25
Probabilities of esotropia and retinoblastoma in a pediatric patient.

	Esotropia	*Retinoblastoma*
Pretest probability based on prevalence and incidence	High: estimated 0.8	Low: estimated 0.1
Reduced acuity monocularly: probability that finding is present in pediatric patients with condition	0.7	0.9
Reduced acuity monocularly: probability that finding is present in pediatric patients without condition	0.3	0.3
Reduced acuity monocularly: positive likelihood ratio	0.7/0.3 = 2.33	0.9/0.3 = 3.00
Reduced acuity monocularly: post-test odds become pretest odds for next test in series	$0.80 \times 2.33 =$ 1.86	$0.10 \times 3.00 =$ 0.30
Apparent tropia on cover test: probability that finding is present in pediatric patients with condition	0.9	0.6
Apparent tropia on cover test: probability that finding is present in pediatric patients without condition	0.1	0.5
Apparent tropia on cover test: positive likelihood ratio	0.9/0.1 = 9.00	0.6/0.5 = 1.20
Apparent tropia on cover test: post-test odds become pretest odds for next test in series	$1.86 \times 9.00 =$ 16.74	$0.30 \times 1.20 =$ 0.36
Leukocoria: probability that finding is present in pediatric patients with condition	0.2	0.9
Leukocoria: probability that finding is present in pediatric patients without condition	0.1	0.1
Leukocoria: positive likelihood ratio	0.2/0.1 = 2	0.9/0.1 = 9
Leukocoria: post-test odds become final odds for the series of tests	$16.74 \times 2 =$ 33.48	$0.36 \times 9 =$ 3.24

REFERENCES

1. Ahlbom A, Norrell S. Introduction to Modern Epidemiology. Chestnut Hill, MA: Epidemiology Resources, 1984.
2. Hennekens CH, Buring JE, Mayrent SL (ed). Epidemiology in Medicine. Boston: Little, Brown, 1987.
3. Sox HC Jr, Blatt MA, Higgins MC, et al. Medical Decision Making. Boston: Butterworths, 1988.
4. Weiss NS. Clinical Epidemiology: The Study of the Outcome of Illness. New York: Oxford University Press, 1986.
5. Schuman SH. Practice-Based Epidemiology: An Introduction. New York: Gordon and Breach Science Publishers, 1986.
6. Newcomb RD, Marshall EC. Public Health and Community Optometry (2nd ed). Boston: Butterworths, 1990.
7. Kini MM, Leibowitz HM, Coiton T, et al. Prevalence of senile cataract, diabetic retinopathy, senile macular degeneration, and open-angle glaucoma in the Framingham eye study. Am J Ophthalmol 1978;85:28–34.
8. U.S. Department of Health and Human Services, National Center for Health Statistics Organization and Activities, November 1988, DHHS pub. no. (PHS) 88-1200.
9. Zadnik K, Satariano WA, Mutti DO, et al. The effect of parental history of myopia on children's eye size. JAMA 1994;271:1323–1327.
10. Mausner JS, Kramer S. Epidemiology—An Introductory Text (2nd ed). Philadelphia: Saunders, 1985.
11. Sugarman JR, Gilbert TJ, Weiss NS. Prevalence of diabetes and impaired glucose tolerance among Navajo Indians. Diabetes Care 1992;15:114–120.
12. National Eye Institute, National Institutes of Health. Don't Lose Sight of Glaucoma. (NIH, pub. no. 91-3251) Bethesda, MD: Public Health Service, U.S. Dept. of Health and Human Services, 1993.
13. Barresi B. Ocular Assessment: The Manual of Diagnosis for Office Practice. Boston: Butterworths, 1984.
14. Bennett GR, Blonden M, Ruskiewicz J. Incidence and prevalence of selected visual conditions. J Am Optom Assoc 1982;53:647–656.
15. Duane TD (ed). Clinical Ophthalmology. Hagerstown, MD: Harper & Row, 1976.
16. Graham PA. Epidemiology of strabismus. Br J Ophthalmol 1974;58:224–231.
17. Ihalainen A. Clinical and epidemiological features of keratoconus: genetic and external factors in the pathogenesis of the disease. Acta Ophthalmol Suppl 1986;178:1–64.
18. Kanski JJ. Ophthalmology. New York: Churchill Livingstone, 1992.
19. Letourneau JE, Ducic S. Prevalence of convergence insufficiency among elementary school children. Can J Optom 1988;50:194–199.
20. Pavan-Langston D. Manual of Ocular Diagnosis and Therapy (4th ed). Boston: Little, Brown, 1995.
21. Petersdorf RG, Adams RD, Braunwald E, et al. Harrison's Principles of Internal Medicine (10th ed). New York: McGraw-Hill, 1983.
22. Sommer A. Epidemiology of eye disease. Epidemiol Rev 1989;11:236–240.
23. Sperduto RD, Siegel D, Roberts J, et al. The prevalence of myopia in the United States. Arch Ophthalmol 1983;101:405–407.
24. Webster's New Collegiate Dictionary. Springfield, MA: G&C Merriam Company, 1981.

25. Greenberg RS. Medical Epidemiology. Norwalk, CT: Appleton & Lange, 1993.
26. Eng C, Li FP, Abramson DH, et al. Mortality from second tumors among long-term survivors of retinoblastoma. J Natl Cancer Inst 1993;85:1121–1128.
27. Hakim RB, Tielsch JM. Maternal cigarette smoking during pregnancy. A risk factor for childhood strabismus. Arch Ophthalmol 1992;110:1459–1462.
28. Risk factors for age-related cortical, nuclear, and posterior subcapsular cataracts. The Italian-American Cataract Study Group. Am J Epidemiol 1991;133:541–553.
29. Lee GA, Williams G, Hirst LW, et al. Risk factors in the development of ocular surface epithelial dysplasia. Ophthalmology 1994;101:360–364.
30. Raskin EM, Speaker MG, McCormick SA, et al. Influence of haptic materials on the adherence of staphylococci to intraocular lenses. Arch Ophthalmol 1993;111:250–253.
31. Rath EZ, Frank RN, Shin DH, et al. Risk factors for retinal vein occlusions. A case-control study. Ophthalmology 1992;99:509–514.
32. Stapleton F, Dart J, Minassian D. Nonulcerative complications of contact lens wear, relative risks for different lens types. Arch Ophthalmol 1992;110:1601–1606.
33. Winsa B, Mandahl A, Karlsson FA. Graves' disease, endocrine ophthalmopathy and smoking. Acta Endocrinol (Copenh) 1993;128:156–160.
34. Fletcher RH, Fletcher SW, Wagner EH. Clinical Epidemiology (2nd ed). Baltimore: Williams & Wilkins, 1988;49.
35. Sackett DL, Haynes RB, Guyatt GH, et al. Clinical Epidemiology (2nd ed). Boston: Little, Brown, 1991.
36. Rosenbaum JT, Wernick R. Selection and interpretation of laboratory tests for patients with uveitis. Int Ophthalmol Clin 1990;30(4):238–242.
37. Rosenbaum JT. Uveitis: an internist's view. Arch Intern Med 1989;149:1173–1176.
38. Desmonts G. Definitive serological diagnosis of ocular toxoplasmosis. Arch Ophthalmol 1966;76:839–851.
39. McCabe R, Remington JS. Toxoplasmosis: the time has come [editorial]. N Engl J Med 1988;318:313–315.
40. Durbridge TC, Edwards F, Edwards RG, et al. An evaluation of multiphasic screening on admission to hospital. Precis of a report to the National Health and Medical Research Council. Med J Aust 1976 May 8;1(19):703–705.
41. Scheiman MM, Rouse MW. Optometric Management of Learning-Related Vision Problems. St. Louis: Mosby, 1994;267–297.
42. Morgan MW. Analysis of clinical data. Am J Optom 1944;21:477–491.

4

Information Access and Management: Biomedical Literature and the Practicing Optometrist

Claudia A. Perry and Robin B. Fogel

SCIENTIFIC INFORMATION EXPLOSION

In recent decades, the health care professions have witnessed an extraordinary increase in the volume of published information essential for the delivery of high quality care. More than 2 million journal articles are published in the biomedical sciences every year, and new journals are established continually. Optometry is no exception to this trend. Major advances in such areas as contact lens materials, refractive surgery techniques, and the treatment of amblyopia have contributed to a surge in vision-related titles. The expansion in the scope of optometric practice and new developments in related fields have vastly broadened the range of topics with which effective practitioners must stay current. Massive changes in the health care system have spurred the publication of specialized newsletters, books, and journal articles assessing and interpreting these changes.

What steps can a busy clinician take to deal with this potential information overload? The goal of this chapter is to outline a practical approach to the problem of information access and management in the clinical setting. We assume that information is a key component in the delivery of quality patient care and in the decision-making process. The clinician has an ethical obligation to provide care that is both appropriate and informed by the latest advances in research and practice. However, the stringent time limitations in the clinical setting make it difficult to find answers to questions unless the practitioner can rely on effective information management skills. Knowing where to start the information search and the subsequent steps to follow can reduce frustration and maximize efficiency in finding answers that may contribute to improving the quality of patient care.

This chapter includes a basic overview of the publication process and the structure of biomedical communication. The characteristics and appropriate uses of different types of information sources (e.g., textbooks, the journal literature) also are addressed. This summary provides a model for the analysis of specific types of questions arising in clinical practice and suggests approaches for answering such questions efficiently. For example, often it is more effective to consult a drug handbook than to search the journal literature when seeking information on ocular side effects of a drug.

The advantages and disadvantages associated with the use of MEDLINE, the online database of the world's biomedical journal literature will be examined. Finally, the special difficulties associated with indexing of the optometric journal literature will be explored. In view of the many different user interfaces available, a tutorial on MEDLINE use is not provided; however, suggestions for further reading are listed for those interested in obtaining further information on this and other topics. Quality issues, reprint management, and electronic access to the Internet are examined as well.

ORGANIZATION OF BIOMEDICAL INFORMATION: TYPES OF INFORMATION SOURCES

Generally, the published biomedical literature is grouped into three categories: primary, secondary, and tertiary. The *primary* literature consists of original accounts presented by authors without interpretation by others, as in a journal article. Other examples include case reports, conference proceedings, patent applications, technical reports, and theses and dissertations. This is the most current published form of information. Developments in electronic publishing hold promise for even greater currency. However, the primary literature usually is extremely specific. One frequently must read more than one journal article to gain sufficient background on a new development. Furthermore, journals usually contain articles on a variety of topics and are issued on a serial basis (e.g., weekly, monthly, or quarterly). Accordingly, finding an article on a particular topic can be a challenge.

The *secondary* literature repackages the primary literature for more efficient or easier access. Authors of textbooks and review articles, for example, have surveyed the literature for the reader, selecting more important developments and highlighting essential points or controversies. Multimedia publications may offer impressive audiovisual presentations of complex procedures or clinical findings. Newspapers and popular magazines report the publication of noteworthy studies or the results of recent research developments, in language geared to a lay audience. Handbooks present essential facts culled from other sources, whereas indexes and abstracts provide subject access to the journal literature. The secondary literature is efficient, compact, and fairly easy to use. However, by its very nature, it is much less current than the primary literature, and may reflect the biases of authors or editors. In the case of articles published in the popular press, information sometimes may be inaccurate, misleading, incomplete, or lacking in detail.

The *tertiary* literature is yet another repackaging, this time of the secondary literature. Examples include guides to the literature, the card catalog, or the online library catalog. The tertiary literature consists of essential "finding tools," but a tertiary source is not material that one normally would read for its own sake. This chapter focuses primarily on the first two categories of biomedical literature.

A final type of information source is not published at all. Clearly people—colleagues, authors, editors, experienced clinicians—are responsible for the intellectual work that generates the biomedical knowledge base. Much essential clinical knowledge is unpublished but resides inside people's minds. Those people (colleagues, mentors, experts) constitute what is sometimes called one's *invisible college*: the group of professional contacts with whom one interacts. Information from the invisible college may be obtained conveniently, and may be current, but it also may be biased, incorrect, or out of date, depending on its source. The quality and timeliness of information obtained from colleagues is directly dependent on whom one knows or can easily contact.

Fortunately, interpersonal consulting may become easier with the advent of electronic mail (e-mail), electronic bulletin boards, listservs, Usenet newsgroups, and the many other features available on the Internet. America Online, CompuServe, Prodigy, and a variety of local service providers offer relatively easy and inexpensive access to the so-called information highway. (See the chapter appendix for contact information.) Many of these companies will provide step-by-step guidance to assist the novice in the installation and configuration of access software. Practitioners equipped with a computer, a modem, and the appropriate online account may contact distant colleagues efficiently—

Table 4.1
Typology and trade-offs of biomedical information sources.

Source	Advantages	Disadvantages
Invisible college (e.g., people)	Convenient, interactive, efficient	Possibly biased or incorrect, depending on whom you know or can contact
Primary literature (e.g., journal articles)	Up-to-date, specific, direct from the author	Overwhelming volume, perhaps too specific
Secondary literature (e.g., textbooks, review articles, newspaper reports, multimedia publications)	Efficient, compact, usable, filtered for a specific audience; may serve an alerting function	More dated; possibly biased, incomplete, insufficiently detailed

even those one has never met—for advice, general background, current awareness information, or answers to specific information needs.

Studies have indicated that clinicians often prefer to use interpersonal sources to answer their questions.[1, 2] Convenience and familiarity appear to be prime reasons for choosing one particular source over another.[3] However, clinicians hoping to maximize their effectiveness would do well to consider all possible options when seeking information in the decision-making process. Clearly, this includes published as well as interpersonal sources. Table 4.1 summarizes the different types of literature and the relative advantages and disadvantages of each category.

The foregoing discussion and table suggest the trade-offs inherent in the information search. Though textbooks can provide important and insightful commentary on the value of research developments for clinical practice, they inevitably lag behind the most current findings published in the journal literature. Multimedia publications provide an immediacy lacking in more traditional sources but require appropriate hardware for their use. Furthermore, few books or multimedia titles are updated more often than every 3–5 years. At the same time, it is clearly impossible to research the journal literature on every subject of potential clinical interest in a practice. Thus, for many topics, the secondary literature is an essential starting point for finding the answer to a question.

Figure 4.1 lists various types of information sources, ranging from people to the library catalog. They are presented in order of gener-

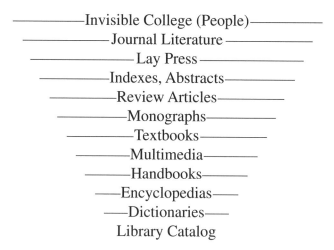

Figure 4.1 Typology of sources. An inverted pyramid illustrates various information sources, with decreasing levels of specificity and currency for sources further down the pyramid. (Copyright ©1995 Claudia A. Perry and Robin B. Fogel.)

ally decreasing specificity and currency, suggesting the progressive distillation of information that takes place at each step. As will be discussed, seeking information at another step on the ladder may prove useful when one's initial information-seeking efforts are unsuccessful.

FINDING INFORMATION: THE SEARCH PROCESS AND TYPOLOGY OF QUESTIONS

The questions that arise in clinical practice can be grouped into categories in much the same way as are information sources. Recognizing a question category permits one to check first in a particular type of source, thus potentially saving time and frustration. Though some question-source pairs are obvious (a dictionary is a logical place to check for the meaning or spelling of a word), others may be less so. Even less clear may be the strategy to follow when one's initial efforts prove unsuccessful. Objectively assessing the nature of one's question may provide additional fruitful places to check with a minimum of wasted effort. Following the typology listed in Table 4.2, strategies are presented for dealing with each type of question.

Table 4.2
General typology of questions.

Does a thing exist? What am I looking for?
  Information needed: a definition of the problem that will point to the
    most likely source for the answer
Who? What? Where?
  Information needed: a definition, quantity, or brief description
Basic overview
  Information needed: the current thinking on a given subject
The latest information
  Information needed: the most recent and innovative studies, which may
    not have been reviewed extensively by others
Comprehensive information on a subject
  Information needed: a detailed overview complemented and updated by
    specific, current articles
Information for a patient (popular works)
  Information needed: materials that assume no prior knowledge of termi-
    nology or process

Does Such a Thing Exist? (Or What Am I Looking For?)

Assuming that you are considering relocating to northern Vermont,
how would you go about researching the competitive environment for
optometrists in that part of the country? Attempting to clarify what
one is looking for or to prove that something exists is in some ways
one of the most difficult types of questions to answer in any setting.
Discussing a problem with a colleague or a reference librarian may provide relevant terminology or a key reference or may refresh one's
memory. This can suggest a subsequent step: to conduct an online catalog or MEDLINE search, retrieve a recommended book or article, or
look in the indexes of a comprehensive textbook.

  Alternatively, consulting with a colleague may suggest that little
material has been published on a topic. For example, no statistics may
be available on the number of optometrists grouped by county or city,
and there may be no point in searching for them. Instead, you may
need to count the number of optometrists listed in the yellow pages of
the phone book. Talking to someone provides important feedback
when what you are seeking is not necessarily clear or when you have
difficulty in getting started or in finding information.

Who? What? Where?

Who is Dr. Green? What is Marfan's syndrome? Where is the Orton
Dyslexia Society located? Usually, the fastest way to find the answer to

an identification-type question is to consult a dictionary, atlas, handbook, textbook, or directory. Directories typically list addresses, phone numbers, and brief descriptions. Dictionaries usually provide a brief definition and pronunciation, whereas an atlas includes numerous illustrations. A handbook or textbook also may provide information on management and references for further reading.

Trade-offs to consider are convenience and size versus the amount of information required. Kanski's *Clinical Ophthalmology*[4] will provide superb photographs and discussion, but the *Wills Eye Manual*[5] can fit in your clinic coat pocket. A useful rule is to try a more convenient source first and to extend your search if greater detail is required. In some cases, it will become apparent that the information being sought is the subject of controversy or has never been established. In this case, it may be necessary to reframe the question, obtain a more general overview, or even determine whether current research is being done on the topic.

Basic Overview

What are the ocular effects of plaquenil? How might a coexisting cardiac condition affect your patient management plan? A textbook, handbook (or a choice among several), or a clinical practice guideline should provide sufficient background information when questions arise concerning the implications of a particular condition or drug. This background then can be integrated with one's clinical knowledge and experience to proceed appropriately.

Clearly, the textbook or handbook consulted should be a fairly recent edition; building one's office collection is not a process that ends with graduation from optometry school. A looseleaf service, such as *Duane's Clinical Ophthalmology*,[6] has the advantage of relative currency despite the burden of regular updating and annual subscription costs. For a group practice, a CD-ROM version of *Duane's* or another comprehensive textbook may be a more convenient alternative to looseleaf updating. Access to a nearby medical or vision science library may reduce the need to update office sources as frequently, but what is close at hand tends to be more frequently used.

Clinicians may want to consider the types of questions that recur frequently when building their office collections and to update or purchase books accordingly. The Association of Vision Science Librarians regularly updates an "Opening Day Collection," which can suggest important reference sources for potential purchase (see the chapter appendix for availability). Consulting with colleagues, reading book reviews, checking conference exhibits, and browsing through library collections also may be useful in selecting books for purchase.

Drug sources constitute an entire specialized category of secondary sources. Although the *Physician's Desk Reference*[7] may be one of the most common sources in the clinical setting, it is far from being the most useful or most objective drug-related reference. Recommendations for augmenting one's collection of drug information sources are included in the Suggested Reading section at the end of the chapter. If a drug is very new or if treatment for a condition is changing rapidly, information obtained from a textbook or handbook may have to be updated by the journal literature.

Although clinical practice guidelines have been available for more than 20 years, they are only now becoming popular among mainstream practitioners. Written under the auspices of professional societies (e.g., the American Optometric Association or the American Academy of Ophthalmology) or by such governmental organizations as the National Institutes of Health, these guidelines represent a distillation of expert thought on a subject. In contradistinction to the other sources discussed here, publishers of clinical practice guidelines try to maximize distribution rather than sales and often provide free materials or charge a nominal fee. The guidelines emphasize diagnosis, treatment, management, and monitoring and often will include a carefully selected bibliography. Selected organizations that prepare these guidelines are listed in the chapter appendix.

The Latest Information

What is the current recommended treatment for CMV retinitis? What are the results of the latest report from the Early Treatment Diabetic Retinopathy Study Research Group? When current data are an important factor, one must consult the journal literature. Knowing where to start is essential. Paging through recent issues is probably the least efficient way to find current information on a specific topic. Checking the cumulative indexes to the *Journal of the American Optometric Association, Optometry and Vision Science,* or similar titles can be useful for those who maintain backfiles of their journal subscriptions. Unfortunately, few can track or subscribe to all the relevant journals that publish articles of potential interest. Creating a personal reprint file has many advantages but poses demands in terms of organization and ongoing management. (Suggestions for maintaining such a collection of journal articles are addressed later in this chapter in the section titled The Office Collection.)

Although a plan to stay current with the literature through a program of ongoing reading is an important part of lifelong learning, memory can be frustrating when it comes to retrieving specific pieces of information. Was that relevant article published in *Optometry Clinics*, or was it in the *Journal of the American Optometric Association*? Searching through the paper or electronic indexes to the journal literature permits one to check multiple potential sources by author, date, and subject much more efficiently than simply by looking at the table of contents of recent issues.

Access to Biomedical Journal Literature

Those with a personal computer and modem, or access to a vision science library, academic library, or even a large public library, are probably best served in the quest for recent information by an electronic database search. MEDLINE, the electronic equivalent of *Index Medicus*, is the primary database indexing the international biomedical literature. MEDLINE is produced by the National Library of Medicine (NLM), and indexes approximately 4,000 current biomedical journals. These include most of the leading English-language ophthalmology titles. Searching MEDLINE is not necessarily easy or intuitive, but its access by author, keyword, journal title, and subject heading constitutes a quantum leap over the access provided by paper indexes. Usually, there is a delay of 2–6 months before a published article is indexed in MEDLINE.

Abstracts are available for approximately 80% of the current references in MEDLINE, or 60% of references in the database overall. Since the introduction of structured abstracts in many major biomedical journals, abstracts often provide substantial guidance concerning the key components of a published paper (e.g., purpose, methods, study design, findings, and implications). If further detail is required, the full paper can be retrieved from one's personal files, requested from the author, or obtained from the library of one's alma mater, the library of the American Optometric Association, or another vision science library (e.g., Southern College of Optometry [SCO]). These latter options sometimes may involve a small fee. Other possibilities include purchase from a document delivery service such as University Microfilms International, the Institute for Scientific Information (The Genuine Article), or EMDOCS. Contact information for selected document providers is listed in the chapter appendix.

MEDLINE is searchable on a dial-in basis via a number of user-friendly interfaces. Hourly connect rates for MEDLINE and related databases average $18.00 per hour if accessed through the NLM. The same databases may cost slightly more if one uses a commercial database vendor, such as DIALOG or OVID Technologies (formerly

Bibliographic Retrieval Services). Grateful Med, developed by NLM, is one commonly used, inexpensive software package to aid in searching MEDLINE. It is particularly suitable for the clinician in a solo practice. Numerous CD-ROM–based versions of MEDLINE are available on a subscription basis and may constitute a viable option for those in a group practice anticipating a fairly substantial level of use. OphthaLine CD-ROM Database for Ophthalmology is a subject-specific subset of the MEDLINE database available from Aries Systems Corporation. Additional information regarding MEDLINE searching is provided in the chapter appendix and in Suggested Reading.

Other databases overlap and complement MEDLINE's coverage. Of primary interest to optometrists is VISIONET, an optometric database discussed later. Others include ERIC (an index to the education literature), PsycInfo (the database version of Psychological Abstracts), Health Planning & Administration, and Excerpta Medica (a biomedical database with a European emphasis). Consultation with a reference librarian is advised when a database other than MEDLINE or VISIONET seems appropriate.

Access to Optometric Journal Literature

Although MEDLINE is the foremost database indexing the international biomedical literature, its coverage of the optometric literature is limited to four journals: *Journal of the American Optometric Association*, *Ophthalmic and Physiological Optics*, *Optometry and Vision Science*, and *Optometry Clinics*. For more comprehensive access to the optometric literature, the primary alternative to MEDLINE is VISIONET, a database compiled at SCO in Memphis, TN (see the chapter appendix). Coverage is very timely and includes indexing of all vision-related articles in the journals received at SCO. Individuals and organizations may establish accounts to search SCO's VISIONET database directly through a dial-up connection or may request individual searches on a specific topic for a reasonable fee. Results are usually mailed on the day of the request. Many vision science libraries subscribe to the paper subject version of VISIONET, but an online search is a far more cost-effective choice when time constraints are considered. CD-ROM access to VISIONET is under development.

For current awareness purposes, a number of specialized sources exist that are geared to the vision specialist (see the chapter appendix). *Ocular Resources* provides monthly copies of the tables of contents of vision-related journals on diskette. *Optometry: Current Literature in Perspective* selectively critiques and abstracts recent articles of potential interest to the optometrist. *Ophthalmic Literature*, an abstracting index of the international journal literature in optometry and ophthalmology, is published quarterly. Its annual index provides an alternative choice to VISIONET and MEDLINE for subject or author searching, but it is not available as an online database.

Comprehensive Information

Suppose you have been asked to address your local optometric association on the role of a doctor of optometry in diagnosing child abuse, or you have encountered an interesting case and would like to submit an abstract for a poster presentation at the next meeting of the American Academy of Optometry. In these instances, neither the latest journal article nor the information available in your office collection is likely to be sufficient. Comprehensive information on a topic is best obtained by consulting a combination of primary and secondary sources. Recent textbooks and looseleaf services, such as *Duane's Clinical Ophthalmology*, can provide an initial overview of a subject. The references cited in chapter bibliographies can suggest older sources to consult for additional detail. Specialized monographs can be identified through a search of your library's online or card catalog. A MEDLINE or VISIONET search is recommended to track recent developments.

Information for Patients (Popular)

Although not strictly related to the clinical decision-making process, a final category of questions is of great importance for the patient-provider relationship. Patients legitimately expect their eye care providers to be well-informed experts who can answer their vision-related questions. Moreover, expanding radio and newspaper coverage of health care topics, and the trend toward a more active patient role in the health care process, is increasing patient interest in and demand for biomedical information.

Articles in the science section of such sources as *The New York Times* may prompt patient questions during the optometric examination. For example, what are the long-term effects of radial keratotomy? Other questions may arise directly from a patient's own concerns and condition: What will be the side effects of this new drug prescription, or how can I find out more about age-related macular degeneration? The ability to provide a relevant pamphlet or to refer patients to appropriate sources of information can be reassuring for patients, improve their confidence in the quality of care they are receiving, and improve patient adherence to treatment recommendations.

Providing a selection of current patient education materials in the waiting room and including at least one patient-oriented reference work in the office (e.g., *Mayo Clinic Family Health Book*[8] or the *American*

Medical Association Family Medical Guide[9]) can be a helpful start in this process. The American Optometric Association, the American Academy of Ophthalmology, the federal government, and numerous other groups publish a variety of patient-oriented brochures at a reasonable cost. Selected sources for obtaining patient education resources are listed in the chapter appendix.

In addition to professional associations and government agencies, organizations such as The Lighthouse, Inc., provide a wealth of popular information. Such library reference sources as *The AFB Directory of Services for Blind and Visually Impaired Persons in the United States and Canada*[10] or the *Consumer Health Information Source Book*[11] list names and addresses of organizations that include information provision among their services. For those practitioners who have the greatest interest in patient education, a variety of more general-purpose health databases for the layperson are available on CD-ROM. One example is the *Health Reference Center*, published by the Information Access Company (see the chapter appendix). These databases have been developed to address a broad variety of health concerns and often include the ability to create handouts specific to a given patient's condition.

THE OFFICE COLLECTION AND KEEPING UP WITH NEW DEVELOPMENTS

Much of the preceding discussion has advocated the development of an office collection for meeting clinical information needs. This may include books, journals, multimedia materials, and electronic resources, both for reference purposes and to maintain currency with new advances. Developments in multimedia software—products that incorporate sound and images with text—have been especially rapid. Reviews and directory listings in such sources as *Eyecare Technology* or *M.D. Computing* may prove helpful in staying current with new offerings and evaluating recently introduced software.

The Internet

The Internet is a voluntary association, a network linking millions of computers around the world. It is a repository of documents, an access route to private information systems, and one of the primary routes for e-mail. To join this network, a user needs a computer, modem, telephone or local area network connection, and a service provider (which may be a local company, an online service, or an organization's information systems department). These choices will multiply in the near future as different sectors of the telecommunications industry begin to offer service and even the ubiquitous cable hookup becomes a gateway to the Internet. For the present, the providers listed in the chapter appendix are reliable service sources.

Once online, the new user will begin to understand why the Internet is often referred to as an *information frontier*. The Internet is constantly changing. The tools used to perform subject searches still are being developed, software is in a rapid state of flux, and service providers frequently go in and out of business. Consequently, valuable information sources found during the course of an intensive search may suddenly become unavailable only to reappear at a new address at some later date. Because the management of the Internet is almost entirely distributed, there is neither a single database nor a standard classification system to organize information. The Internet thus stands in stark contrast to traditional published information services.

Despite its immaturity, the Internet offers a great deal of potentially useful information. Government and educational organizations are particularly rich sources to tap, although users may be frustrated by overpatronage at many sites. This heavy use may lead to long connect times and sometimes unreachable computers, especially during peak usage hours. As the Internet develops, commercial applications also are multiplying. An ever-increasing number of individual optometrists, optical suppliers, drug companies, associations, and publishers have established a presence on the World Wide Web (WWW), the most popular and user-friendly feature of the Internet. The network may be used to contact such businesses, view the schedule of an upcoming conference, download software updates, or even display a review of the latest computer system.

The WWW (or simply, the Web) is a subset of Internet-connected computers running software that may be read by PCs, Macintoshes, and other computer platforms. Web documents may contain text, pictures, sound, and even video clips. These documents also typically use the powerful link feature. Linking creates direct connections between any information source on the Web, so that documents no longer need to be in close physical proximity to be read together. Users find their way around the Web with the aid of browsing software such as Netscape, Internet Explorer, or Mosaic. These Web browsers use graphical user interfaces (GUIs) allowing users to make selections with a mouse. Starting at a welcome screen known as a *home page*, the user simply clicks on a link with a mouse in order to jump to another page of potential interest. Pointers embedded in the home page include the network address of the computer running the selected link, the log-in commands, and the path or region on the computer where the linked file is stored. This information is used by the browsers to locate and display the chosen file. The Web can be flexible and relatively easy to use, even for computer neophytes, but the heavy use of graphics on many home pages may slow the display of the information retrieved.

Many colleges of optometry, vision science researchers, and optometrists have established Web home pages. The NASA-sponsored Vision Science Web virtual library (as of this writing, located at http://vision.arc.nasa.gov/VisionScience/VisionScienceContent.html) provides a catalog of many of these sources. The page lists numerous links to research groups, institutes, university departments, organizations, conferences, software, journals, and other sources of vision science information. Because the Web is so fluid, this source could be located at a different address by the time this book is published. To locate a new address or to search for new sites, use one of the many Web search databases that allow location of Internet information by subject. Two particularly powerful databases are Alta Vista (http://altavista.digital.com) and Excite (http://www.excite.com). Use Alta Vista to perform a comprehensive search; use Excite to pinpoint the location of a popular page.

An earlier generation of finding tools on the Internet include Gopher and Veronica. Gopher software allows system administrators to organize textual information into hierarchic menus for ease of retrieval. Gophers at different sites are each unique, providing customized menus of the information of local importance. Resources need not be lodged on the same computer displaying the menu; like Web browsers, Gophers provide access to global information stored on computers separated by thousands of miles. Gopher software allows the Internet user to follow the trail of related documents, while Veronica provides keyword searches of Gopher titles. Over time, the use of text-based tools like Gopher is likely to be eclipsed by those programs using a GUI.

The Internet is still in its infancy, but it is growing quickly. Today, access may be slow and the identification of useful information is frequently a multistep procedure. However, as use of e-mail increases familiarity with networks, the technology matures, and the software becomes incorporated into everyday productivity packages, the uses for Web communication or its successors will explode. For now, Internet users should be flexible and willing to learn.

Journal Literature

A regular program of journal reading is probably the preferred way for most clinicians to stay current with developments relevant to their practice. This activity includes several components: selecting journals to receive on subscription, selecting journals to scan (either at a vision science library or through a current awareness source), and obtaining copies of articles. Association memberships often result in journal subscriptions that may or may not be of interest for a regular program of journal reading. Targeting specific journal titles for reading on the basis of their quality and relevance to one's own practice is probably the most effective approach from a clinical and time management perspective. One might consider, for example, a general clinically oriented journal (e.g., *Clinical Eye and Vision Care, Optometry Clinics*), a research journal (e.g., *Optometry and Vision Science*), a current awareness source (e.g., *Optometry: Current Literature in Perspective*), and a specialty journal based on one's particular interests (e.g., *Journal of Behavioral Optometry, International Contact Lens Clinic*). Whatever the mix, you should not feel constrained about changing titles based on your own perceptions of utility and quality. A journal subscription is of little use unless it is read. Beyond reading to stay current with new developments, the next step in one's use of the journal literature is to consider retaining and organizing articles of lasting value for future reference.

Managing Reprint Collections

Articles you wish to retain for future reference may be identified in your reading and through literature searches, by the scanning of article bibliographies or current awareness sources, and through referrals from colleagues (notoriously inaccurate!). Some clinicians regularly tear articles of interest from their subscription copies. After reading or identifying articles of particular lasting interest and value, the next steps are to request or copy, organize, and store them. Collecting articles without some basic organizational scheme is likely to be a waste of both time and paper. The goal is a usable scheme that permits ready retrieval of reprints when needed, with a relatively minimal time commitment.

Articles may be organized by date, by author, by subject, or by various other schemes. Filing by arbitrarily assigned number is possible if one maintains an author or subject index, perhaps using computer software. A general textbook outline or thesaurus (e.g., NLM's *Medical Subject Headings* or *MeSH*) may be used to create a standardized list of headings under which to file articles. This can help to avoid filing similar articles in multiple locations. Alternatively, for smaller collections you may be willing to tolerate some filing redundancy for the flexibility of creating headings as needed.

The availability of reference management software can simplify the organization of reprints, the compilation of bibliographies, and the identification of needed references. Using such programs as Reference Manager, EndNote Plus, or Papyrus, one can import citations downloaded from CD-ROM or online databases or can enter references manually. Keywords can be assigned for rapid retrieval by subject, and reference lists can be reformatted easily to meet the style requirements of a specific journal. Additional information about obtaining these programs is listed in the chapter appendix. McCarthy's book on personal filing systems[12] provides detailed guidance for creating information retrieval systems using a personal computer. Articles by Miller[13] and Blumenthal and Gilad[14] compare the relative merits of leading software programs. For those with substantial reprint collections or a regular publishing schedule, bibliographic software can be of invaluable assistance.

Special Skills Needed for Effective Use of the Literature: Quality and Selection

Information management skills are not limited to rapid retrieval of data. In view of the potential quantity of information in existence, its cost, and the limited availability of time in the clinical setting, selection issues are also extremely important. The ability to assess available sources both for relevance and quality is an essential skill for the effective clinician. This is true either in building one's own collection or in deciding what to read.

In evaluating information sources, one must consider the bias and expertise of the author. A book or review paper written by a specialist clinician may have an approach different from one written by a researcher, but either is likely to be more authoritative than that written by a generalist clinician. An optometrist may have a different perspective than a physician. It may be useful to read articles or chapters with contrasting viewpoints to obtain a fully balanced overview. A matter of particular concern for optometry relates to what has been excluded (e.g., in the MEDLINE database).

Although a detailed discussion of selection, critical review, and statistical analysis is beyond the scope of this chapter, it is necessary to remind readers of the controversial nature of the cutting edge. A study may not have been repeated or even reviewed by leading scientists in the field when it is first published and may be disproved within the next month or year. Certain simple tactics are helpful when making quality decisions; the reputation of the journal or the author is particularly important. Knowing also the editorial policy of a journal—

Table 4.3
Quality issues.

Qualifications and reputation of author (any particular expertise in the topic)

Possible biases of the author (medical, surgical, optometric, behavioral, other)

Reputation of the publisher and editor (established press, other books or journals in the field)

Standard source, multiple editions (sources published in multiple editions are more likely to have stood the tests of time)

References to support text (for tracking past research on a topic and suggesting a more scholarly approach)

Ease of use (e.g., indexes, table of contents); important for efficiency in finding needed information

Quality and types of illustrations (supporting the text; for atlases, a possible primary focus)

Peer review (no guarantee of quality, but some measure of outside expert assessment)

Cost (especially for office collections, possibly an overriding concern)

---

specifically whether articles are peer-reviewed as part of the selection process—will help to determine how much weight should be given to a new article.

Peer-reviewed (or *refereed*) articles are read by authorities in the field, who review the validity of the study's assumptions, methodology, results, and conclusions and who then recommend accepting, rejecting, or provisionally accepting the study. Peer review alone is no guarantee of the value of a paper, but it suggests that some quality filtering has taken place. The *instructions to authors* section often will indicate whether a given journal is peer reviewed. Basic library reference sources such as *Ulrichs International Periodical Directory* or the *Serials Directory* provide lists of selected peer-reviewed journals but are not necessarily comprehensive in their inclusion of optometric journal titles. Readers also are referred to the article by Zadnik in the suggested reading list at the end of this chapter for a primer on critical assessment of the journal literature. The series by Oxman, Sackett, and Guyatt provides useful guidance in judging the quality of published articles as well (see Suggested Reading).

Table 4.3 may be used as a checklist to assist in evaluating information sources, whether for purchase, consultation, or regular reading. For practitioners who consider modifying their current practice on the basis of the results of recently published studies, quality issues are a special concern.

Table 4.4
Factors in the search process.

Nature of Information	Nature of Query
Amount of information available	Amount of information needed
Rate of change of topic	Need for currency
Type of topic (e.g., medical, optometric)	Purpose of inquiry
Quality of information available	Quality of information required (quick and dirty?)
Level of treatment available	Level desired (e.g., popular, expert)
Time required to search	Time available to search
Availability of technology	Skills in using technology
Cost	Resources willing to spend or use

IMPLICATIONS OF INFORMATION STRUCTURE: SUMMARY

We have presented the most common categories of knowledge-based questions that may arise in the clinical setting, along with the types of sources one might wish to consult to answer them and organizational strategies to prepare for what one might encounter. Although the nature of the question is an important basis for selection, it is certainly not the only one. Other factors of potential relevance have been mentioned in passing and are summarized in Table 4.4. These items include the volume of information on the topic, its currency, the rate of change in the field, and the nature of the information required.

For example, there is an enormous quantity of information on the acquired immunodeficiency syndrome (AIDS) and related topics, and new developments are being reported all the time. This rapid rate of change suggests that, although a textbook could provide useful background information on ocular manifestations of AIDS, it would be appropriate to update this information with current journal articles found by using a MEDLINE search. On the other hand, information on refraction techniques changes relatively slowly, and one is likely to find relatively little published on refraction in the recent journal literature.

Other considerations involve the trade-offs between the costs (e.g., time, money, frustration) involved in obtaining information and the quality and quantity of information required. At times a "quick-and-dirty" search of the resources at hand will provide sufficient information to proceed. At other times, the potential implications of outdated or erroneous information will require greater care in finding the best information available. Individual preference also plays a role: Clinicians comfortable with technology may be more likely to seek out electronic resources, whereas others may wish to rely on personal contacts or printed materials.

Finally, care in selecting information resources for future reference is likely to make the search process much easier when questions do arise. The model presented here cannot claim to eliminate the continuing pressure all clinicians face in the handling of biomedical information. However, it should provide a means for dealing efficiently with many routine questions and for developing the information management skills so essential to the process of lifelong learning and the delivery of high-quality patient care.

REFERENCES

1. Covell DG, Uman GC, Manning PR. Information needs in office practice: are they being met? Ann Intern Med 1985;103:596–599.
2. Stinson ER, Mueller DA. Survey of health professionals' information habits and needs. Conducted through personal interviews. JAMA 1980;243:140–143.
3. Northup DE, Moore-West M, Skipper B, et al. Characteristics of clinical information-searching: investigation using critical incident technique. J Med Educ 1983;58:873–881.
4. Kanski JJ. Clinical Ophthalmology: A Systematic Approach (3rd ed). Oxford: Butterworth-Heinemann, 1994.
5. Cullom RD, Chang B (eds). The Wills Eye Manual: Office and Emergency Room Diagnosis and Treatment of Eye Disease (2nd ed). Philadelphia: Lippincott, 1994.
6. Tasman W, Jaeger EA (eds). Duane's Clinical Ophthalmology. Philadelphia: Lippincott, 1995.
7. Physician's Desk Reference (50th ed). Montvale, NJ: Medical Economics, 1996.
8. Larson DE (ed). Mayo Clinic Family Health Book (3rd ed). New York: W Morrow, 1996.
9. Clayman CB (ed). American Medical Association Family Medical Guide. New York: Random House, 1994.
10. The AFB Directory of Services for Blind and Visually Impaired Persons in the United States and Canada (24th ed). New York: American Foundation for the Blind, 1993.
11. Rees AM (ed). Consumer Health Information Source Book (4th ed). Phoenix: Oryx, 1994.
12. McCarthy S. Personal Filing Systems: Creating Information Retrieval Systems on Microcomputers. Chicago: Medical Library Association, 1988.
13. Miller MC. Reference management software: a review of Endnote Plus, Reference Manager, and Pro-Cite. MD Comput 1994;11:161–168.
14. Blumenthal EZ, Gilad R. Storing a bibliographic data base on your PC: a review of reference-management software. N Engl J Med 1993;329:283–284.

SUGGESTED READING

Brizuela BS, Hesp JA. Drug Information. In AR Gennaro (ed), Remington's
Pharmaceutical Sciences (18th ed). Easton, PA: Mack Publishing, 1990;49–59.

Read pages 49–50 and introductions to lists of specific sources. Skim descriptions of specific titles for an overview of individual sources. Although geared to the practicing pharmacist, comments concerning journals and newsletters (p. 57) provide useful background information for any clinician interested in drug sources.

Frisse ME. Acquiring information management skills. Acad Med 1994;69:803–806.

Notes the importance of information and computer-related skills for the clinician.

Lowe HJ, Barnett GO. Understanding and using the Medical Subject Headings
(MeSH) vocabulary to perform literature searches. JAMA 1994;271:1103–1108.

A fairly technical overview for the highly motivated searcher.

McKibbon KA, Walker-Dilks CJ. How to harness MEDLINE to solve clinical problems. ACP Journal Club 1994;120(suppl 2):A10–A12.

Provides guidance on various means to access the MEDLINE database.

Oxman AD, Sackett DL, Guyatt GH. Users' guides to the medical literature. I. How
to get started. The Evidence-Based Medicine Working Group. JAMA
1993;270:2093–2095. (See also other articles in the series.)

A primer on evaluating scientific evidence for incorporation into one's clinical practice.

Zadnik K. Critically reviewing the ophthalmic literature. Optom Vis Sci
1994;71:254–258.

A guide to understanding research. Essential reading for those seeking to stay abreast of current clinical advances.

APPENDIX: SOURCES OF FURTHER INFORMATION

Association of Vision Science Librarians "Opening Day Collection"

Archived at: http://spectacle.berkeley.edu/~library/pubs.htm
Contact: Maureen Watson
Reading Room
College of Optometry
Ferris State University
Big Rapids, MI 49307
(616) 592-2394

Clinical Practice Guidelines

American Academy of Ophthalmology
Quality of Care Committee
P.O. Box 7424
San Francisco, CA 94120-7424

American Optometric Association
AOA Clinical Guidelines Coordinating Committee
243 North Lindbergh Boulevard
St. Louis, MO 63141-7881

U.S. Department of Health and Human Services
Public Health Service
Agency for Health Care Policy and Research
Executive Office Center, Suite 501
2101 East Jefferson Street
Rockville, MD 20852

Document Delivery Providers

UMI Article Clearinghouse
University Microfilms, Inc.
P.O. Box 1346
300 North Zeeb Road
Ann Arbor, MI 48106-1346
(800) 248-0360

EMDOCS
469 Union Avenue
Westbury, NY 11590
(800) 282-2720
Internet: dds@work4u.artx.com

The Genuine Article
Institute for Scientific Information
3501 Market Street
Philadelphia, PA 19104
(215) 386-0100

International Library, Archives, and Museum of Optometry
243 North Lindbergh Boulevard
St. Louis, MO 63141
(314) 991-0324; 991-4100

Access to the MEDLINE Database, Grateful Med Software

MEDLARS Service Desk; Grateful Med
National Library of Medicine (#38/4N-421)
8600 Rockville Pike
Bethesda, MD 20894
(800) 638-8480
Internet: mms@nlm.nih.gov

OphthaLine CD-ROM Database for Ophthalmology (a subset of
MEDLINE)
Aries System Corporation
200 Sutton Street
North Andover, MA 01845
(508) 975-7570

VISIONET Database and Thesaurus (Document Delivery also available)

Ms. Nancy Gatlin, Library Director
Southern College of Optometry
1245 Madison Avenue
Memphis, TN 38104
(901) 722-3237

Current Awareness

Ophthalmic Literature
Elsevier Science Inc.
660 White Plains Road
Tarrytown, NY 10591-5153

Optometry: Current Literature in Perspective
Mosby–Year Book
200 North LaSalle Street
Chicago, IL 60601

Selected Sources of Information for Patients (e.g., brochures)

American Optometric Association
243 North Lindbergh Boulevard
St. Louis, MO 63141
(314) 991-0324; 991-4100

American Academy of Ophthalmology
Free brochure (enclose a self-addressed, stamped envelope)
P.O. Box 7424
San Francisco, CA 94120
(415) 561-8540

Information Access Company
(Health Reference Center)
362 Lakeside Drive
Foster City, CA 94404
(800) 227-8431

National Eye Health Education Program
National Institutes of Health
2020 Vision Place
Bethesda, MD 20892-3655
Internet: 2020@b31.nei.nih.gov

Internet Service Providers

America Online (800) 827-6364
CompuServe (800) 848-8199
Prodigy (800) 776-3449

Internet Service Providers Database:
http://www.yahoo.com/Business_and_Economy/Companies/
   Internet_Services/Internet_Access_Providers/

Bibliographic Management Software

EndNote Plus
Niles and Associates
800 Jones Street
Berkeley, CA 94710
(510) 559-8592

Papyrus
Research Software Design
2718 Southwest Kelly, Suite 181
Portland, OR 97201
(503) 796-1368

Reference Manager
Research Information Systems
2355 Camino Vida Roble
Carlsbad, CA 92009
(800) 722-1227

5

Ethical Clinical Decision Making

Ellen Richter Ettinger

In this book, we examine the issues involved in clinical decision making. It is important to realize that clinical decision making is based on more than scientific knowledge and observations; many clinical decisions involve ethical dilemmas.

Answers to the questions facing optometrists are not always as simple as choosing among one *outstanding* correct decision and several clearly wrong ones. Sometimes there are several acceptable alternatives, and the clinician has to determine which is the best. To help the clinician make ethical decisions, this chapter investigates the principles of ethics that impact on clinical care.

Ethics can be described as an examination of moral values, an investigation of the distinction between right and wrong, or a study of human character and conduct.[1] It also has been defined as "the study of principles or moral values which govern principled relationships between individuals."[2] Medical ethics is a branch of the study of ethics and moral philosophy that has been applied to the clinical environment.[3]

DePender and Ikeda-Chandler[4] emphasize that ethics relates to making choices and involves considering the results of our actions. It has been said that ethics involves choosing, from a set of alternatives, what one "ought to do."[2, 5] If clinical care were an exact science and there were only one answer for each clinical situation, the study of medical ethics would be much less intriguing. That medical care involves uncertainty and requires the doctor to choose the *best* choice from a group of possible actions makes the study of biomedical ethics much more complex.

A study of clinical ethics is not meant to serve as a cookbook on a professional's conduct.[6] The possible situations encountered by a clinician over the course of his or her career are too numerous to outline, and an analysis of choices, concerns, and patient's needs must be made

Table 5.1
Principles of biomedical ethics.

Nonmaleficence (to do no harm)
Beneficence (to do good)
Respect for autonomy (respecting the decision-making capacities of
    patients)
Justice (fairness in the distribution of clinical care)

Source: Based on TL Beauchamp, JF Childress. Principles of Biomedical Ethics. New York: Oxford University Press, 1994.

on an individual basis. Examining ethical principles, however, can provide the clinician with a better understanding of how decisions are made and how they affect the patient.

Four principles of biomedical ethics have been identified (Table 5.1). First, *nonmaleficence* is the principle often cited in the clinical maxim: "Above all (or first) do no harm."[7] This principle reminds the doctor that clinical intervention should never be used to cause harm or injury.

Second, the principle of *beneficence* maintains that clinical care should benefit and contribute to the welfare of the patient. It has been said that beneficence requires more of the clinician than nonmaleficence, because the former requires the doctor to take actual, positive steps to help the patient, not just to refrain from harming the individual.

The third principle, *autonomy*, reminds the clinician that patients must be given appropriate information and that they must be allowed to make up their own minds. To this end, the doctor must educate the patient about clinical problems and management options, give the patient an opportunity to express decisions, and *listen carefully* to the patient's desires. Campbell et al.[3] refer to this practice as a "respectful" dialogue between the doctor and the patient, with a goal of combining the patient's values and the doctor's expertise to produce benefit. They point out that both the patient and the doctor must be prepared to listen to one another for this to occur.

Fourth, *justice* refers to fairness in distributing clinical care and resources. Justice reminds the clinician to treat people fairly in the allocation of clinical services, without discriminating with respect to age, gender, ethnicity, social status, sexual orientation, and other factors. Campbell et al.[3] discuss an example of unfair discrimination, citing the case of two people who have equal and comparable needs for a particular treatment and are treated quite differently on the basis of bias in favor of wealth or race.

It has been pointed out that, although nonmaleficence and beneficence have played a central role in the history of medical ethics, auton-

Table 5.2
American Optometric Association's code of ethics.

It shall be the ideal, the resolve, and the duty of the members of the
   American Optometric Association:
To keep the visual welfare of the patient uppermost at all times;
To promote in every possible way, in collaboration with this Association,
   better care of the visual needs of mankind;
To enhance continuously their educational and technical proficiency to the
   end that their patients shall receive the benefits of all acknowledged
   improvements in vision care;
To see that no person shall lack for visual care, regardless of his [or her]
   financial status;
To advise the patient whenever consultation with an optometric colleague
   or reference for other professional care seems advisable;
To hold in professional confidence all information concerning a patient and
   to use such data only for the benefit of the patient;
To conduct themselves as exemplary citizens;
To maintain their offices and their practices in keeping with professional
   standards;
To promote and maintain cordial and unselfish relationships with members
   of their own profession and of other professions for the exchange of
   information to the advantage of mankind.

Source: Reprinted from American Optometric Association. Code of Ethics.
J Am Optom Assoc 1994;6:front cover.

omy and justice have become more prominent in recent times, as the
rights of patients have received heightened attention.[7]

Numerous codes of ethics have been developed for health care professionals.[8–11] It is the intent of this chapter not to redefine these principles of ethics but to show how they relate to decision making.

THE PATIENT'S BEST INTERESTS

To make ethical clinical decisions, the clinician must have the *best*
interests of the patient in mind. All the previously mentioned clinical
codes of ethics refer to the patient's interests as a priority in deliver-
ing clinical care. The American Optometric Association's Code of
Ethics refers to the need to "keep the visual welfare of the patient
uppermost at all times" (Table 5.2). A statement in the introduction
to the American Medical Association's Principles of Medical Ethics
states that its ethical code is developed "primarily for the benefit of

the patient."[10] Similarly, an introduction to the Principles of Ethics and Code of Professional Conduct of the American Dental Association states that the ethical code of the dental profession has "always held as their primary goal the benefit of the patient."[11] The needs of many individuals and groups can be considered in the scope of health care: the doctor, insurance companies, managed care plans, professional organizations, government agencies, political forces, pharmaceutical companies, medical equipment companies, consumer groups, and individual patients. Examinations of all these viewpoints affect the complexity of the ethical situation. Decisions made in the clinical setting include choosing procedures to perform, setting fees, making referrals, using and prescribing drugs, advising the patient when to return for further care, and other recommendations. Although it is interesting to note the interests of each of these constituents and how their interests may affect the delivery of care, it must be the needs of the patient that provide the best guidance. No other constituent can surpass the patient's own interests in determining the best actions for the patient.

UNDERSTANDING THE PATIENT

Ethical clinical decisions require that clinicians understand the concerns, needs, and priorities of their patients. To act in patients' best interests, doctors must get to know their patients well enough to understand their needs, values, and priorities. A doctor must be a good listener and must ask appropriate questions. Good communication skills are imperative for patient-centered clinical care.[12] Effective interviewing and case history skills are an essential component to good clinical decision making. There is no substitute for an effective doctor-patient interaction as part of good, ethical clinical care.

COMPASSIONATE CARE GIVING

To make ethical clinical decisions, the clinician must provide humane, compassionate, patient-centered care. Taking the time to provide such care conveys an attitude of respect and sensitivity toward the patient that affects the clinical environment and the delivery of clinical care in a very positive way. Putting patients at ease may help them respond more ably during the testing sequence, which can result in better, more comprehensive clinical data. Providing compassionate care is part of building a strong, effective interaction with the patient. Doctors who deliver care of this caliber convey a message that they truly are dedicated to the patient's interests. Respectful care can make patients more receptive to doctors and to their delivery of clinical services. Developing positive listening attitudes and demonstrating empathy for patients are important aspects of this component of clinical care.[12] Treating patients well (e.g., ethically) is a fundamental step that helps to build the foundation for ethical clinical decision making.

MAINTAINING PROFESSIONAL PROFICIENCY

Making ethical clinical decisions demands that clinicians be life-long learners, continually updating their knowledge base and clinical proficiency so that their delivery of care is optimal and their decisions are based on the most current knowledge and clinical standards. Health care is changing rapidly, with the standards of clinical care advancing as technology permits. To make good decisions, clinicians must be knowledgeable about the options currently available for a patient, and they must be able to determine the best choice. By not staying up-to-date, a clinician may overlook a testing procedure or therapy that is in the patient's interest. The notion that a clinician will know everything needed for a full career when he or she graduates from a clinical training program is unrealistic; this is especially true in light of the rapid gains and changes occurring in the health care delivery system. An excellent clinician can remain excellent only by staying up-to-date with the latest standards of care.

REFERRAL SKILLS

To make ethical decisions, the clinician must make appropriate referrals, always choosing a referral source that will serve the patient's best interests. When a clinician determines that the services required for a patient are beyond the scope of his or her abilities or that a patient is better served by the care of another professional, a referral is indicated. The choice of referral must be in the best interests of the patient, to the best qualified person, regardless of personal, financial, political, and other pressures.

To facilitate referrals, the referring doctor should communicate the purpose of the referral in some way, either written or oral. Some doctors like to send a letter with information about the patient's status, and some prefer to transmit the information by telephone. These forms of communication facilitate effective referrals in which the receiving doctor understands why the patient was sent and what services are needed. They also improve continuity of care by providing relevant information from previous clinical findings and by preventing unnecessary repetition of tests and procedures.

The initial doctor should be specific in terms of what is expected of the other clinician: *consultation* (for special tests or an expert opinion, after which the patient returns to the initial doctor), *referral* (for management of a problem for which the referral doctor's care usually lasts for an extended period), or *comanagement* (in which two or more health care providers work *together* in caring for a patient). To avoid confusion or misunderstanding, this intention should be made clear to both the patient and the referring doctor. Health care professionals who receive referrals should provide timely feedback to the referring doctors, with detailed information regarding the patient's clinical status. If the scope of the problem eliciting the referral is completed, the patient should be referred back to the initial doctor. Effective referrals clearly are in the best interests of the patient, using their time and expenditures on health care optimally.

PROVIDING APPROPRIATE INFORMATION TO THE PATIENT

Clinicians also must provide the patient with appropriate information. This service helps patients to make good decisions for themselves. Educating patients adequately about the need for tests and therapies can help to improve patient compliance. For example, if a patient understands the need for glaucoma medications and the risk of not adhering to appropriate recommendations, he or she may be more likely to comply. Other examples can be seen in educating patients about when to use distance and near glasses, when and how to use medications, and how to use and care for contact lenses properly. Patients are entitled to informed consent.[13] Good patient education also promotes good health care behaviors, such as motivating patients to return for future care.

Forrow et al.[5] commented that optimal clinical decision making occurs when "the doctor and patient each contribute their own special knowledge to the decision making process." The doctor provides scientific information relevant to diagnosis and treatment, calling on clinical knowledge, training, and experience. The patient provides insights into the overall effects of treatment on personal well-being, with information on how well a particular intervention is likely to meet his or her goals, values, and needs. Each individual brings to the relationship a special understanding and perspective that enhances the decision-making process.

Doctors make many decisions, but ultimately it is the *patient* who must return for testing procedures, take medications, and follow other therapeutic modalities. Providing appropriate patient education and information supplies a framework from which patients can make good decisions for themselves.

PATIENT CONFIDENTIALITY

Ethical clinical decision making requires the clinician to protect the confidentiality of the patient. The concept of patient confidentiality is based on the premise that a patient who is not assured that personal information will remain private and confidential is less likely to reveal personal details to a health care worker.[14] This is true especially of intimate or sensitive information, such as details about sexually transmitted diseases, psychiatric conditions, drug or substance abuse, and serious medical illnesses (e.g., cancer). Patient confidentiality must be protected and respected. Clinicians also must be certain to train staff members about the confidentiality of such sensitive information in their access to patients' clinical records. By ensuring patient confidentiality, clinicians reassure patients that sensitive information is secure and that their privacy is maintained. This can help to make patients more open in discussing details important to the decision-making process.

AVOIDANCE OF PREJUDICE

Ethical decision making calls for the clinician to provide care to patients without bias with regard to age, gender, race, ethnicity, social or financial status, sexual orientation, disability, or other factors. The basis for this rule is the principle of justice, ensuring that patients will not face discrimination. This does not mean that appropriate patient-centered differences in care are not acceptable; in fact, research to examine the needs of diverse groups of patients has helped clinicians understand how to provide better care. For example, studies have been helpful in learning about useful testing and treatment modalities for patients with disabilities; other studies have focused on recommendations for testing and treatment procedures that address cultural and ethnic factors. These differences are used to provide better care. Differences should be based on sound epidemiologic, scientific, and clinical knowledge. To make ethical clinical decisions, the clinician must not discriminate in the delivery of clinical care.

The clinician also must be conscious of removing obstacles to good clinical care. Economics is a major barrier to good care, and is an example of the ethical dilemmas that exist in contemporary optometric practice.[15] Health care professionals should work to eliminate barriers "caused by economic, geographic, language, cultural and other factors."[16] They also must remember that it is unethical to use third-party reimbursement availability as a primary motivation for performing procedures or services.[17] Although finances for health care are a challenge beyond the scope of this chapter, it is important to remember that it is a patient's need—not finances—that should be the primary factor in determining which tests and procedures a patient should receive. Clinicians must work to ensure that health care services are available to those who need them.[18]

PATIENT INDIVIDUALITY

To make ethical clinical decisions, the clinician must recognize each patient as an individual and make patient-centered decisions. Two patients with the same clinical profile may require two significantly different management plans. What is best for one patient may not be best for another. Clinicians must recognize and respect patients as individuals and find appropriate solutions for their unique sets of clinical findings, problems, concerns, and priorities.

ETHICAL CONSISTENCY

Ethical clinical decision making must be maintained on a regular basis. The process by which one makes clinical decisions is not altogether different from the process used in making other lifetime decisions. DePender and Ikeda-Chandler say "Ethics isn't just a public display of concern for right and wrong. It's a process of working toward consistently excellent choices."[4] It is hoped that the information and discussions presented in Part I of this book will help students and clinicians make consistently excellent decisions.

REFERENCES

1. Webster's Dictionary. Baltimore, MD: Ottenheimer Publishers, 1986.
2. Beauchamp GR, Bettman JW, Stromberg CD. Ethics in Ophthalmology: A Practical Guide. San Francisco: American Academy of Ophthalmology, 1986;3.
3. Campbell AV, Gillett G, Jones G. Practical Medical Ethics. Auckland: Oxford University Press, 1992.
4. DePender W, Ikeda-Chandler W. Clinical Ethics: An Invitation to Healing Professionals. New York: Praeger, 1990.
5. Forrow L, Wartman SA, Brock DW. Science, ethics, and the making of clinical decisions. Implications for risk factor intervention. JAMA 1988;259:3161–3167.
6. American Academy of Ophthalmology Ethics Committee. The Ethical Ophthalmologist: A Primer. San Francisco: American Academy of Ophthalmology, 1993.
7. Beauchamp TL, Childress JF. Principles of Biomedical Ethics (4th ed). New York: Oxford University Press, 1994.
8. Code of Ethics of the American Optometric Association. St. Louis: American Optometric Association, 1944.
9. Code of Ethics of the American Academy of Ophthalmology. San Francisco: American Academy of Ophthalmology, 1993.
10. American Medical Association Principles of Medical Ethics. Chicago: American Medical Association, 1992.
11. Principles of Ethics and Code of Professional Conduct of the American Dental Association. Chicago: American Dental Association, 1992.
12. Ettinger ER. Professional Communications in Eye Care. Boston: Butterworth-Heinemann, 1994.
13. Classe JG. Legal Aspects of Optometry. Boston: Butterworths, 1989.
14. Classe JG. To hold in professional confidence all information concerning a patient and to use such data only for the benefit of the patient. J Am Optom Assoc 1994;65:404–405.
15. Werner DL. Ethics in the optometric curriculum. Optom Educ 1996;21:124–125.
16. Bailey RN. To promote in every possible way, in collaboration with this association, better care of the visual needs of mankind. J Am Optom Assoc 1994;65:391.
17. Haffner AN. Issues of optometric ethics and values for the '90s. J Am Optom Assoc 1991;62:780–791.
18. Hopping RL. Ethics: a professional challenge revisited. J Am Optom Assoc 1990;61:345–351.

II

Clinical Practice

Introduction

Part II is unique in that it presents clinical decision making within the context of expert clinicians solving the underlying cause of a series of entering patient complaints. These case scenarios use 18 common or challenging clinical conditions to illustrate the decision-making process.

We have not identified the diagnosis in the title of the case scenarios, and we have not presented the cases in a particular order according to topic, because we wanted to simulate the way that patients actually present to a doctor's office: with unknown diagnoses that require a doctor's insight and decision-making skills. We have also avoided naming cases by diagnoses or topics (e.g., anterior segment diseases or binocular vision disorders) because we wanted to refrain from the conscious or unconscious compartmentalized, departmental, fragmentary thinking that often comes from working in a clinical training setting. We want the reader to approach the case as a challenge from the primary eye care practitioner's perspective. We have provided a summary of the primary and secondary diagnoses or topics for each case scenario, in the Appendix, if the reader wants to review a single case or a series of cases rather than the total 18.

A specific case or a series of cases can serve as the basis for discussion in a clinical decision-making course lecture or seminar series. We believe the 18 cases in Part II present the common decision-making strategies in the most frequent types of cases seen by eye care professionals. Additional cases can be constructed by the instructor or students to expand topic areas. The format in Part II is an excellent method for students to use in summarizing clinical encounters. It requires students to review why they made certain decisions in a particular case or series of cases: Why did I ask that particular question? What information was I looking for? Why did I think that test was problem-specific? What database or baseline data did I forget to address?

For each case scenario the expert clinician does the following:

1. Presents an entering clinical scenario
2. Provides the case history interaction
3. Develops a working hypothesis list
4. Discusses the thinking that leads to selecting problem specific data to rule in or out each hypothesis
5. Explains why certain other data are needed for database or baseline evaluation
6. Identifies the final diagnostic summary and management plan

The entire clinical decision process is summarized in a flow chart at the end of each case. Readers of this book may find this flowchart format helpful in summarizing their own clinical cases, and in gaining insights into their own clinical decision-making strategies.

Michael W. Rouse
Ellen Richter Ettinger

Case Scenario 1

Susan A. Cotter

PATIENT BACKGROUND

CS is a 5-year-old kindergarten girl, accompanied to the optometric examination by her mother.

DOCTOR: What brings you in today for an eye examination?

MOTHER: My daughter came home from kindergarten last week with a form saying she failed the vision screening at school.

DOCTOR (*thinking*): *The chief complaint is that this child failed the vision screening at school. The local schools test only distance visual acuity (unaided and then with the plus-sphere test using +1.75 D lenses) and "muscle balance"; therefore, there's a high probability that she has reduced distance visual acuity or that a high phoria or a strabismus is present. However, it also is possible there is no vision problem at all. It's common for children this age to fail school vision screenings because they do not know their letters well enough, they do not understand what is expected of them, they are too shy to answer, or the duration of the testing exceeds their attention span. I can obtain more insight into possible vision problems by determining why the child failed the screening.*

DOCTOR: Do you know why your daughter failed the vision screening, or do you have the form that the school sent home?

MOTHER: Yes, I have the form right here in my purse. It says she failed "visual acuity."

DOCTOR (*thinking*): *The cutoff for failing distance visual acuity is 20/40 or worse. There are many conditions that might cause a visual acuity reduction such as this. Knowing whether the acuity problem is unilateral or bilateral will help formulate my diagnostic hypotheses.*

DOCTOR: Could I please see the form to see whether she failed visual acuity for one eye or both eyes? (*The form, however, does not specify this information.*)

DOCTOR (*thinking*): *No helpful information there. However, if a significant visual acuity deficit is present bilaterally, it is possible that the parents may have noticed some behavioral signs such as CS sitting close to the television, squinting to see at distance, or holding her reading material close. I'll ask some questions to explore whether there are any signs or symptoms that might suggest bilaterally reduced visual acuity.*

DOCTOR: Have you noticed anything unusual about her eyes or any behavior that might indicate she is not seeing well?

MOTHER: Not at all. We've never had any indication that she doesn't see clearly. Actually, she sits farther away from the television than her 7-year-old brother, and she has no problem coloring or playing video games at home.

DOCTOR: Have you noticed her squinting to see, or that one of her eyes turns inward or outward, or that she is holding her reading or coloring books too close?

MOTHER: No, nothing unusual.

DOCTOR: Has she ever said anything to you about her eyes or vision?

MOTHER: No, she hasn't.

DOCTOR: Has she ever had an eye examination?

MOTHER: No, this is her first.

DOCTOR: CS, do you see OK? *(Child just shrugs her shoulders.)*

DOCTOR *(thinking)*: *Because the parents have not noticed any behavioral signs of decreased vision, it's unlikely that CS has a high degree of isoametropic myopia. However, the lack of observed signs does not necessarily rule out significant myopia, hyperopia, or moderate to high astigmatism. Although aberrations of behavior and observed signs sometimes are of value in identifying children with vision problems, they are not related necessarily to specific types of vision problems, nor to the magnitude of such problems.[1] In fact, I have seen a number of children who have significant uncorrected refractive error (e.g., −10.00 D OU) and whose parents have denied observing behaviors suggestive of decreased vision.*

The first thing I need to determine is whether an acuity deficit is indeed present and, if so, to investigate the cause of reduced vision. However, before I proceed to my diagnostic testing, I need to complete the history. I'll inquire about the family eye history and the presence of visual conditions that are genetically determined or familial that might be related to reduced vision.

DOCTOR: Are there any visual conditions or eye diseases that run in your family?

MOTHER: I wear contact lenses for my nearsightedness, and nearsightedness runs in my side of the family. My husband wears glasses for astigmatism, and he has a lazy eye.

DOCTOR *(thinking)*: *Myopia is familial, and there is an increased incidence in children with two myopic parents.[2] I wonder whether the father also has myopia. That would increase the likelihood that CS is myopic and that myopia is the reason for decreased vision. In addition, I would like to know exactly what the mother means by "lazy eye." Some lay people use the term to mean strabismus and others use the term to describe amblyopia. I would like to know whether the father has strabismus or ambly-*

opia, because a positive family history is a risk factor for the development of strabismus and amblyopia in offspring.[3]

DOCTOR: Do you know whether your husband is nearsighted or far-sighted?

MOTHER: I don't think he is either; he just has a lot of astigmatism and can't see without his glasses.

DOCTOR (*thinking*): *Although that tells me that the father probably has a moderate to significant amount of astigmatism, I do not know whether it is myopic or hyperopic astigmatism. I still need to investigate the "lazy eye."*

DOCTOR: When you say your husband has a "lazy eye," do you mean that it turns, such as wandering outward or crossing inward, or do you mean that the eye does not see well?

MOTHER: He doesn't see well out of his left eye even when wearing his glasses. I know that he wore a patch over one eye when he was young. His eyes look straight—I don't think he has crossed eyes.

DOCTOR (*thinking*): *On the basis of being patched as a child and having poor vision in one eye, it sounds as if the father may have amblyopia. Because the eyes appear straight, it's possible that it could be anisometropic amblyopia. However, the father could have a strabismus that is not apparent cosmetically and therefore have strabismic amblyopia. I'd like to investigate the family eye history a little farther.*

DOCTOR: Are there any other eye conditions that run in your family, or are there other family members who have vision loss?

MOTHER: No, not that I know of.

DOCTOR (thinking): *Good. It doesn't sound as if there are any hereditary eye diseases that might cause decreased vision by CS's age (e.g., Best's vitelliform macular degeneration, juvenile retinoschisis, dominant optic atrophy), or mom would probably be aware of them. To complete my understanding of the patient's case and to collect database information, I'll investigate the patient's and family's medical history.*

DOCTOR: How is her general health? Have there been any significant illnesses, or has she ever been hospitalized?

MOTHER: No, she is very healthy. In fact, she just saw her pediatrician for a kindergarten physical, and everything was fine.

DOCTOR: Does she have any allergies or take any medication?

MOTHER: She is allergic to penicillin and bee stings, and only takes a daily vitamin.

DOCTOR: How about your family and your husband's family? Are there any health problems such as diabetes or high blood pressure?

MOTHER: The only person who has any health problems is my father; he takes medication for high blood pressure.

DOCTOR: How is CS doing in kindergarten? Any problems?

MOTHER: No, she is doing just fine.

DOCTOR: In terms of general development, were there any delays, such as when CS first crawled or walked, or when she first started drawing or writing?

MOTHER: No, not that I know of.

DOCTOR: Were there any delays in speech and language skills, such as when CS said her first words? Was her speech easily understood?

MOTHER: No, in fact she has always been a little ahead of others of her age in speech and language skills.

DOCTOR (*thinking*): *The patient's and the family's medical histories are rather unremarkable and do not provide any new information for formulating my diagnostic hypotheses.*

DIAGNOSTIC HYPOTHESES

On the basis of the case history, the initial hypothesis list is as follows.

1. *Uncorrected unilateral or bilateral refractive error.* Statistically, uncorrected refractive error is the most likely cause of decreased visual acuity in children[4]; therefore, it is highest on the list of diagnostic hypotheses. Myopia is the most likely refractive error to cause reduced distance vision, with a prevalence of 5–9% at CS's age.[4, 5] As a general guideline, one would expect myopia to be –0.75 D or greater, hyperopia to be +5.00 D or greater (children usually can accommodate to compensate for mild to moderate amounts), and astigmatism in certain combinations to be –1.75 D or greater, before visual acuity would be reduced to 20/40 or worse in a child this age.[6] However, if CS passed unaided distance visual acuity with 20/20 and then read 20/20 viewing through the plus-sphere test (i.e., +1.75 D), hyperopia of a lesser amount (approximately +1.25 D) might be present (assuming CS did not memorize the 20/20 line she read previously).

2. *Functional amblyopia (strabismic, anisometropic, isoametropic).* After uncorrected refractive error, amblyopia (with a prevalence of approximately 2% in preschool and school-age children),[7, 8] is the most likely cause of reduced vision in children.[4] Strabismic, anisometropic, or unilateral-form deprivation amblyopia would cause a monocular decrease in vision and isoametropic or bilateral-form deprivation amblyopia would cause a bilateral decrease in visual acuity.

It is unlikely that CS has unilateral- or bilateral-form deprivation amblyopia, because form deprivation amblyopia is caused by an obstacle that physically blocks or occludes the visual axis during the sensitive period from birth to approximately age 6–8. We would expect that CS's parents or pediatrician previously would have observed any of the typical ocular conditions (e.g., congenital cataract, ptosis, cloudy cornea) that cause this type of amblyopia. Therefore, unilateral- and bilateral-form deprivation amblyopia were not included in the initial list of hypotheses.

For two reasons, it is more likely that CS has strabismic or anisometropic amblyopia than isoametropic amblyopia: First, strabismic and anisometropic amblyopia are more common,[8] and second, a unilateral vision decrease is more likely to remain undetected than is a bilateral decrease, because the child sees well with both eyes open and therefore usually does not complain or demonstrate aberrations in behavior. However, because isoametropic amblyopia results in a bilateral acuity loss typically in the range of 20/30–20/70, it could account for the absence of observed signs of decreased vision.

3.   *Vision screening over-referral (i.e., false-positive finding).* CS might belong in the category of a vision screening over-referral (i.e., one who fails the vision screening, yet on professional examination is found not to have a vision problem). A practitioner's rapport with youngsters on a one-to-one basis is often better than that established with vision screening personnel. Therefore, the data collected during a practitioner's evaluation is often more reliable. Although CS might have been able to see the test target perfectly, she might have given an unsatisfactory response during the vision screening if any of the following conditions occurred: poor understanding of what was expected, shyness preventing her from speaking or participating fully, or testing duration exceeding her attention span.

4.   *Malingering or psychogenic vision loss (i.e., ocular hysteria).* The child malingerer or the child with psychogenic vision loss typically presents with bilaterally reduced visual acuity, and it is often difficult for the practitioner to distinguish one condition from the other. CS might be a malingerer and might have failed the vision screening purposely in an effort to gain attention or because she wants a pair of spectacles. (Perhaps an older sibling or friend recently received spectacles, and now CS wants them also.) A less likely cause would be psychogenic vision loss, which has an emotional or psychological basis. Although juvenile-onset psychogenic vision loss is reported to be most common in children from ages 8–14, it can affect any individual regardless of age.[9]

5.   *Anterior or posterior segment pathology.* Although it is the least likely cause of reduced vision in this age group,[4] it is possible that a congenital anomaly or ocular disease is the cause of the decreased vision. Posterior segment pathology is a more likely cause than is anterior segment pathology. Anterior segment pathology usually is detected early in life because it is obvious to the parents, whereas posterior

segment pathology might not be discovered until later in childhood. If CS does have ocular pathology, a unilateral condition (e.g., retinal detachment, optic nerve hypoplasia, coloboma) would be more likely than would a bilateral condition, because CS's performance in school and elsewhere have not been affected.

DIAGNOSTIC TESTING

The diagnostic testing is presented in a decision-making format, not in the exact order in which I conducted the examination. I did, however, begin with visual acuity testing for several reasons. First, there are medical and legal reasons for measuring entering visual acuity before further testing is performed. Second, measuring visual acuity would confirm whether the reason for referral (i.e., decrease in visual acuity) was correct. Assuming that a decrease in vision was present, this would rule out the hypothesis of a vision screening over-referral. Third, I could narrow down my hypotheses on the basis of whether the decrease in visual acuity was unilateral or bilateral.

Of the five diagnostic hypotheses, uncorrected anisometropic refractive error, amblyopia (strabismic or anisometropic), or unilateral ocular pathology would result in a unilateral decrease in vision. If the decreased visual acuity is bilateral, the hypotheses can be narrowed to bilateral uncorrected refractive error, isoametropic amblyopia, malingering or ocular hysteria, or bilateral ocular pathology.

To arrive at a definitive diagnosis, I started with the most likely hypothesis and gathered all the clinical data either to confirm or to deny its relationship to the entering complaint of decreased vision. I then continued through the list of clinical hypotheses.

To rule out the initial hypothesis of uncorrected refractive error, I collected the following problem-specific clinical data: (1) entering visual acuities (Snellen) at distance and near (using a single-line versus a full-chart presentation because it is usually easier for young children), (2) static retinoscopy with distance visual acuities, and (3) cycloplegic retinoscopy with distance visual acuities.

The clinical data are presented in Table CS1.1. Static retinoscopy revealed significant anisometropic refractive error and decreased best-corrected visual acuity (BVA) in the eye with the greater ametropia. The decision to conduct a cycloplegic refraction was made immediately after finding the significant refractive error; however, the cycloplegic evaluation was postponed until completion of all clinical testing that needed to be administered without cycloplegia. A subjective refraction was not performed because of the patient's young age.

Table CS1.1
Hypothesis 1 (uncorrected refractive error): problem-specific testing results.

Entering visual acuities (Snellen single-line) at 6 m and 40 cm
  OD 20/20
  OS 20/100
Static retinoscopy and visual acuities
  OD +1.00 DS (20/20)
  OS +5.50 −2.25 × 180 (20/100)
Cycloplegic retinoscopy and visual acuities
  OD +2.50 DS (20/20)
  OS +6.75 −1.75 × 180 (20/100)

DS = diopter sphere.

Based on the refractive testing, I ruled out the first hypothesis of uncorrected refractive error as the cause of reduced visual acuity. Because optical correction of the ametropia did not improve the left eye's visual acuity (even under cycloplegia when accommodation could not interfere with plus acceptance), some other condition was causing the decreased vision. Additionally, I also was able to rule out malingering and psychogenic vision loss on the basis of finding a unilateral decrease in vision.

The second diagnostic hypothesis on my list was amblyopia (strabismic, anisometropic, or isoametropic). Isoametropic amblyopia was eliminated as a possibility as soon as I determined that the visual acuity decrease was unilateral. To make the diagnosis of anisometropic or strabismic amblyopia, both of the following conditions were necessary: a unilateral reduction in BVA in the absence of any obvious structural or pathologic anomalies of the eye, and amblyogenic anisometropia or a constant unilateral strabismus during the critical period (i.e., birth to ages 6–8).

The magnitude of uncorrected hyperopic anisometropia found (approximately 4.25 D) is associated invariably with anisometropic amblyopia,[10] and CS was only 5 years old; therefore, the second condition was met. Thus, I was rather certain at this point that anisometropic amblyopia accounted for at least part (if not all) of the left eye's vision loss. However, I needed to gather the remainder of problem-specific clinical data that would either confirm that my hypothesis alone was correct or would suggest that the decreased vision had a combined etiology. Uncorrected refractive error had been ruled out, but coincidental ocular congenital anomalies or eye disease that might contribute to the decreased vision had not been evaluated yet. In addition, it was important to investigate the possi-

Table CS1.2
Hypotheses 2 (anisometropic or strabismic amblyopia) and 5 (anterior or posterior segment pathology): problem-specific testing results.

Cycloplegic retinoscopy and aided visual acuity
OD +2.50 DS (20/20)
OS +6.75 −1.75 × 180 (20/100)
Pupil testing
PERRL, −APD
Biomicroscopy
Media: clear; no apparent pathology present OU
Dilated fundus evaluation
Media: clear OU
ONH: healthy pink; margins distinct OU
Cup-to-disc ratio: 0.2/0.2
Macula: homogeneous, clear OU
Background and periphery: no holes, tears, flat 360 degrees OU
Vessels: A/V ratio 4/5; normal crossings OU
Unilateral cover test with static retinoscopy results trial-framed
Distance: no movement
Near: no movement
Visuoscopy
OD: central and steady
OS: central and unsteady

DS = diopter sphere; PERRL = pupils equal, round, reactive to light; −APD = no afferent pupillary defect; ONH = optic nerve head; A/V = arteriovenous.

bility of strabismus because of the frequent occurrence of combined strabismic-anisometropic amblyopia.

To rule out congenital ocular anomalies and eye disease, I collected the following problem-specific clinical data:

- Pupil testing
- Biomicroscopy
- Dilated fundus evaluation

Further, to rule out the hypothesis of associated strabismic amblyopia, I collected additional problem-specific clinical data using the unilateral cover test (UCT) at distance and near, and visuoscopy.

These clinical data are presented in Table CS1.2. No strabismus was seen on the UCT (performed with the patient wearing her refractive correction as determined by static retinoscopy). The absence of movement on the UCT, however, did not rule out completely the presence of a strabismus. It was possible that a microtropia was present, where the angle of eccentric fixation is the same magnitude and in the same direction as the angle of strabismus (e.g., constant left esotropia of 2Δ with 2Δ of nasal eccentric fixation in the left eye). Because microtropic patients fixate with the same retinal area under monocular and binocular viewing conditions, no movement was seen on the UCT. Therefore, I evaluated CS's monocular fixation status by using visuoscopy. I found that CS had central fixation in each eye. My conclusion, then, was that because no strabismus was seen on the UCT and central fixation was present in each eye, strabismic amblyopia was very unlikely. (It is possible that I could have missed a $1-2\Delta$ strabismus because of less-than-perfect fixation in the amblyopic eye or measurement error.) Additionally, because no coincidental congenital anomalies or ocular disease were present, ocular pathology was eliminated from the hypotheses list. Thus, the diagnosis of anisometropic amblyopia was confirmed. The need to conduct further testing to rule out malingering was considered unnecessary.

The following additional clinical data were collected for baseline or database purposes:

- *Keratometry to obtain an objective measure of the cornea's anterior surface curvature.* This was used because this was CS's first vision examination and I wanted a baseline measure and other objective supplemental refractive information.
- *Baseline version testing.* This allowed determination of whether there were any overacting or underacting extraocular muscles.
- *Color vision (Ishihara) testing.* This test serves as a rapid screener for a color vision deficiency and as a baseline test administered at the first office visit.
- *Intraocular pressures (IOPs).* This test establishes baseline measures and determines whether the child might be at risk for glaucoma.
- *Stereopsis (Randot Stereotest) at near.* This was conducted with CS using prescription lenses, as determined by static retinoscopy, worn in a trial frame. Baseline measure was important because this was her first eye examination and the results could be used to monitor binocularity improvement during amblyopia treatment.

The clinical results from this testing are presented in Table CS1.3. Testing revealed normal color vision, normal IOPs, and full range of movement on versions. The keratometry readings correlated well with the magnitude and axis of astigmatism found on retinoscopy. (I considered keratometry baseline data instead of problem-specific data because I was confident of my retinoscopy results.) I was unable to obtain a measure of stereopsis on the Randot Stereotest, which was not surprising considering that the patient had anisometropic amblyopia of 20/100. Some doctors might collect additional baseline data such as:

Table CS1.3
Additional database testing results.

Keratometry
OD 42.00 @ 180, 42.00 @ 090
OS 42.00 @ 180, 44.00 @ 090
Versions
Full range of movement OD and OS
Color vision: Ishihara plates
Passed all plates OD and OS
Intraocular pressure (noncontact)
OD 17 mm Hg
OS 16 mm Hg
Stereopsis (Randot Stereotest) at 40 cm
No forms identified; 0/10 on circles

- Baseline accommodative amplitude and facility measures because reduced accommodative ability is found in amblyopic eyes
- Ocular motility testing to evaluate CS's monocular pursuit and saccadic ability
- Worth's four-dot test at distance and near to evaluate CS's sensorimotor fusion.

I felt that in this case there was little clinical uncertainty regarding the diagnosis. Though the previous tests would serve as useful baseline measures for amblyopia treatment, they would not provide any critical information needed for diagnostic purposes. In addition, the data would be more meaningful after the patient had worn her ametropic correction for a time. Therefore, I decided that I would collect this data at the next office visit if the patient elected to undergo amblyopia treatment.

DIAGNOSTIC SUMMARY

CS was found to have anisometropic amblyopia that caused reduced visual acuity identified at the school vision screening. The level of diagnostic certainty was very high. Anisometropic amblyopia, resulting in unilateral vision loss, usually produces little handicap and few symptoms or signs that might be noted by parents or teachers, because the patient typically has good visual acuity in the nonamblyopic eye. Parents often are surprised when anisometropic amblyopia is diagnosed because usually they have been completely unaware that there was a loss of vision in one eye. This was true in CS's case.

TREATMENT OPTIONS

The best treatment approach for CS's anisometropic amblyopia was a sequential treatment plan consisting of (1) full correction of the refractive error, (2) part-time occlusion, and (3) active vision therapy.[11] Because CS was not esotropic, I did not feel it necessary to prescribe the full hyperopic prescription associated with cycloplegia (thus, I cut the prescription by 1.00 D in each eye). I did, however, prescribe the full amount of anisometropia and astigmatism correction. A spectacle prescription of OD +1.50 DS and OS +5.75 −1.50 × 180 was ordered and dispensed that day. CS was rescheduled for follow-up and to begin amblyopia therapy 3 weeks later.

CS returned to the office 4 weeks later. Her mother reported that CS had been wearing her spectacles full-time with no complaints. Corrected visual acuity was still 20/100 in the left eye. Part-time total occlusion using a translucent occlusion foil was prescribed for the right eye. CS was to wear the occluder for all waking hours except those at school (approximately 4–6 hours per day). In addition, I prescribed active vision therapy procedures designed to improve monocular function in the amblyopic eye. These activities were primarily designed to improve accommodative efficiency and form recognition (discrimination). As acuity improved and reached the 20/50 level, antisuppression therapy was prescribed. CS attained 20/25 visual acuity in the left eye after 4.5 months of treatment.

REFERENCES

1. Blum HL, Peters HB, Bettman JW. Vision Screening for Elementary Schools: The Orinda Study. Berkeley: University of California Press, 1959.
2. Gwiazda J, Thorn F, Bauer J, et al. Emmetropization and the progression of manifest refraction in children followed from infancy to puberty. Clin Vis Sci 1993;8:337–344.
3. Francois J. Heredity in Ophthalmology. St. Louis: Mosby, 1961;239–269.
4. Scheiman M, Gallaway M, Coulter R, et al. Prevalence of vision and ocular disease conditions in a clinical pediatric population (abstract). Optom Vis Sci 1992;69(suppl):108.
5. Goss DA, Eskridge JB. Myopia. In JF Amos (ed), Diagnosis and Management in Vision Care. Boston: Butterworths, 1987;121–171.

6. Peters HB. The relationship between refractive error and visual acuity at three age levels. Am J Optom Arch Am Acad Optom 1961;38:194–198.
7. Ciuffreda KJ, Levi DM, Selenow A. Amblyopia: Basic and Clinical Aspects. Boston: Butterworths, 1991;36–37, 415–458.
8. Flom MC, Neumaier RW. Prevalence of amblyopia. Public Health Rep 1966;81:329–341.
9. Maino JH. Ocular Hysteria and Malingering. In JF Amos (ed), Diagnosis and Management in Vision Care. Boston: Butterworth, 1987;409–429.
10. Tanlamai T, Goss DA. Prevalence of monocular amblyopia among anisometropes. Am J Optom Physiol Opt 1979;56:704–715.
11. Wick B, Wingard M, Cotter S, et al. Anisometropic amblyopia: is the patient ever too old to treat? Optom Vis Sci 1992;69:866–878.

Appendix: Case Scenario 1

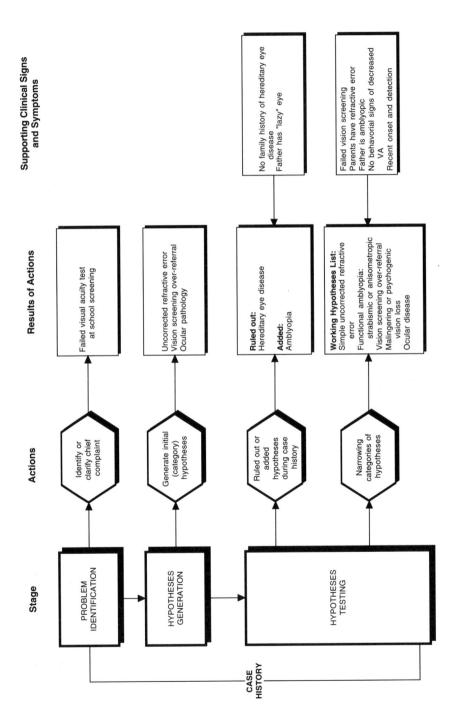

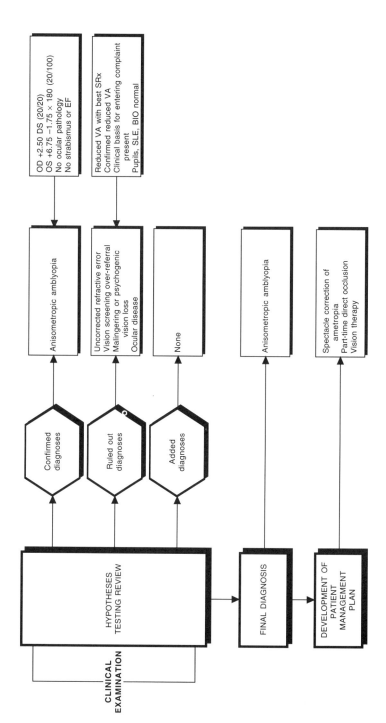

Case Scenario 1 decision-making summary. (VA = visual acuity; DS = diopter sphere; EF = eccentric fixation; SRx = spectacle Rx; SLE = slit-lamp examination; BIO = binocular indirect ophthalmoscopy.)

Case Scenario 2

Joel A. Silbert

PATIENT BACKGROUND

DG is a 32-year-old white woman who presents for her initial ocular examination in my office. Prior to this examination, she has not had her eyes examined in the past 5 years.

DOCTOR: I see it's been quite some time since you had your eyes examined. How can I be of assistance?

PATIENT: Well, my vision's pretty good. The reason I'm here is that my eyes are always irritated. They itch and burn a lot, and people are always telling me that my lids and eyes are red.

DOCTOR (*thinking*): *This woman's chief complaint revolves around an anterior segment disorder causing general physical discomfort and an abnormal appearance of the adnexa. A fairly broad range of conditions could cause these symptoms; therefore, I will need to ask more questions about other possible signs and symptoms beyond those she offered, in addition to questions regarding time of day and use of topical or systemic medications. As I'm questioning her, I'm also observing her eyes, lids, and lashes, which are indeed red and somewhat scaly and edematous, and making a general observation of her skin and scalp (both of which are clear, without dandruff or unusual dermatologic presentation).*

DOCTOR: Have you had problems with mattering on your lashes or difficulty in opening your eyes in the morning?

PATIENT: I have no problem opening my eyes when I wake up, but I've always noticed these crusty scales on my lashes. I try to remove them, but they don't brush off. Sometimes, I can get them off, but then my lashes come out with them, which is awful. The crusting has been worse than usual lately.

DOCTOR: How do your eyes feel in the morning, compared to other times of the day?

PATIENT: Oh, they bother me a lot in the morning. The burning and itching are much more noticeable when I wake up and for a couple of hours afterward but not so bad during the rest of the day.

DOCTOR: Because you came in wearing glasses, is it safe to assume that you're not a contact lens wearer? Also, are you taking any med-

ications, either prescription or over-the-counter, or putting anything in your eyes?

PATIENT: You're right . . . I don't wear contacts. I tried them several
times in the past but could never tolerate them, even the soft
kind. And the redness in my eyes always got worse after wearing
them. I'm not taking any medicines, except for some of those eye
drops that "get the red out." They really haven't helped at all.

DOCTOR: Have you had any long-standing problems with your skin or
scalp, such as with dandruff or dry skin? Also, have there been
any problems in the past with styes or small lumps in your lids?

PATIENT: I haven't had any dandruff, but all through my childhood I can
remember getting styes periodically. They stopped when I was in
my 20s. There were a couple of occasions when I would get a small
lump in my upper lid after a particularly bad stye, but it would gradually decrease in size once the stye was treated by my doctor.

DOCTOR (*thinking*): *It's pretty evident that DG has an underlying chronic lid
condition that's making her lids red, with scaling and associated symptoms. However, burning and itching are common symptoms that do not
point specifically to a diagnosis. Besides the obvious lid inflammation, the
cornea and conjunctiva also could also involved, and dry eyes are certainly
also associated with these symptoms. Though I can rule out contact lens
solution effects, DG has admitted to using topical vasoconstrictors that
could be causing a rebound injection or medicamentosa effect. Still, this
wouldn't really account for the lid scaling or morning symptoms. A viral
or bacterial corneal infection is pretty unlikely, in the absence of watery
or mucopurulent discharge, and she has no complaints of pain, photophobia, or visual decrement. Though she reports some itching, it seems to
be associated with the morning burning, and she reports no stringy mucus
discharge, thereby reducing the likelihood of an allergic etiology.*

DIAGNOSTIC HYPOTHESES

DG's initial history and brief presentation suggest some form of blepharitis or blepharoconjunctivitis. However, both of these related conditions can be caused by many things and have numerous associations
at which I will need to look to make not only a definitive diagnosis but
also to direct my management plan. Blepharitis also could be a secondary finding to a broader underlying problem, so I will have to consider this in my differential hypotheses.

On the basis of the case history, the following initial hypothesis list
is possible.

1.   *Marginal staphylococcal blepharitis.* This is a very common condition, and the underlying lid hyperemia, scaling at the base of the lashes, and complaints of burning and itching are entirely consistent with this etiology. The complaints of morning symptoms are strongly suggestive, because bacterial exotoxins given off by the staphylococcal bacteria tend to concentrate in the lower cul-de-sac during sleep hours.[1] These would be diluted once the eye has opened and blinking ensues, a condition consistent with the patient's reports of feeling better later in the day. If staphylococcal blepharitis is the cause, generally it is quite chronic and would be expected to present with other signs (often affecting the inferior cornea). Signs of chronicity, such as loss of lashes and thickened or irregular lid margins, and scales tightly adherent to the lashes (sometimes leading to a small bleeding ulcer when removed) point strongly to marginal staphylococcal blepharitis. In addition, signs of staphylococcal toxin hypersensitivity including micropannus, inferior corneal staining and infiltrates, phlyctenulosis, or marginal keratitis may be found.[2]

2.   *Dry eye.* Chronic hyperemia of the conjunctiva with complaints of burning, dryness, low-grade itching, and foreign-body sensation in a middle-aged woman could be suspected as a possible etiology here. Keratoconjunctivitis sicca (KCS) can vary widely in its symptoms and presentations and could be an underlying condition in DG's case, with blepharitis occurring secondarily. However, dry-eye symptoms often become worse as the day wears on, whereas DG's symptoms are most pronounced in the morning. Dry eye itself does not explain the crusting at the base of her lashes.

3.   *Seborrheic blepharitis.* Though this form of marginal blepharitis also can produce crusting and symptoms similar to DG's, the lid margins are less inflamed than in staphylococcal blepharitis. The lids would be expected to have a greasy or waxy appearance, with lashes clinging together. The crusts (or scurf) are softer, are not concentrated around the base of the lashes, and do not leave an ulcer when removed. However, patients can develop secondary meibomianitis, leading to symptoms of burning and foreign-body sensation, also worse in the morning.

4.   *Demodicosis.* Often considered a great mimic of staphylococcal blepharitis, *Demodex folliculorum*, a mite infestation of the lash follicles producing tubular collarettes along the base of the lashes, could be the source of DG's problem. The morning symptoms of burning and itching would be more exacerbated and intense with demodicosis than with staphylococcal blepharitis.

5.   *Acne rosacea, with secondary staphylococcal blepharitis and dry eye.* Here, an underlying dermatologic disorder is present, leading to vari-

able episodes of symptoms consistent with those presented by DG. Rosacea often is associated with dry eye and blepharitis and can lead to pronounced conjunctival hyperemia, keratitis, and corneal pannus.[3] Because rosacea affects patients older than 30 (especially those of Celtic descent) and is exacerbated with exposure to temperature extremes and alcohol,[4] these disorders will have to be explored in DG's case and considered in our hypotheses.

6. *Lice infestation.* Although we may not want to think about it, pediculosis (or infestation of the lashes with lice) is another diagnostic possibility to be ruled out when a patient presents with blepharitis, conjunctivitis, itching, and mattering on the lashes. *Phthiriasis palpebrum*, or pubic lice infestation of the cilia, is an increasing public health problem in certain parts of the country, frequently presenting as blepharitis and conjunctivitis, with intense itching and the presence of crablike lice and egg nits in the lashes. Pubic lice can be considered one of the sexually transmitted diseases and are most often seen among male homosexuals with multiple partners.[5] Given these parameters, it can be seen that this condition is the least likely to affect DG and can be ruled out easily by gross observation and examination of the lashes.

DIAGNOSTIC TESTING

In making a diagnosis, the clinician should always consider the most likely etiology on the basis of the history and age of the patient and presenting signs. Clinical data and observations are documented or ruled out to help confirm or deny the diagnostic associations. Although the clinician may have a strong clinical suspicion or intuition regarding one or two of the most likely diagnostic hypotheses, it is nevertheless important to consider them all and, by clinical observation and examination, to rule out quickly those of least likelihood. With the subtleties in varieties and etiologies of blepharitis, this rule-out technique is both rapid and valuable in preventing the clinician from making a hasty diagnosis and thereby initiating a management regimen that may be ineffective.

To confirm the lack of disturbance of the condition to the patient's vision and to establish medicolegally the visual capability of the patient presenting for examination, I initially measured DG's visual acuity, pupillary reflexes, and field of vision, through the following quick steps:

- Habitual visual acuities, distance and near
- Pinhole acuities or refraction to best visual acuity, if reduced
- Pupillary reflexes, ruling out an afferent defect
- Confrontation fields

Table CS2.1
Diagnostic database testing results.

Habitual visual acuities at far and near
   20/20 OD, OS at 6 m; 20/20 OD, OS at 40 cm
Pupil reflexes: PERRLA, –APD
Field of vision: confrontation fields full OD, OS

PERRLA = pupils equal, round, reactive to light and accommodation; –APD = no
afferent pupillary defect.

Table CS2.2
Problem-specific testing (via observation and biomicroscopy) for all hypotheses.

Lids and lashes
   Active blepharitis, scaling flat and irregular, debris scattered on various
      portions of the lash and lid margins OU
   Lid hyperemia and slight lid swelling OU
   Madarosis OU
   Crusty brittle exudate, not in tubular sleeves OU
   Leathery lid margins OU
   Nits and lice absent OU
   Normal meibomian gland appearance OU
Conjunctiva: generalized injection OU
Cornea
   Inferior corneal punctate staining
   Active vascularization observed in inferior cornea (micropannus)
Anterior chamber: grade 4 OU, clear and quiet OU, no cells or flare OU
Iris: brown and clear OU
Lens: clear OU
Vitreous: clear OU

    The clinical data for patient DG are presented in Table CS2.1, confirming good visual acuity in each eye, absence of afferent pupillary defects, and full field of vision. These rapid assessments allowed me subsequently to focus on the correlation between symptomatology and anterior segment findings.

    As with any anterior segment workup involving complaints of discomfort or the potential for infection, inflammation, or trauma, my initial biomicroscopic scan looked at the cornea to rule out rapidly any abrasion, foreign bodies, infiltrates, vascularization, and endothelial disturbance to provide a qualitative assessment of the bulbar and palpebral conjunctivae and anterior chamber (Table CS2.2). The absence of folliculosis and papillae helped narrow the field of clinical possibilities by lessening the likelihood of a viral or allergic etiology. This initial scan with low magnification was able to provide an enormous amount of information within seconds. In DG's case, the scan proved negative except for significant changes in the inferior cornea, which further heightens the clinical suspicion for the primary diagnostic hypothesis of marginal staphylococcal blepharitis.

In DG's case, we might have had a primary pathologic condition or an underlying problem on which is superimposed a secondary condition that accounted for the patient's distress. As previously noted, in assessing a patient with presenting signs and symptoms of obvious blepharitis of undetermined origin, it often is helpful first to rule out the least likely conditions in our hypothesis list. Basic gross inspection and observation of the patient for signs of underlying dermatologic conditions is the most obvious example and can rule out or help to define whether the patient has rosacea or lice. I ruled out lice by examination of the patient's lashes and brows, where it was evident immediately that the scaling on the lashes was simply scales and crusts and not nits. Similarly, DG neither presented with papules or pustular lesions of the face nor demonstrated a hyperemic and telangiectatic skin condition suggestive of acne rosacea. The woman was not of Celtic origin and denied experiencing changes in skin appearance or in symptoms when experiencing temperature extremes, drinking hot beverages, or when drinking alcohol.

Ruling out demodicosis would not be quite so simple, however. Again, a careful examination with biomicroscope is imperative in establishing the nature and characteristics of the exudate. In *Demodex* infestations, the organisms are not readily visible to the examiner as they are miniscule and transparent and live in the lash follicles (*D. folliculorum*) or in the sebaceous and meibomian glands (*D. brevis*).[6] Inspection of the exudate, however, can be very revealing, as *Demodex* produces collarettes that are tubular, creating a sleeve or debris collar of approximately 0.5 mm upward from the base of the lashes. Chronic irritation can lead to edematous, boggy lids with madarosis or loss of lashes, although this is not pathognomonic for *Demodex* (madarosis also occurs with other forms of chronic blepharitis). Where suspicion for *Demodex* is high, a definitive diagnosis can be made by epilating a few lashes and searching for the eight-legged, transparent parasite attached to a lash follicle under the oil-immersion microscope.[7] DG's lashes did not reveal any tubular collarettes. The scaling and crusting on her lashes was flatter and more irregular, with some adherent debris scattered on various portions of the lash and lid margins.

To assist in discovering whether DG had an underlying dry eye (or KCS), I included in my biomicroscopic examination an evaluation

Table CS2.3
Hypothesis 2 (dry eye): problem-specific testing results.

Cornea
Inferior corneal punctate staining
Negative rose bengal staining
Positive fluorescein staining: inferior corneal punctate staining
Tear film
Tear meniscus: full and thick
Schirmer I: >15 mm wetting in 5 mins

of the patient's cornea, conjunctiva, and tear film, with the assistance of sodium fluorescein and rose bengal (Table CS2.3). Staining with both these vital dyes would be expected in the presence of KCS. Staining patterns in KCS tend to be across the middle third of the cornea, due to exposure and breakup of the tear film from bacterial lipase activity.[8] Rose bengal staining of desiccated and devitalized cells may be present in both the corneal and bulbar conjunctival epithelium. The results of these clinical observations (seen in Table CS2.3) show that DG had staining only in the inferior corneal regions, inconsistent with a dry-eye diagnosis. The tear film meniscus was assessed and found to be normal (it will be very thin or absent in aqueous-deficient dry eye, and there will be more solid matter in an aqueous-deficient tear film). Additionally, tear breakup time (TBUT) and Schirmer testing are performed easily. The Schirmer I test (for aqueous tear production) resulted in normal age-related values for DG (>15 mm in 5 minutes). This test can be helpful in identifying mild to moderate KCS (5–10 mm wetting) and severe KCS (<5 mm wetting). The Schirmer II modification also can be accomplished easily, with addition of a topical anesthetic. The TBUT is a more qualitative test of the ability of the tear film to stay as a complete, unbroken film over the anterior corneal surface. A TBUT of less than 10 seconds after instillation of fluorescein implies an abnormal tear film, consistent with mucin deficiency.[9] However, the test is poorly reproducible, and the results are unreliable whenever there is any compromise to the cornea, as there was in DG's case, with inferior punctate staining present. Thus, the TBUT was not performed in this particular workup.

This leaves the two varieties of uncomplicated blepharitis, staphylococcal or seborrheic, as the most likely etiologies for DG's symptoms. Qualitative differences in the appearance of the lash exudate can be helpful in differentiating staphylococcal from seborrheic forms of ble-

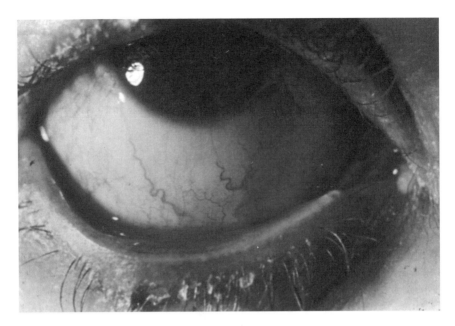

Figure CS2.1 Marginal chronic staphylococcal blepharitis. Note loose, brittle crusts and scales on the lashes. (Reprinted with permission from GE White. Dermatologic Complications. In JA Silbert [ed], Anterior Segment Complications of Contact Lens Wear. New York: Churchill Livingstone, 1994.)

pharitis. Examination of the meibomian glands and looking for signs of foamy tears and retained meibomian secretions are important in making a definitive diagnosis of seborrheic blepharitis.[10] As most patients with seborrheic blepharitis also demonstrate forms of seborrheic dermatitis, signs of scalp dandruff or seborrhea of the brows or nasolabial folds should be investigated. My examination of DG's lids and lashes showed that there was no scurf or greasy appearance on the lashes. Also, there was no foam in the tears, nor was there evidence of meibomianitis or clogged meibomian glands. DG denied having dandruff of the scalp, and I could observe no evidence of seborrhea of the brows, glabellar, or malar areas. Seborrheic blepharitis is also more common in patients over 50, whereas DG was in her early 30s.

On the other hand, DG's lashes did manifest a good deal of scaling and adherent crusting, although an absence of tubular sleeves (Figures CS2.1 and CS2.2). Her morning symptoms were correlated highly, however, with the observation of inferior superficial punctate staining of the cornea, a few tiny sterile infiltrates in the same region, and more pronounced micropannus, all signs of staphylococcal exotoxin hypersensitivity. Her lids

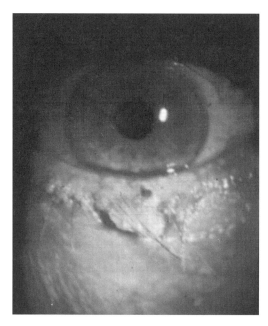

Figure CS2.2 Chronic staphylococcal blepharitis, with tightly adherent exudative scaling. Removal may cause lash loss. (Reprinted with permission from GE White. Dermatologic Complications. In JA Silbert [ed], Anterior Segment Complications of Contact Lens Wear. New York: Churchill Livingstone, 1994.)

were hyperemic and slightly swollen, the lids appeared somewhat leathery, and the lower lids showed evidence of a few missing lashes. There were no signs of styes or chalazia at the time of examination. Her history of previous styes throughout childhood and her inability to tolerate contact lenses shed some interesting light on the chronicity of the condition and point to chronic staphylococcal blepharitis as my definitive diagnosis.

The balance of the ocular examination was unremarkable, with DG demonstrating no significant refractive error or binocular anomalies, intraocular pressures of 15 mm Hg by Goldmann applanation tonometry, and a dilated ophthalmoscopic examination revealed no abnormalities in either eye (Table CS2.4).

DIAGNOSTIC SUMMARY

DG was found to have chronic staphylococcal blepharitis. There was a high correlation found between presenting symptoms and signs of chronic lid erythema, conjunctival hyperemia, and lash exudate. Of great importance in the diagnosis were the associated corneal findings of staphylococcal exotoxin hypersensitivity, including inferior corneal staining, marginal infiltrates, and micropannus (vasculariza-

Table CS2.4
Additional database testing results.

Cover test
Unilateral: no movement far and near
Alternate: orthophoria at 6 m, 3Δ exophoria at 40 cm
Stereopsis: 20 secs of arc Randot Stereotest
Subjective refraction: +0.25 DS OD, OS
Dilated fundus examination
Cup-to-disc ratio: 0.3/0.3
ONH margins: distinct OU
A/V ratio: 2/3 OU
Macula: positive foveal reflex OU, clear OU
Periphery: no holes, tears, and flat 360 degree OU
Goldmann tonometry: 15 mm Hg OD, OS

ONH = optic nerve head; A/V = arteriovenous.

tion). The compromised cornea and the presence of staphylococcal toxins give rise to the feeling of discomfort, gritty foreign-body sensation, burning, and itching, all made worse in the morning by the concentration of toxins in the cul-de-sac during the sleep hours.[11] It is this concentration of toxins that also accounts for the particular location of the corneal signs. Dilution of toxins with the open eye, with blinking and lid wiping, account for the improvement in symptoms as the day wears on (opposite to the dry-eye situation). Though dry eye often is accompanied by blepharitis, there was no evidence in this case of an underlying KCS or signs of seborrhea, rosacea, or parasitic involvement.

TREATMENT OPTIONS

I prescribed the following treatment regimen for DG's chronic staphylococcal blepharitis:

1. *Patient education.* Patients with staphylococcal blepharitis need to be educated regarding the need for ongoing self-treatment. The chronicity of the condition is typically lifelong, with waxing and waning of signs and symptoms.

2. *Warm compresses.* These were prescribed for 5–10 minutes, 2–4 times daily. The compresses loosen crusty, scaly debris and exudate from the lashes and loosen meibomian secretions.

3.   *Lid hygiene.* I recommended daily lid scrubs, using either baby shampoo (diluted 50% with warm water) or commercially available lid cleansing kits (containing gauze pads and a bottle of lid cleanser solution, or individually wrapped premoistened pads). The cleansing and debridement reduce the bacterial and toxin load on the lids and the crusty debris from the lids and lashes. DG was advised to use the scrubs at least once daily, after warm compresses had been applied, and to continue them for 1–2 weeks or until the lid condition had improved greatly. Then, the frequency of the scrubs could be reduced to twice weekly or to whatever level able to maintain lid control.

4.   *Topical antibiotic-steroids.* When patients have an active case of uncomplicated staphylococcal blepharitis, I prescribe a topical antibiotic ointment to be rubbed liberally into the lid surface after lid hygiene. Bacitracin is the drug of choice, as it has excellent activity against staphylococci. Polysporin ophthalmic ointment also is fairly effective, as it contains both bacitracin and polymyxin B. For those patients sensitive to either of these antibiotics, erythromycin ointment is a good substitute. Aminoglycoside ointments are best reserved for more acute conditions, such as acute blepharoconjunctivitis or a concern for corneal infection.[3]

In DG's case, I decided to use a steroid-antibiotic ointment instead of the antibiotic ointment alone, because DG was presenting with frank signs of staphylococcal exotoxin hypersensitivity. As hypersensitivity is an inflammatory response to the presence of the toxins and is not a result of the bacteria per se, these signs will respond favorably to the judicious use of topical steroids. However, they are best used in combination with an antibiotic for short-term treatment and should be monitored closely. As the signs of inferior corneal staining, infiltration, and micropannus lessen, the steroid-antibiotic should be tapered, followed by a switch to the antibiotic ointment alone and, ultimately, to simple maintenance with lid hygiene.

REFERENCES

1. Silbert JA. Microbial Infection in Contact Lens Patients. In MG Harris (ed), Contact Lenses and Ocular Disease. (Problems in Optometry vol. 2, no. 4) Philadelphia: Lippincott, 1990;571–583.
2. Smolin G, Okumoto M. Staphylococcal blepharitis. Arch Ophthalmol 1977; 95:812–816.
3. Browning DJ, Proia AD. Ocular rosacea. Surv Ophthalmol 1986;31:145–158.
4. Wilkin JK. Oral thermal-induced flushing in erythematotelangiectatic rosacea. J Invest Dermatol 1981;76:15–18.
5. Wroblewski JJ. Spread the word on pediculosis. Drug Topics 1983;127:54–58.

6. Heacock CE. Clinical manifestations of demodicosis. J Am Optom Assoc 1986;57:914–919.
7. Fulk GW, Clifford C. A case report of demodicosis. J Am Optom Assoc 1990;61:637–639.
8. Snyder C. Anomalies of the Tears and the Preocular Tear Film. In JA Silbert (ed), Anterior Segment Complications of Contact Lens Wear. New York: Churchill Livingstone, 1994;1–11.
9. Vanley GT, Leopold IR, Gregg TH. Interpretation of tear film breakup. Arch Ophthalmol 1977;95:445–448.
10. White GE. Dermatologic Complications. In JA Silbert (ed), Anterior Segment Complications of Contact Lens Wear. New York: Churchill Livingstone, 1994;193–201.
11. Silbert JA. Contact lens-induced microbial infections. Pract Optom 1994;5:99–104, 128.

Appendix: Case Scenario 2

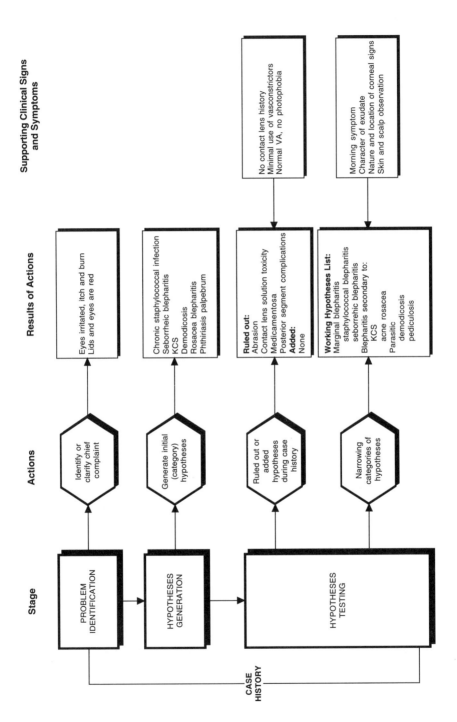

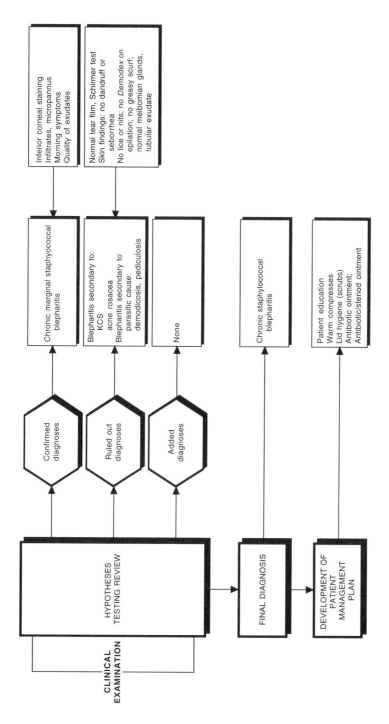

Case Scenario 2 decision-making summary. (KCS = keratoconjunctivitis sicca; VA = visual acuity.)

Case Scenario 3

Dennis W. Siemsen

PATIENT BACKGROUND

WA is a 78-year-old white man, a retired mechanic. He is accompanied to the examination by his wife.

DOCTOR: What brings you into the office for an eye examination today?

PATIENT: I think I need a new pair of glasses. I can't seem to get these adjusted right, and I'm having some problems seeing when I drive. The street signs are so blurry that I have to get right up on top of them to see them.

WIFE: He makes me so nervous when he drives. It's like he can't see anything anymore.

DOCTOR *(thinking)*: *With a patient this age, there are a variety of problems that can occur. Cataracts come immediately to mind, but there also may be macular changes, vitreal liquefaction, corneal clouding, or simply, a change in the refraction. If his complaints are of a recent onset, I would lean toward a retinal etiology. If it's a more gradual onset, a refractive or lens opacity would be a more likely cause. Other areas to explore are whether the complaint of blurred vision is bilateral in nature or only present when he's driving, or whether other activities are affected.*

DOCTOR: How long have you noticed this problem? Did this come on all of a sudden, or has this been a gradual change?

PATIENT: I used to be able to see everything clearly at a distance, even without my glasses. Now it's blurry.

WIFE: I think this has been a slow change. I've noticed it for several months now. He didn't seem to notice at first, but now he agrees that he can't see as well as I do.

DOCTOR *(thinking)*: *This doesn't sound like an acute onset of, say, a macular hole or wet maculopathy. I still can't rule out another retinal component, such as dry maculopathy or retinal pigment epithelium changes, however.*

DOCTOR: Are both eyes about the same now? Has the vision always been about the same in each eye?

PATIENT: The right eye is a little better now than the left; in the past, they always were about the same, though.

DOCTOR *(thinking)*: *With the information of a gradual onset, I can now rule out more severe causes, such as a retinal vascular occlusion. Now I'm thinking that this is almost certainly cataract or uncorrected refractive error, with some potential for retinal involvement.*

DOCTOR: How is your vision at other times? Do you have any problems in reading?

PATIENT: I notice now that I have to have more light than I used to, to be able to read.

DOCTOR: What kind of reading do you do?

PATIENT: I read the newspaper, and I do crossword puzzles.

DOCTOR: What kind of lamp do you use?

PATIENT: Oh, just a regular table lamp.

DOCTOR *(thinking)*: *His need for extra light suggests an etiology that decreases the amount of light getting to the retina. That strongly points toward a cataract. If this were solely a refractive problem, the light would be less of a problem, and the positioning of the reading material would be more critical.*

DOCTOR: Is it more difficult for you to see at night? Do you drive at night?

PATIENT: No, I don't drive at night, I just can't see as well as during the day.

WIFE: I do the driving at night. He drives during the day.

DOCTOR *(thinking)*: *This supports my suspicion of the cataract. Of course, a good refraction may improve his visual function, and a thorough fundus examination is in order to rule out other disease, but the cataract seems like the most logical primary cause for the vision loss.*

DOCTOR: How is your general health?

PATIENT: Well, I have high blood pressure, and I take two pills a day.

WIFE: He takes one Aldoril in the morning and one again at night.

DOCTOR: Have you had any other serious medical problems?

PATIENT: Well, I had brain surgery 3 years ago.

DOCTOR: Why did you have brain surgery?

PATIENT: I had a brain aneurysm.

DOCTOR *(thinking)*: *WOW! This puts an entirely different slant on the situation. He could have a variety of visual-field problems, including a scotoma, a peripheral constriction, or a generalized field depression secondary to optic nerve atrophy. There could also be another aneurysm that's compressing any of a number of points on the visual pathway.*

DOCTOR: Was the surgery successful?

WIFE: Yes, the surgery was successful. The aneurysm was clamped off, but he wasn't himself for almost 3 months after the surgery. And he had a droopy eyelid on the side they did the surgery for about 6 weeks.

DOCTOR *(thinking)*: *This suggests that there was some third-nerve involvement that has resolved. I'll have to do a cranial nerve assessment to rule out any residual damage from the surgery.*

Doctor: Does your family have any history of cataracts, glaucoma, or blindness? Any other serious family medical problems?

Patient: My family all wore glasses, but no one ever had cataracts or glaucoma. My sister died from a cerebral hemorrhage.

Doctor *(thinking)*: *A vascular etiology can't be overlooked here. With a strong personal and family history, I have to be careful. I wonder whether he has had any transient ischemic attacks.*

Doctor: Have you had any situations where you completely lost your vision but had it come back later? Have you had any dark spots that came and went?

Patient: No, I haven't had anything like that.

Doctor *(thinking)*: *Well! We're part-way home if he hasn't had any loss of vision.*

Doctor: Have you had any double vision before or after the surgery?

Patient: No, never had it before. I don't remember much right after surgery, but I don't think so. I haven't seen double since the surgery.

Doctor *(thinking)*: *He's still a candidate for a stroke, with his history of hypertension. I wonder whether . . .*

Doctor: Since your surgery, have you had any headaches or weakness in your arms or legs?

Patient: The only headache I ever had in my life was the day I went to the doctor and they found the aneurysm. Everything's been fine since.

DIAGNOSTIC HYPOTHESES

On the basis of the history, the initial hypothesis list includes several possibilities.

1. *Cataracts.* In this age group, almost everyone will have some lens opacity. The symptoms he has given also point to cataracts. He says that he needs more light to read and that his night driving is getting worse.

2. *Shift in refractive error.* This could give similar symptoms, as extra light can help overcome some minor refractive errors. The change in refraction, if there is one, could be secondary to any lens changes as well, so there could be a combination etiology.

3. *Early maculopathy.* Once again, in the early stages, loss of contrast sensitivity and minor decrease in visual acuity are the hallmarks of the disease.

4. *Visual-field loss secondary to trauma from brain surgery or new vascular etiology.* Over and above the previous hypotheses, there could be some residual vision loss from vascular or surgical causes.

Table CS3.1
Hypotheses 1 (cataract) and 2 (uncorrected refractive error): problem-specific testing results.

Unaided, habitual, and pinhole acuities
   VA sc: 20/200 OD; 20/200 OS; 20/200 OU
   VA cc: 20/40 OD; 20/30 OS; 20/30⁺ OU
   Pinhole: no improvement
   VA cc at near: 20/30 OD; 20/25 OS at 30 cm
   Habitual Rx:
      OD +3.00 −1.25 × 015
      OS +3.25 −1.25 × 090
      +2.50 add OU
Static retinoscopy
   Dull reflex OU
   OD +3.00 −1.25 × 180 (20/30)
   OS +3.25 −1.00 × 090 (20/30)
Subjective refraction to best visual acuity
   OD +2.75 −1.25 × 175 (20/25)
   OS +3.00 −1.00 × 095 (20/25⁺)
   +2.50 Add OU
   Pinhole: no improvement

VA = visual acuity; sc = without correction; cc = with correction.

DIAGNOSTIC TESTING

Even though this patient has a significant medical history possibly contributing to his complaint, he reports that the condition is stable and is being followed by his family physician and his neurologist. This would tend to downplay any acute neurologic situation that has to take precedence at this time. In other words, an experienced clinician would continue with a normal optometric evaluation and would reserve any sophisticated medical or neurologic workups for later. A novice clinician might, on the other hand, jump at the medical history and fail to rule out the simpler causes of the apparent visual loss. Because of this, I'll rule out the simpler of the potential causes with tests that are already part of the routine data gathering.

To test hypotheses 1 (cataracts) and 2 (uncorrected refractive error), the diagnostic testing begins with the refractive sequence, which includes:

- Unaided, habitual, and pinhole visual acuities at distance and near
- Static retinoscopy
- Subjective refraction to obtain best visual acuity

The clinical data (Table CS3.1) do indicate some impairment of the visual acuity and a slight subjective improvement with the new refrac-

Table CS3.2
Hypotheses 1 (cataract) and 3 (early maculopathy):
problem-specific testing results.

Brightness acuity test, medium setting:
VA OD 20/40; OS 20/50
Amsler's grid test (habitual near Rx, held at 13 in.): lines straight and complete, all four corners visible
Vistech 6500 contrast sensitivity testing (see also Figure CS3.1)
Normal range contrast sensitivity function with spatial frequencies of 0.5 and 1 cycles/degree
Low-contrast sensitivity function in frequencies of 2, 4, 6 cycles/degree

VA = visual acuity.

tion. These findings alone do not explain the patient's complaints, as he reports better vision in the daytime than at night. If the problem were due solely to refractive error, he would have problems at either time of day. Nor do the findings immediately support or rule out the other hypotheses; yet, having this information is invaluable. Why? As clinicians gain experience, one of the subjective evaluations they must make is the matching of visual acuity and visual function to the physical findings. In this case, a careful refraction followed by multiple pinhole visual acuities has ruled out simple refractive error. It also has allowed me to concentrate on other, potentially more serious conditions. So, while gathering database information, I am also applying the data to my hypotheses.

The next set of tests applies further to hypothesis 1 (cataracts) and addresses the patient's complaint of poor vision for night driving. The tests also begin to address hypothesis 3 (maculopathy). Usually, 20/25 Snellen acuity would be adequate for most visual tasks, so other tests must be used to simulate the glare and reduced contrast experienced at night. In addition, a simple test for metamorphopsia secondary to macular changes is indicated. The tests performed at this point are:

- Brightness Acuity Test
- Amsler's grid test
- Contrast sensitivity testing

The data are found in Table CS3.2, and the contrast sensitivity function (CSF) recording chart is shown in Figure CS3.1. Consistent with the patient's complaint, the acuity is reduced under glare conditions, and there is a drop-off in high-frequency CSF.[1, 2] Although the CSF reduction could be caused by either an early maculopathy or cataracts, the reduction in acuity secondary to glare is more a hallmark of cataract formation.[3, 4] The Amsler's grid test results were unremarkable.[5]

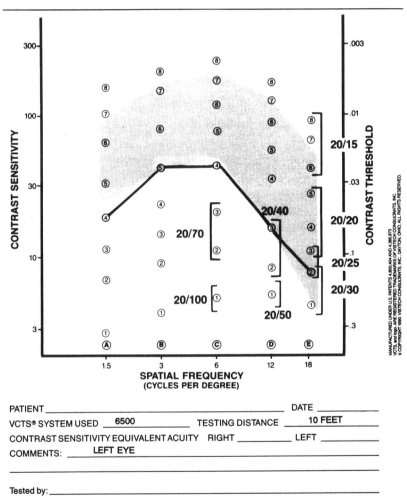

Figure CS3.1 Contrast sensitivity function (CSF), Vistech 6500 (Vistech Consultants, Dayton, OH). A. Left eye. Patient's CSF is on the bottom of the normal scale for almost all spatial frequencies and falls below normal for two spatial frequencies.

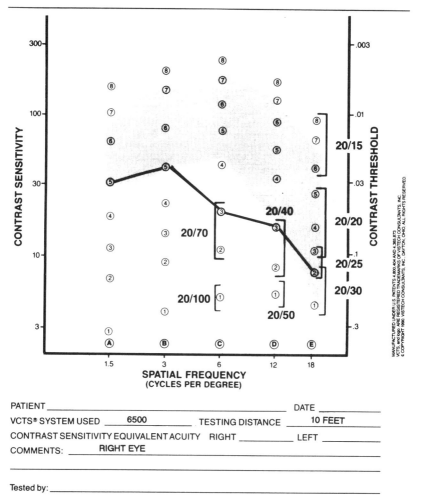

VISTECH CONSULTANTS, INC.

Contrast Sensitivity

EVALUATION FORM

PATIENT _____ DATE _____

VCTS® SYSTEM USED _____6500_____ TESTING DISTANCE ____10 FEET____

CONTRAST SENSITIVITY EQUIVALENT ACUITY   RIGHT _____ LEFT _____

COMMENTS: _____RIGHT EYE_____

Tested by: _____

The normal range of contrast sensitivity is shown in the gray area. The normal range is only relevant if proper lighting is used as described in the Instruction Manual. It is provided to help AID in the diagnosis of optical, neurological, or pathological disorders and should not be used as a sole criterion for diagnosis and treatment. In some cases, depressed contrast sensitivity is due strictly to normal variation and not to an optical, neurological, or pathological problem. For this reason, contrast sensitivity should be used in conjunction with other diagnostic techniques.

Figure CS3.1 B. Right eye. Patient's CSF for the right eye also is on the bottom of the normal scale for almost all spatial frequencies and falls below the norm in one spatial frequency.

Table CS3.3
Hypothesis 4 (visual-field loss secondary to brain surgery):
problem-specific testing results.

Pupils: PERRL, –APD
Oculomotor: full motion in all positions of gaze; no apparent ptosis
Strabismus: no apparent tropia on unilateral cover test at far or near
Carotid auscultation: no bruits detected

PERRL = pupils equal, round, reactive to light; –APD = no afferent pupillary defect.

Next, evaluation of the extraocular muscles, fusion, and pupil response was performed in response to hypothesis 4 (secondary visual-field loss). If positive, these tests might point to other neuro-ocular problems secondary to either vascular compromise or surgical intervention. Some practitioners would do these before the refraction, but because the pupil testing requires a bright source to detect slight pupil function loss (as in a binocular indirect ophthalmoscope), the possibility of slow glare recovery from the source might interfere with our refraction. Hence, these tests have been deferred until now; their findings appear in Table CS3.3. There appears to be no damage to the cranial nerves or the areas of the brain that control pupils, ocular motility, or fusion.[6, 7] This finding argues against permanent effects from trauma secondary to the brain surgery. Carotid auscultation was performed to rule out carotid artery stenosis, but no bruits were detected.[8]

At this point, other anterior-segment eye health procedures (gross external examination, external slit-lamp examination, anterior chamber evaluation, and applanation tonometry) are added to complete the patient's baseline database (Table CS3.4). The findings are consistent with a normal 78-year-old man. There is nothing to contraindicate pupil dilation, so this is the next phase of the evaluation. The dilation will provide database information and data needed for hypotheses 1 and 3.

Pupils were dilated to 6 mm to allow easy evaluation of the lens. The lenses showed 2+ brunescent nuclear changes OU. Although there were some cortical spokes present, they were well out of the optical axis of the eye. The lens opacities would account for the fact that the acuity is good for most situations but that, in compromised lighting conditions, the amount of light reaching the retina through the cloudy lens is reduced more so than in a normal patient and thus the level of visual functioning is reduced as well.

Evaluation of the posterior pole (included in Table CS3.4) revealed no unusual findings. Though the macula did not demonstrate a bright foveal reflex, good visualization of the macula was accomplished with

Table CS3.4
Hypotheses 1 (cataract) and 3 (early maculopathy):
problem-specific testing results.

External biomicroscopy (database information)
    Lids: clear OU
    Cornea: 1+ arcus OU
    Conjunctiva: 1+ injection OU
    Anterior chamber: clear OU
    Angles: 3+ OU
Dilated fundus examination (database and problem-specific information)
    Lens: 2+ brunescent nuclear cataracts OU
    Vitreous: intact, clear OU
    ONH: rim margins clear OU, normal central pallor, 0.4/0.4 cup-to-disc
      ratio OU
    Macula: dull reflex, some retinal pigment epithelium dropout OU
    Vessels: narrowed arterioles, no plaques evident OU
    Periphery: no apparent breaks, tears, or holes, flat 360 degrees OU

ONH = optic nerve head.

a 78 D lens. There was some clumping of the retinal pigment epithelium; otherwise the macula looked healthy.[9] This finding ruled out hypothesis 3 (early maculopathy). My observation of the optic nerve head showed that some normal central cup pallor existed, but its appearance did not suggest optic neuropathy.[9] On the whole, the posterior pole looked capable of 20/25 visual acuities.

Although the testing until now pointed strongly toward the cataracts as the primary cause for the decrease in visual function, one last test needed to be carried out. A threshold visual-field test should tell us whether there is any post–brain surgery trauma altering the patient's visual field. The results show no scotomas or hemianopic visual-field loss. This and other neuro-ocular testing ruled out hypothesis 4 (secondary visual-field loss). The general depression in sensitivity is consistent with a 78-year-old with nuclear cataracts.[10]

DIAGNOSTIC SUMMARY

My original suspicion of cataracts confirmed the apparent cause of the patient's functional complaints. The routine eye examination for elderly patients (refraction, dilated fundus examination, CSF testing) confirmed my hypothesis. This information was necessary before I began to rule out more serious causes for the patient's complaint.

There was some subjective change in the patient's refractive error. This change could be a contributing factor in his decreased visual performance and could be associated with the developing cataracts.

I ruled out maculopathy through Amsler's grid test and physical examination. This is a potential cause of concern for the future, but not at this point.

The visual-field, pupil, and oculomotor tests showed no lasting effects of the brain surgery or other cerebrovascular defects. There also was no sign of any vision loss from new vascular compromise.

TREATMENT OPTIONS

Because the cataracts are the primary source of vision loss, surgery to remove the crystalline lenses and replace them with intraocular lenses is an option. Although the risks attendant to this surgery have been reduced dramatically in the past 10 years, complications can and do occur, and 20/25 acuity is still adequate to pass the driver's test in this state. As long as the patient has good visual acuity and unless the cataracts cause a significant alteration of lifestyle, a cataract extraction may not be necessary. Once the options had been discussed with the patient, he decided to take a conservative approach and wait. His wife was willing and able to drive at night, and they are comfortable with that arrangement.

Because he needed a new pair of glasses anyway (the old ones are in bad shape and hurt his nose), I prescribed the new refraction. The cataracts reduce the amount of light reaching the retina; thus, he also was instructed as to the importance of proper lighting when reading.

Finally, a decision on re-examination had to be made. Given the situation with nuclear lens opacities (unlikely to change very rapidly) and the relatively stable condition of other aspects of eye health, a return visit in 1 year was appropriate unless the patient noticed changes in his vision sooner. He also was instructed in identifying signs and symptoms of further cerebrovascular disease. He was instructed to contact me or his physician if he experienced symptoms such as sudden vision loss, double vision, headache, dizziness, or abrupt muscular weakness.

REFERENCES

1. Patogris CJ. Glare Testing. In JB Eskridge, JF Amos, JD Bartlett (eds), Clinical Procedures in Optometry. Philadelphia: Lippincott, 1991;487–492.
2. Cink DE. Quantification of the reduction of glare disability after standard extracapsular cataract surgery. J Cataract Refract Surg 1992;18:385–390.

3. Patogris CJ. Contrast Sensitivity. In JB Eskridge, JF Amos, JD Bartlett (eds), Clinical Procedures in Optometry. Philadelphia: Lippincott, 1991;498–503.

4. Elliott DB, Whitaker D. How useful are contrast sensitivity charts in optometric practice? Case reports. Optom Vis Sci 1992;69:378–385.

5. Amsler Grid Test. In M Fingeret, L Casser, HT Woodcome (eds), Atlas of Primary Eyecare Procedures. Norwalk, CT: Appleton & Lange, 1990;218–221.

6. Walsh TJ. Pupillary Abnormalities. In TJ Walsh (ed), Neuro-Ophthalmology: Clinical Signs and Symptoms (3rd ed). Philadelphia: Lea & Febiger, 1992;52–75.

7. Wilson-Pauwels L, Akesson EJ, Stewart PA. Cranial Nerves: Anatomy and Clinical Comments. Philadelphia: BC Decker, 1988;26–28.

8. Walsh TJ (ed). Neuro-Ophthalmology: Clinical Signs and Symptoms (3rd ed). Philadelphia: Lea & Febiger, 1992;438–444.

9. Alexander LJ. Primary Care of the Posterior Segment. Norwalk, CT: Appleton & Lange, 1994;145–150, 288–299.

10. Anderson DR. Perimetry With and Without Automation. St. Louis: Mosby, 1987;128.

Appendix: Case Scenario 3

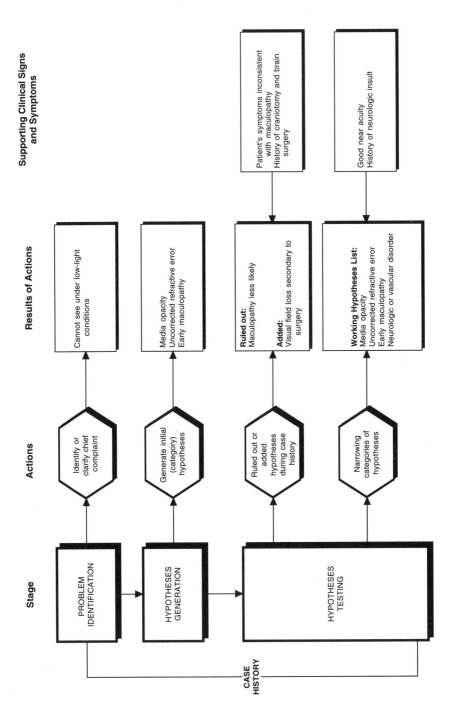

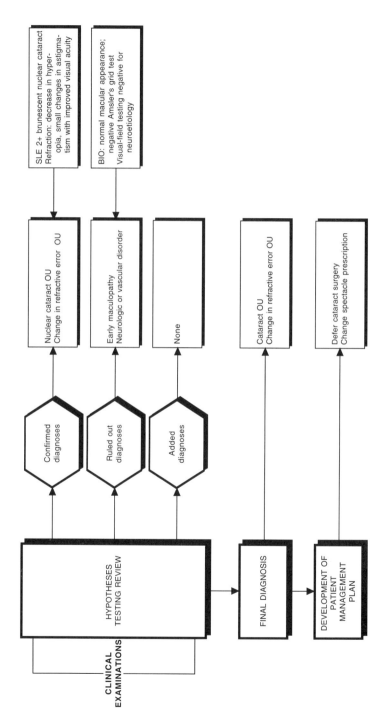

Case Scenario 3 decision-making summary. (SLE = slit-lamp examination; BIO = binocular indirect ophthalmoscopy.)

Case Scenario 4

Ellen Richter Ettinger

PATIENT BACKGROUND

PV is a 47-year-old male bus driver who presents for his first examination at this office. His last eye examination was 2 years ago. His chief complaint is a red eye.

DOCTOR: What brings you in for an examination today?

PATIENT: My eye has been red recently. It's been irritated, too, and bothering me. I figured I should get it checked out.

DOCTOR *(thinking)*: *Eye red and irritated. Sounds like a possible case of conjunctivitis. I'll ask some questions to rule out more serious problems, such as a narrow-angle glaucoma attack or iritis, that also present with a red eye.*

DOCTOR: Have you noticed any decrease in your vision?

PATIENT: No, I'm seeing fine.

DOCTOR: How about any pain?

PATIENT: My eye has been itchy, but there's not really any pain that I've noticed.

DOCTOR *(thinking)*: *A narrow-angle attack and iritis usually are accompanied by intense pain. This patient doesn't sound like he is in any pain. Also, there usually is a decrease in vision with a narrow-angle attack and sometimes with iritis. I'll check the patient's visual acuity during my examination, but with no intense pain and no decrease in visual acuity, it sounds more like one of the varieties of conjunctivitis. I'm going to ask some more questions now to distinguish between the types of conjunctivitis: bacterial, viral, and allergic.*

Factors to investigate to help differentiate between the three types of conjunctivitis include whether the problem is unilateral or bilateral, whether there has been a discharge (and the type of discharge), and whether there are any associated problems (e.g., recent upper respiratory infection [URI]). Bacterial conjunctivitis usually is unilateral, although it may spread to the other eye.[1] Allergic conjunctivitis usually is bilateral because allergens (e.g., pollen, animal danders, dusts) usually are accessible to both eyes,[2] and whatever causes one eye to become red usually irritates the other eye as well. Viral may be either unilateral or bilateral.[3] The presence and type of discharge is a particularly distinguishing factor among the three types of conjunctivitis.[1-5] A sticky, mucopurulent discharge on awakening is a common finding in cases of bacterial conjunctivitis.[5] Recent URIs are common in cases of viral conjunctivitis.[3] The doctor can use questions about these factors at this point in the case history to help determine the type of conjunctivitis.

DOCTOR: Is it one eye that is red, or have both eyes been red?

PATIENT: No, just one eye. Just my left eye.

DOCTOR: Have you noticed any type of discharge around your eyes? Any material that you've noticed on your eyelid?

PATIENT: Yes, I'm getting some sticky, stretchy yellow stuff on my lid.

DOCTOR (thinking): *Sounds like a mucopurulent discharge. Sometimes allergic conjunctivitis produces mucoid strands that may appear similar to a mucopurulent discharge,[3, 4] so I need to follow up on this more.*

DOCTOR: Do you notice the discharge more at any particular time of the day?

PATIENT: Yes, especially in the morning.

DOCTOR: What happens in the morning?

PATIENT: My lids are stuck together. They get very sticky in the mornings.

DOCTOR (thinking): *This is sounding more like a bacterial conjunctivitis and less like any of the other possibilities. To further my understanding of the patient's situation, I'll ask some typical follow-up questions.*

DOCTOR: How long have you had this problem?

PATIENT: It's been 2 weeks already.

DOCTOR: Has it gotten any better or worse?

PATIENT: I've noticed that my eye has gotten more red and irritated in the last couple of days.

DOCTOR (thinking): *The problem does not seem to be resolving by itself, and the patient is remaining symptomatic. Although acute bacterial conjunctivitis is sometimes self-limited, resolving in 7 days to 2 weeks,[1, 2] this man's problem is lasting. To investigate whether this is a chronic problem, I need to ask now whether he has had this problem before and whether it had to be treated.*

DOCTOR: Have you ever had this problem before?

PATIENT: Yes, I had a red eye like this about 3 years ago, but it went away after a few days. This time it seems to be staying red and irritated.

DOCTOR (thinking): *A problem that resolved on its own 3 years ago, with no repeat episodes, does not suggest a chronic problem.*

DOCTOR: Do you have any allergies?

PATIENT: No, no allergies.

DOCTOR *(thinking)*: *Patients with allergic conjunctivitis frequently report a history of allergies.*[6] *No sign of allergies here.*

DOCTOR: Have you had a cold recently?

PATIENT: No, fortunately not. No colds lately.

DOCTOR *(thinking)*: *I have found evidence in the case history supporting a hypothesis of conjunctivitis—specifically, bacterial conjunctivitis. I also have gathered some information that helps to rule out some of the other possible diagnoses that present with a red eye, such as a narrow-angle glaucoma attack, iritis, and the two other types of conjunctivitis conditions (allergic and viral). To complete my understanding of this patient's case and identify any other accompanying problems, I will continue by investigating the patient's previous eye and medical history, and family eye and medical history.*

DOCTOR: When was your last eye examination?

PATIENT: My last eye exam was 2 years ago.

DOCTOR: Do you see clearly at distance?

PATIENT: Yes, everything is clear.

DOCTOR: Do you wear any glasses for distance?

PATIENT: No, only reading glasses.

DOCTOR: Do you see clearly with your reading glasses?

PATIENT: I see okay, but small print is not as clear as it used to be when I first got my glasses.

DOCTOR: When did you get your reading glasses?

PATIENT: I got them when I had my last eye examination, 2 years ago.

DOCTOR *(thinking)*: *Because the patient is 47 years old and has had his near prescription for 2 years, he may need a change in his near Rx. He is a presbyope, and it is therefore important for me to check whether he needs a change in his near prescription.*

DOCTOR: Do you ever get headaches?

PATIENT: No, I don't get any headaches.

DOCTOR: How about double vision? Do you ever see two when you know there is only one object?

PATIENT: No, I never see double.

DOCTOR: Do you ever experience eye pain?

PATIENT: No, no pain at all in my eyes.

DOCTOR: Do you ever see bright flashes of light?

PATIENT: No, I never notice anything like that.

DOCTOR: How about little floating dots?

PATIENT: No. I know my wife has mentioned those, but I don't see anything like that at all.

DOCTOR: Do your eyes tear at all?

PATIENT: No, no tearing.

DOCTOR: How about any burning?

PATIENT: No, I never feel my eyes burning.

DOCTOR: Have you ever been told that you have any eye diseases, like glaucoma?

PATIENT: No, fortunately I have never had any problems like that.

DOCTOR: Have you ever had any eye surgery?

PATIENT: No, I've never had surgery at all, fortunately.

DOCTOR: Have you ever had any vision therapy?

PATIENT: No, I've never had that.

DOCTOR: I always ask what kind of work my patients do, so I know how they use their eyes at work. Are you currently working?

PATIENT: Yes, I drive a bus.

DOCTOR: Do you experience any problems with your eyes at work?

PATIENT: No, everything is fine.

DOCTOR: What kinds of hobbies do you have?

PATIENT: I like to watch television and read.

DOCTOR: Any problems in these activities?

PATIENT: No, none when I watch television. Reading is fine, except that very small print is not as clear as it used to be.

DOCTOR *(thinking)*: *I notice that the patient is mentioning difficulty with small print again. I definitely will look at the near findings to determine whether he needs a change in his near prescription. I'll ask some other history questions now before I start the testing sequence.*

DOCTOR: How is your general health?

PATIENT: It's excellent. I just saw my doctor about a month ago.

DOCTOR: Do you have any medical conditions, such as diabetes or hypertension?

PATIENT: No, I don't have any medical problems.

DOCTOR: Are you taking any medications?

PATIENT: No, no medications.

DOCTOR *(thinking)*: *I have gathered a lot of information about the patient's ocular and medical history. Now I can collect some information about the patient's family ocular and medical history.*

DOCTOR: Does anyone in your family have any eye diseases, like glaucoma?

PATIENT: No, my grandmother had cataracts, but no one has glaucoma.

DOCTOR: Is there any history of blindness or any other significant vision problems in your family?

PATIENT: No, no blindness in my family.

DOCTOR: Does anyone in your family have any medical problems, like diabetes or hypertension?

PATIENT: My grandfather had hypertension, and my mother's brother is diabetic. Everyone else in my family is healthy, and there are no other medical problems that I know about.

DIAGNOSTIC HYPOTHESES

On the basis of PV's case history, the initial hypothesis list contains the following items:

1.   *Bacterial conjunctivitis.* The patient complains of a red, irritated eye. He describes a mucopurulent discharge in the morning, a characteristic finding for bacterial conjunctivitis. These symptoms are consistent with a diagnosis of bacterial conjunctivitis.

2.   *Allergic conjunctivitis.* The patient complains of a red, irritated eye, which is also common in allergic conjunctivitis. Mucopurulent discharges, found in bacterial conjunctivitis, sometimes are confused with mucous strands, which frequently are found in cases of allergic conjunctivitis. Allergic conjunctivitis, however, frequently is found bilaterally, because whatever is causing the allergic symptoms in one eye usually would be accessible to the other eye, too (e.g., pollen or environmental factors, make-up).

3.   *Viral conjunctivitis.* The patient complains of a red eye, although he does not report a recent URI, which is common in cases of viral conjunctivitis.

4.   *Narrow-angle glaucoma.* The patient complains of a red, uncomfortable eye. The problem also is unilateral, which is consistent with a narrow-angle attack. However, he does not appear to be in extreme pain, which is typical of a narrow-angle attack, and he does not report any decrease in visual acuity.

5.   *Iritis.* As with the previous hypothesis, the patient presents complaining of a red eye, but he does not appear to be in significant discomfort, and he does not report a decrease in visual acuity. Although hypotheses 4 and 5 are remote possibilities because of the symptoms, they must be considered seriously in the presence of a red eye because of their potentially severe consequences.

6.   *Presbyopia.* The patient is 47 years old and currently wearing a near correction. He complains that near vision with his current glasses is not as clear as it used to be, so he may need a change in his prescription.

DIAGNOSTIC TESTING

To arrive at the definitive diagnosis, I started with the most likely hypothesis and gathered all the related clinical data to either confirm or rule out its presence. I then continued through the hypothesis list to collect data to rule in or rule out the other hypotheses.

Table CS4.1
Hypotheses 1 (bacterial conjunctivitis), 2 (allergic conjunctivitis), and 3 (viral conjunctivitis): problem-specific testing results.

Entering visual acuities at far and near
  20/20 OD, OS, OU at 6 m
  20/25 OD, OS; 20/25⁺ OU at near with current near vision Rx (at 40 cm)
Biomicroscopy
  Lids: clear OU
  Lashes: clear OU
  Conjunctiva: OD clear; OS moderate hyperemia (nasal>temporal), mild
    mucopurulent discharge
  Cornea: clear OU; no staining with fluorescein OU
  Anterior chamber: grade 4 OU; clear and quiet OU; no cells or flare OU
  Iris: brown and clear OU
  Lens: clear OU
  Vitreous: clear OU

To investigate the presence of the most likely hypothesis, bacterial conjunctivitis, I collected problem-specific clinical data: entering visual acuities at far and near, in both eyes, and biomicroscopy (presented in Table CS4.1). With no reduction in visual acuities and with moderate hyperemia observed on biomicroscopy, my consideration of conjunctivitis as the diagnosis (hypothesis 1, 2, or 3) is supported. The observation of a mucopurulent discharge is consistent with my hypothesis of a bacterial conjunctivitis (hypothesis 1). With no follicles seen on the patient's eyelids and with no report of any recent URI, the probability of a viral infection (hypothesis 3) is decreased. (If I still considered the possibility of a viral conjunctivitis, I could have checked for preauricular nodes,[3] but as I was confident of the likelihood of bacterial conjunctivitis, I decided that this was not necessary in this case.) The observation of a unilateral red eye with no history or knowledge of allergies reduces the likelihood of allergic conjunctivitis (hypothesis 2).

The presence of moderate hyperemia on biomicroscopy reduces the probability of a narrow-angle glaucoma attack or iritis, as these two conditions usually are associated with more severe redness. The absence of cells and flare further reduces the likelihood of iritis.

To eliminate further the possibility of a narrow-angle glaucoma attack (hypothesis 4) and iritis (hypothesis 5), I collected some additional data: pupil testing and tonometry (Table CS4.2). The findings of normal pressures and pupillary findings helped rule out the possibility of a narrow-angle glaucoma attack or iritis.

Table CS4.2
Hypotheses 4 (narrow-angle glaucoma) and 5 (iritis):
problem-specific testing results.

Pupil testing: PERRL, –APD
Tonometry (Goldmann applanation) @ 10:30AM
    OD 16 mm Hg
    OS 18 mm Hg

PERRL = pupils equal, round, reactive to light; –APD = no afferent pupillary defect.

Table CS4.3
Hypothesis 6 (presbyopia): problem-specific testing results.

Retinoscopy
    OD +0.25 DS
    OS +0.25 –0.25 × 180
Subjective refraction and visual acuities
    OD +0.25 DS (20/20)
    OS plano –0.25 × 180 (20/20)
    +1.50 add OU; 20/20 OD, OS, OU (at 40 cm) (add determined by plus
      build-up)
Habitual near Rx (lensometry)
    OD +1.25 DS
    OS +1.00 DS

DS = diopter sphere.

To examine the hypothesis of presbyopia (hypothesis 6), I collected further information (provided in Table CS4.3). If the patient were highly symptomatic as a result of the conjunctivitis, I might have brought him back to complete these tests; however, because the patient was comfortable and able to respond appropriately and was not seeing as well at near as he previously had, I felt that at this examination it was useful to perform the following tests:

- Retinoscopy
- Subjective refraction (including near testing)
- Lensometry of patient's current near correction

My refractive testing revealed that the patient did not have a significant distance corrective error and did not require glasses for distance. A change in the near prescription found during the examination resulted in improved visual acuities at near.

Table CS4.4
Additional database testing results.

Oculomotor testing: pursuits full, equal, smooth, accurate
Confrontation visual-field testing: full OD, OS
Binocular testing
    Unilateral and alternate cover test at near and far
        Orthophoria at far
        ~10Δ XP at near
    Near point of convergence: 12 cm break (OD out, diplopia), 17 cm
      recovery
    Phorometry phoria and vergence ranges at near
      van Graefe phoria at far 1Δ XP (no vertical far or near) at near 10Δ XP
      Negative fusional convergence at near x/20/16
      Positive fusional convergence at near x/10/6
Dilated fundus examination
    Cup-to-disc ratio: 0.25 OD; 0.20 OS
    ONH margins: distinct OU
    A/V ratio: 2/3 OU
    Macula: + foveal reflex OU, clear OU
    Periphery: no holes, tears, and flat 360 degrees OU

XP = exophoria; ONH = optic nerve head; A/V = arteriovenous.

Then I collected some additional baseline information to rule out any additional coexisting problems (Table CS4.4). As with the set of diagnostic tests in Table CS4.3, if the patient had been highly symptomatic as a result of the conjunctivitis, I might have rescheduled him to complete these tests; however, because he was comfortable and able to respond appropriately and had not had an examination in 2 years, I opted to gather an optimal database at this visit. These tests included:

- Oculomotor testing
- Confrontation visual-field examination
- Binocular testing
- Dilated fundus examination to evaluate the health and integrity of the retina (using tropicamide and phenylephrine hydrochloride as dilating agents)

Tests such as confrontations were not specific to the patient's presenting complaints but were performed as part of the complete database to rule out any additional problems. No abnormalities in oculomotor testing or confrontation visual-field testing were found.

The findings from the binocular testing revealed an additional problem (convergence insufficiency) that I did not detect during the case history, because at no time did the patient mention any symptoms of asthenopia, visual discomfort, headaches, or any other symptoms related to convergence problems. After obtaining these findings, I went back and asked the patient some additional questions to probe whether he had any symptoms. During this discussion, the patient again expressed that he is asymptomatic. Additional ocular health testing, including a dilated fundus examination, did not reveal any unusual or remarkable findings.

DIAGNOSTIC SUMMARY

This patient was found to have bacterial conjunctivitis. Given PV's symptoms and the related clinical findings, the level of certainty for this diagnosis was high. The magnitude of the redness, along with the patient's symptoms, suggested to me that this was a moderate case.

The patient's binocular findings were supportive of a diagnosis of convergence insufficiency. The patient's clinical data, which show a high exophoria at near, with a decreased near point of convergence and positive fusional convergence, fit the pattern observed in cases of convergence insufficiency.[7]

PV is presbyopic and reported that his vision at near is not as clear as it once was. A change in his reading prescription improved his visual acuities at near.

TREATMENT OPTIONS

Acute bacterial conjunctivitis can be caused by a variety of organisms. The more common ones include *Staphylococcus aureus*, *Streptococcus pneumoniae*, and *Hemophilus influenzae*; others include *Moraxella* and other streptococcal species.[1, 2, 8, 9] Acute bacterial conjunctivitis tends to be a self-limiting infection,[1, 2, 8] but when it is severe, chronic, or nonresolving, treatment is necessary. Conjunctival cultures can be used to identify the particular bacteria and to analyze antibiotic sensitivities, but a broad-spectrum topical antibiotic usually is prescribed prior to culture results, because in many cases the condition is resolved by the time culture results are available.[3] Although cultures do not always affect the course of treatment in isolated cases of acute conjunctivitis, they are essential in chronic and severe cases and cases that are not responding to treatment.[10] This patient's case was moderate and acute, not chronic, so I opted to start treatment with an antibiotic without obtaining a culture, knowing that if the problem did not resolve, I would be able to have him return to perform a culture later.

Erythromycin and bacitracin are common topical antibiotics and are effective against the gram-positive organisms frequently involved in bacterial conjunctivitis. Sometimes antibiotic combinations are used to broaden the spectrum of drug therapy. Polymyxin B combinations (e.g., polymyxin B–bacitracin [Polysporin] and polymyxin B–trimethoprim [Polytrim]) and neomycin combinations (Neomycin-polysporin-bacitracin [Neosporin, AK-Spore]) have a broad range of activity, addressing the common causes of acute bacterial conjunctivitis.[8] Gentamicin, tobramycin, and chloramphenicol also are effective against a broad range of offending organisms.

In this case, gentamicin, 0.3% drops, was prescribed to be instilled every 4 hours. Warm compresses also were recommended to improve circulation to the ocular area. The patient was educated to refrain from touching both eyes consecutively without washing his hands, to prevent spreading the infection from one eye to the other. The patient was told to return in 1 week, or sooner if he noticed any increased symptoms. He returned in 1 week, reporting that he had been free of symptoms for 3–4 days. Biomicroscopy showed that the eye was clear and healthy and free of any signs of injection or inflammation. PV was told that the condition had resolved and that he should discontinue using the eye drops.

Plans for the patient's binocular and refractive status were made at his initial visit. As a result of the diagnosis of convergence insufficiency identified at that visit, the patient was educated about frequent rest breaks. He also was educated about options for vision therapy if any symptoms were to occur. As he is presbyopic, I recommended a change in his prescription to improve his near visual acuities. The patient's new near prescription, corresponding to my examination findings, was OD +1.75 DS, OS +1.50 −0.25 × 180.

REFERENCES

1. Mannis MJ. Bacterial Conjunctivitis. In W Tasman (ed), Duane's Clinical Ophthalmology, Vol 4. Philadelphia: Lippincott, 1993;ch5:1–7.
2. Pavan-Langston D, Foulks GN. Cornea and External Disease. In D Pavan-Langston (ed), Manual of Ocular Diagnosis and Therapy (3rd ed). Boston: Little, Brown, 1991;67–123.
3. Catalano RA. Ocular Emergencies. Philadelphia: Saunders, 1992.
4. Jennings B. Mechanisms, diagnosis, and management of common ocular allergies. J Am Optom Assoc 1990;61(suppl 6):S32–S41.
5. Foulks GN. Bacterial Infections of the Conjunctiva and Cornea. In DM Albert, FA Jakobiec (eds), Principles and Practice of Ophthalmology: Clinical Practice. Philadelphia: Saunders, 1994;1:162–171.

6. Abelson MB, Udell IJ, Allansmith MR, et al. Allergic and Toxic Reactions. In DM Albert, FA Jakobiec (eds), Principles and Practice of Ophthalmology: Clinical Practice. Philadelphia: Saunders, 1994;1:77–100.
7. Rouse MW. Optometric Management of Visual Efficiency Problems. In MM Scheiman, MW Rouse (eds), Optometric Management of Learning-Related Vision Problems. St. Louis: Mosby, 1994;267–297.
8. Bartlett JD, Jaanus SD. Clinical Ocular Pharmacology (3rd ed). Boston: Butterworth–Heinemann, 1995.
9. Chandler JW, Sugar J, Edelhauser HF. External Diseases: Cornea, Conjunctiva, Sclera, Eyelids, Lacrimal System. London: Mosby, 1994.
10. Haesaert, SP. Clinical Manual of Ocular Microbiology and Cytology. St. Louis: Mosby–Year Book, 1993.

Appendix: Case Scenario 4

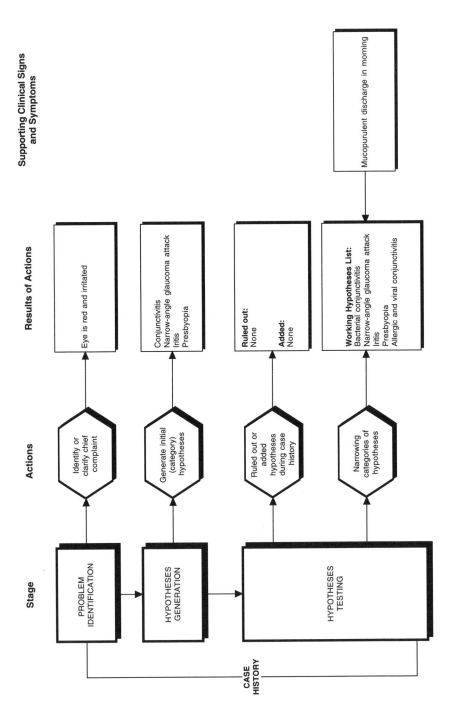

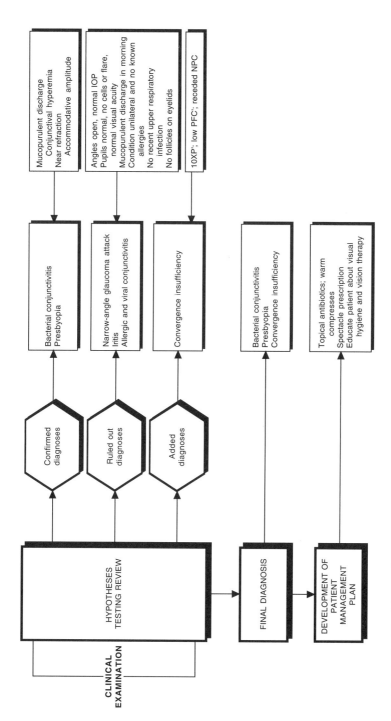

Case Scenario 4 decision-making summary. (IOP = intraocular pressure; XP' = exophoria at near; PFC' = positive fusional convergence at near; NPC = near point of convergence.)

Case Scenario 5

Jerry D. Cavallerano

PATIENT BACKGROUND

MM is a 59-year-old black woman accompanied by her sister-in-law. MM requests an examination for the purpose of replacing her present reading glasses, which are badly scratched and nearly 3 years old.

DOCTOR: I understand you would like an eye examination because you want to replace your scratched reading glasses. Are you having any eye or vision problems?

PATIENT: My glasses are nearly 3 years old and they're badly scratched. Other than needing new glasses, everything is fine.

DOCTOR *(thinking)*: *This patient's presentation seems uncomplicated because she has no real complaints other than the need to replace scratched glasses. I'll investigate her ocular history to see how comfortable her vision is.*

DOCTOR: When did you last have your eyes examined?

PATIENT: That was 3 years ago when I got these glasses.

DOCTOR: What kind of work do you perform on a regular basis?

PATIENT: I'm retired from the telephone company. I was an operator for 25 years. I read the newspaper every day, I do some knitting and sewing, and I'm an avid reader. I can do most everything I need to up close with my glasses on, but I don't use them for television or movies. I don't drive, so that's not a problem.

DOCTOR *(thinking)*: *She appears to have comfortable and clear vision for her needs. I will investigate more of her ocular history for any particular signs, symptoms, or risk factors of which I should be aware. On the basis of her age and race, she has a higher risk of glaucoma.*

DOCTOR: Have you ever had any injuries to your eyes?

PATIENT: No.

DOCTOR: Or any operations on your eyes?

PATIENT: No.

DOCTOR: Were you ever told you have any eye disease or eye disorder of any kind?

PATIENT: No.

DOCTOR: Were you ever told that you have a "lazy eye"?

PATIENT: No.

DOCTOR: Or cataracts or glaucoma?

PATIENT: No.

DOCTOR: Do you ever notice anything unusual with your eyes such as black floating spots in your view?

PATIENT: No.

DOCTOR: Or flashing lights, like lightning or a strobe light in your view?

PATIENT: No.

DOCTOR: Do you ever see double?

PATIENT: No.

DOCTOR: Or have any other problem with your eyes?

PATIENT: No.

DOCTOR *(thinking)*: *There do not appear to be any current signs, symptoms, or risk factors based on her history, although on the basis of her age and race and my observation that she is approximately 40 pounds overweight for her height, I need to investigate her medical history for the use of medication and systemic conditions that might affect her vision, specifically diabetes mellitus and hypertension. I'll also ask some baseline data questions.*

DOCTOR: Do you take any prescribed medications or other medications on a regular basis?

PATIENT: No.

DOCTOR: Are you allergic to any medications that you know of?

PATIENT: No.

DOCTOR: As far as your general health, do you have any chronic illness that's monitored on a regular basis?

PATIENT: No.

DOCTOR: Were you ever told you have diabetes?

PATIENT: No.

DOCTOR: Or high blood pressure?

PATIENT: No.

DOCTOR: Were you ever told you have any kind of heart disease?

PATIENT: No.

DOCTOR: Or any other kind of disorder?

PATIENT: No.

DOCTOR: When did you last have a physical examination?

PATIENT: That was about 2 years ago. I had a terrible flu, and I went to the doctor, and she gave me some antibiotics, but it took me almost a month to shake that cold.

DOCTOR *(thinking)*: *Her general health appears to be normal, although it has been 2 years since her last physical examination. I'll ask some questions about her family ocular and medical histories to see whether there are any particular ocular or systemic risk factors present.*

DOCTOR: Did anyone in your family ever have any kind of eye disease that you know of, such as glaucoma?

PATIENT: No.

DOCTOR: Or retinal detachment?

PATIENT: No.

DOCTOR: Or macular degeneration?

PATIENT: No.

DOCTOR: Did anyone in your family ever go blind from any cause?

PATIENT: No.

DOCTOR: Did anyone in your family ever have any chronic disease, such as high blood pressure?

PATIENT: No.

DOCTOR: Or heart disease?

PATIENT: No.

DOCTOR: Did anyone in your family ever have diabetes?

PATIENT: Yes. My father had diabetes before he died, but he never took any insulin. Also, my older brother has a touch of diabetes, but he doesn't take any insulin either.

DOCTOR *(thinking)*: *This patient's presentation seems uncomplicated because she has no real complaints other than the need to replace scratched glasses, but there are important issues to investigate during the examination. The patient has not had a recent physical examination, and because of her age, race, and family history, she is at risk of diabetes mellitus, hypertension, and glaucoma.*[1–4] *As part of her routine, comprehensive eye examination, each of these issues must be considered.*

DOCTOR: Other than the scratches on your glasses, do you have any problems with your eyes?

PATIENT: No.

DOCTOR: Is there anything else about your eyes or anything you think I should know before we start your eye examination?

PATIENT: No.

DIAGNOSTIC HYPOTHESES

On the basis of MM's case history, the initial hypothesis list includes the following:

1. *Emmetropia and presbyopia.* MM has no distance vision complaints. She is comfortable at near, and she has no ocular or visual symptoms. It is possible that her ocular and physical health are fine, and she requires only a prescription to update the condition and style of her present reading glasses.

2. *Undiagnosed diabetes mellitus.* Blacks are at a greater risk for developing non–insulin-dependent diabetes mellitus (NIDDM) than are whites.[1–7] MM's mild obesity is an additional risk factor for NIDDM.[8] A

positive family history of NIDDM is a further risk factor for NIDDM.[4] The fact that she has no ocular symptoms or symptoms of NIDDM is not unusual, because the onset of NIDDM is usually insidious, and there may be a prolonged period of disease without any clinical signs.

3. *Undiagnosed systemic hypertension.* Blacks have a greater risk for developing hypertension than do whites.[9–13] Obesity and NIDDM, if present, are additional risk factors for hypertension.[7–10] The fact that MM has not had a recent physical examination leaves unresolved the question of her medical status. Furthermore, her last physical examination may have been problem-specific and may not have investigated general physical status, such as blood glucose levels.

4. *Undiagnosed open-angle glaucoma (OAG).* Blacks have a greater risk for developing OAG than do whites.[14, 15] Age and untreated hypertension are additional risk factors for OAG.[14, 15] The likelihood of OAG is greater in people with NIDDM, and diabetes is a recognized risk factor for OAG.[16–19] Like NIDDM and hypertension, OAG causes few, if any, symptoms in the early stages of the disease.

5. *Other possible hypotheses.* Although not indicated necessarily by the history or chief complaint, a comprehensive eye examination will screen for other eye disorders such as ocular surface disease, cataract, age-related macular degeneration, or other visual or ocular health disorders. These other hypotheses are related to MM's age.

DIAGNOSTIC TESTING

Diagnostic testing results and history update during the examination directed the course of the ocular examination. Establishing one diagnosis (e.g., emmetropia-presbyopia) did not rule out other possible diagnoses, such as NIDDM, hypertension, or other ocular disorders.

To investigate the hypotheses of uncorrected refractive error or presbyopia associated with her chief complaint, the following data were collected:

- Uncorrected entering visual acuities
- Near visual acuity with present glasses
- Neutralization and examination of present glasses
- Static refraction-retinoscopy
- Subjective distance and near refraction with visual acuities

The results of this testing are shown in Table CS5.1.

The uncorrected visual acuities of 20/25 OD and OS and 20/25[+] OU suggest emmetropia, and near visual acuities with present glasses of

Table CS5.1
Hypothesis 1 (emmetropia and presbyopia):
problem-specific testing results.

Unaided Snellen visual acuity at 6 m
   20/25 OD, OS
   20/25$^+$ OU
Visual acuity at near with habitual Rx (+2.75 OU)
   14/14 OD, OS, OU
Refraction and visual acuities
   OD +0.75 DS (20/20)
   OS +0.75 DS (20/20)
   Near add: +2.50 (plus build up to best visual acuity)
   14/14 OD, OS

DS = diopter sphere.

14/14 OD, OS, and OU indicate that the near glasses allow for reasonable near vision. Distance and near refraction and visual acuity measurements support the hypothesis that MM has virtual emmetropia and presbyopia, with normal visual acuity levels.

To establish baseline data on visual function and anterior eye health (and rule out age-related hypotheses of cataract and ocular surface disease), the data collected included:

- Pupil evaluation
- Ocular motility
- Cover test
- Finger-counting confrontation visual fields
- Biomicroscopic evaluation of the anterior segment

The results of this testing are shown in Table CS5.2.

The pupil evaluation, tests of ocular motility, confrontation visual fields, and anterior segment evaluation suggested no ocular or systemic disorder. The mild degree of lens opacity was consistent with MM's age, dismissing the hypothesis of clinically relevant cataract.

To investigate the possibility of hypotheses 2–5 (glaucoma, diabetes mellitus, and hypertension), the following data were collected (and shown in Table CS5.3):

- Intraocular pressure by applanation tonometry
- Fundus evaluation through dilated pupils using binocular indirect ophthalmoscope, direct ophthalmoscope, and 78 D lens with the biomicroscope
- Sphygmomanometry

Table CS5.2
Additional database testing results.

Pupils
  PERRL, −APD
Ocular motility: full and smooth
Confrontation fields (finger counting): full OD and OS
Slit-lamp examination
  Cornea: arcus OD and OS
  Anterior chamber: deep and clear OD and OS
  Iris: flat OD and OS
  Lens: 2+ nuclear sclerosis with anterior cortical haze OD and OS

PERRL = pupils equal, round, reactive to light; −APD = no afferent pupillary defect.

Table CS5.3
Hypotheses 2–5: problem-specific testing results.

Intraocular pressure (applanation tonometry)
  OD 14 mm Hg
  OS 13 mm Hg
Fundus evaluation through dilated pupils using binocular indirect ophthal-
    moscope, direct ophthalmoscope, and 78 D lens with the bio-
    microscope
  Cup-to-disc ratio: ~0.35 horizontally and vertically OU with healthy rim
    tissue and color
  Macula: scattered hemorrhages and microaneurysms of a moderate
    degree, with hard exudates greater than 500 μm from the center of the
    macula; no evidence of macular edema in either eye
  Retinal vessels: normal without evidence of venous beading or narrow-
    ing; no evidence of neovascularization or intraretinal microvascular
    abnormalities; vessels without evidence of caliber changes
Blood pressure: 154/98 mm Hg

Applanation tonometry provided readings in the statistically normal range. The optic nerve appearance was healthy, with a cup-to-disc ratio of approximately 0.35 horizontally and vertically OU and with healthy nerve color and rim tissue, suggesting there is no OAG.

The presence of hemorrhages and microaneurysms in the posterior pole of each eye suggests undiagnosed diabetes mellitus (Figures CS5.1 and CS5.2). The blood pressure reading of 154/98 mm Hg at the conclusion of the examination suggests the possibility of hypertension. Referral for medical evaluation for diabetes mellitus and hypertension was warranted on the basis of these examination findings.

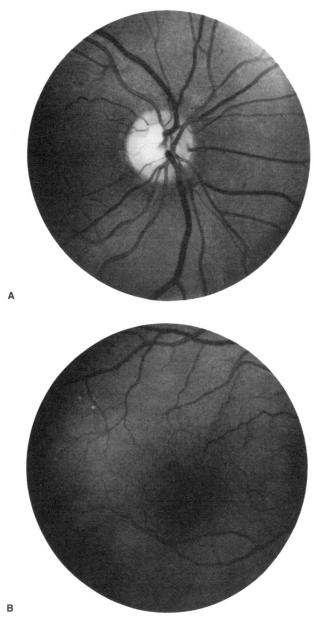

Figure CS5.1 Fundus of the right eye. A. In field 1, centered on the optic nerve, there are two hemorrhages-microaneurysms (H-Ma) nasally, and one H-Ma at the 1 o'clock position. B. In field 2, centered on the macula, one blot hemorrhage and several H-Ma can be seen peripherally at approximately the 9 o'clock position and at the 11 o'clock position. There are several hard exudates at the 10 o'clock position within the temporal vascular arcades. (*continued*)

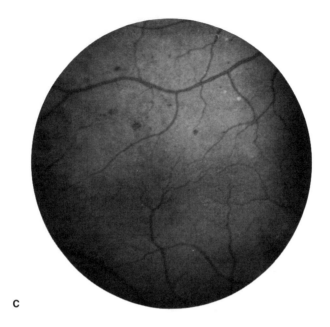

C

Figure CS5.1 (*continued*) C. In field 3, temporal to the macula, more extensive H-Ma are present. (Photographs courtesy of Denis Fleming and Robert Cavicchi, C.R.A., Beetham Eye Insitute, Joslin Diabetes Center, Photo Department.)

Other nonspecific hypotheses are ruled out by the eye examination. There is no sign of age-related macular degeneration or other disorders.

DIAGNOSTIC SUMMARY

The collected data suggest that MM has mild hyperopia and presbyopia, immature cataracts of no clinical significance, undiagnosed diabetes mellitus with mild nonproliferative diabetic retinopathy, and possible systemic hypertension.

MM had mild hyperopia and presbyopia, consistent with her age, case history, and the eyeglass prescription she was wearing. She had immature cataracts in each eye, once again consistent with her age. These cataracts were not of clinical significance, although they should be discussed with MM.

More significantly, MM had retinal signs of diabetes mellitus, although diabetes had not been diagnosed. Similarly, her blood pressure was elevated slightly. Referral to an internist or family practitioner was indicated.

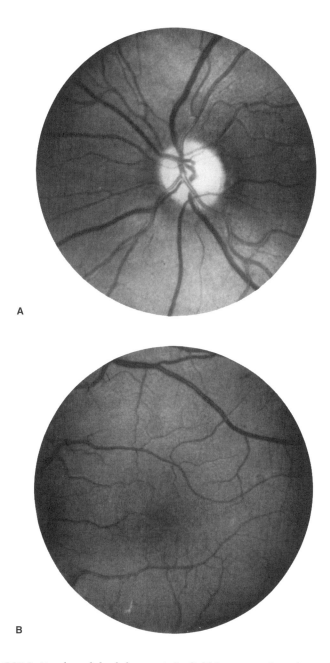

Figure CS5.2 Fundus of the left eye. A. In field 1, centered on the optic nerve, there are hemorrhages-microaneurysms (H-Ma) temporally at approximately the 2 o'clock position. B. In field 2, centered on the macula, H-Ma can be seen peripherally at approximately the 1–2 o'clock position. There is some hard exudate inferiorly. (*continued*)

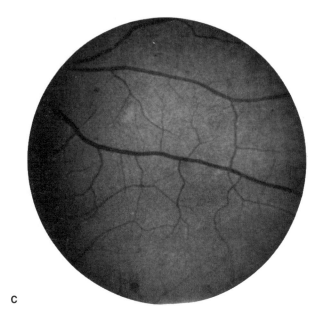

C

Figure CS5.2 (*continued*) C. In field 3, temporal to the macula, more extensive H-Ma are present. (Photographs courtesy of Denis Fleming and Robert Cavicchi, C.R.A., Beetham Eye Insitute, Joslin Diabetes Center, Photo Department.)

TREATMENT OPTIONS

A significant portion of the treatment plan for MM involved patient education. Because she began the examination with no subjective complaint, any unfavorable diagnosis was unexpected and likely to be upsetting. The need for spectacle correction was expected, and she could continue with no distance prescription if she desired. Her mild, immature cataracts were of no clinical consequence.

The likely diagnosis of diabetes mellitus required referral and consultation with an internist and discussion with MM. The fact that already there were ocular complications from diabetes required additional education and counseling. If oral hypoglycemic agents were initiated by MM's internist, a lowering of blood glucose levels might have affected the final refraction, and there might be increased hyperopia and presbyopia following a lowering of blood glucose levels.

MM's blood pressure was 154/98 mm Hg at the conclusion of her examination. In view of her mild obesity and the likelihood of NIDDM, follow-up evaluations and possible treatment by her internist were considered.

The remainder of MM's eye examination ruled out glaucoma and other ocular disease that might be revealed by a comprehensive eye examination. The treatment options for MM were as follows:

1.   *Prescription of new reading glasses.* This option was acceptable, but delay of purchasing new glasses was advisable pending treatment for diabetes mellitus by diet, exercise, oral hypoglycemic agent, or insulin. A suggested near prescription of +3.25 DS OU may have been inappropriate, especially if a reduction of blood glucose levels led to a greater degree of hyperopia.

2.   *Referral to an internist for evaluation of blood glucose levels and blood pressure:* This option had to be pursued, and a letter to the internist summarizing eye examination findings was indicated.

MM was seen by her internist for a routine examination. Fasting blood glucose levels were greater than 140 mg/dl on two successive visits. Her blood pressure readings were 138/98 and 135/95 mm Hg on two successive visits. MM's doctor suggested consultation with a nutritionist to establish a suitable meal plan and will continue to monitor MM to evaluate her blood pressure level and the possible need for oral hypoglycemic agents. No medications were prescribed.

Three months later, MM had lost 10 pounds by strict adherence to a meal plan in conjunction with her nutritionist. She also had initiated an exercise plan of lap swimming four times per week. MM's internist continued to monitor her blood glucose levels and blood pressure but did not initiate pharmacologic treatment for diabetes control or blood pressure control at this time. When seen for repeat refraction, MM's distance and near refraction remained unchanged. She indicated she felt better physically and was pleased that she had taken steps to improve her physical well-being. A near prescription of +3.25 D was given to MM, and she was advised to have eye examinations every 12 months, or sooner if she noticed any eye changes or abnormalities.

REFERENCES

1. Appiah AP, Ganthier R Jr, Watkins N. Delayed diagnosis of diabetic retinopathy in black and Hispanic patients with diabetes mellitus. Ann Ophthalmol 1991;23:156–158.
2. Trilling JS. Screening for non–insulin-dependent diabetes mellitus. Prim Care 1988;15:285–295.
3. Wilson PW, Anderson KM, Kannel WB. Epidemiology of diabetes mellitus in the elderly. The Framingham Study. Am J Med 1986;80(5A):3–9.
4. Warram JH, Rich SS, Krolewski AS. Epidemiology and Genetics of Diabetes Mellitus. In CR Kahn, GC Weir (eds), Joslin's Diabetes Mellitus (13th ed). Philadelphia: Lea & Febiger, 1994;201–215.

5. Harris MI, Hadden WC, Knowler WC, et al. Prevalence of diabetes and impaired glucose tolerance and plasma glucose levels in U.S. population aged 20–74 yr. Diabetes 1987;36:523–534.

6. Diabetes 1991 Vital Statistics. Alexandria, VA: American Diabetes Association, 1991.

7. Niffeneger J, Fong D, Cavallerano J, et al. Diabetes Mellitus. In DM Albert, FA Jakobiec (eds), Principles and Practice of Ophthalmology. Philadelphia: Saunders, 1994;5:2925–2936.

8. Flier JS. Obesity. In CR Kahn, GC Weir (eds), Joslin's Diabetes Mellitus (13th ed). Philadelphia: Lea & Febiger, 1994;351–362.

9. Klein R, Klein BE, Moss SE, et al. Blood pressure and hypertension in diabetes. Am J Epidemiol 1985;122:75–89.

10. Statement on hypertension in diabetes mellitus. Final report. The Working Group on Hypertension in Diabetes. Arch Intern Med 1987;147:830–842.

11. Sowers JR. Antihypertensive Therapy. In HE Lebovitz (ed), Therapy for Diabetes Mellitus and Related Disorders (2nd ed). Alexandria, VA: American Diabetes Association, 1994;204–212.

12. Christlieb AR, Krolewski AS, Warram JH. Hypertension. In CR Kahn, GC Weir (eds), Joslin's Diabetes Mellitus (13th ed). Philadelphia: Lea & Febiger, 1994;817–835.

13. Douglas JG. Hypertension and diabetes in blacks. Diabetes Care 1990;13:1191–1195.

14. Javitt JC, McBean AM, Nicholson GA, et al. Undertreatment of glaucoma among black Americans. N Engl J Med 1991;325:1418–1422.

15. Wilson MR, Hertzmark E, Walker AM, et al. A case-control study of risk factors in open angle glaucoma. Arch Ophthalmol 1987;105:1066–1071.

16. Armstrong JR, Daily RK, Dobson HL, et al. The incidence of glaucoma in diabetes mellitus: a comparison with the incidence of glaucoma in the general population. Am J Ophthalmol 1960;50:55–63.

17. Becker B. Diabetes mellitus and primary open-angle glaucoma. The XXVII Edward Jackson Memorial Lecture. Am J Ophthalmol 1971;71:1–16.

18. Mapstone R, Clark CV. Prevalence of diabetes in glaucoma. Br Med J (Clin Res Ed) 1985;291:93–95.

19. Klein BEK, Klein R, Jensen SC. Open-angle glaucoma and older-onset diabetes. Ophthalmology 1994;101:1173–1177.

Appendix: Case Scenario 5

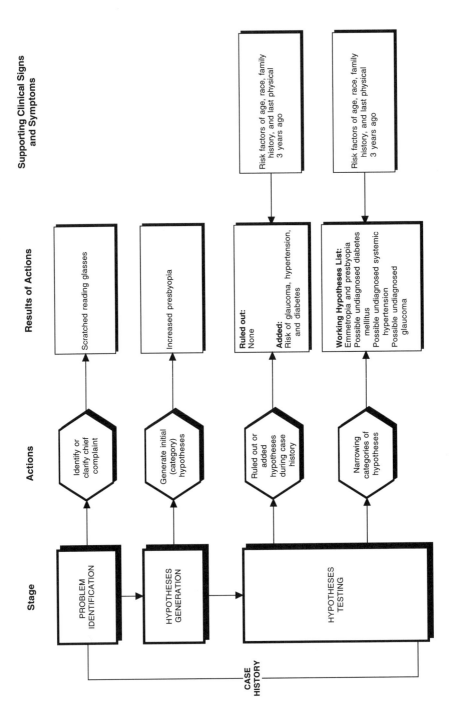

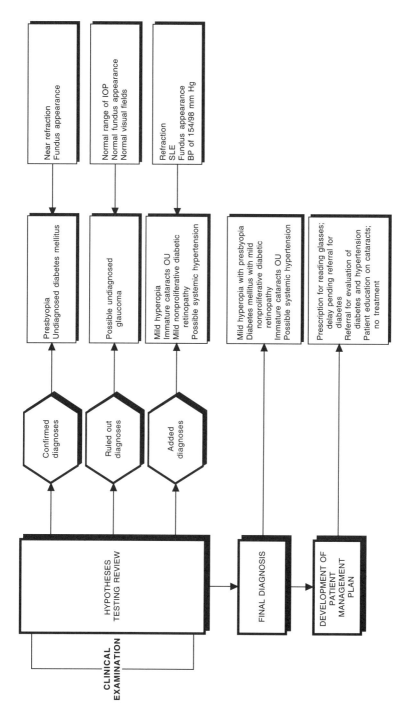

Case Scenario 5 decision-making summary. (IOP = intraocular pressure; SLE = slit-lamp examination; BP = blood pressure.)

Case Scenario 6

Gerald E. Lowther

PATIENT BACKGROUND

ML is a 48-year-old woman appearing for a comprehensive optometric examination. She has not been seen in this office previously.

DOCTOR: Are you having any problems with your eyes or vision?

PATIENT: I feel that my vision while reading is not quite as clear as it used to be and it tends to be worse at some times than others. My eyes often feel gritty or like I have some sand in my eyes. I also have some excessive tearing.

DOCTOR (*thinking*): *The patient seems to be reporting two or three problems: blurred near vision, ocular discomfort, and excessive tearing. There could be a number of causes of these complaints. The near vision problem could be due to an undercorrection for presbyopia. The ocular discomfort could be eyestrain due to improper correction, a binocular vision problem, allergies, a dry-eye problem, or a foreign body under the lid. The excessive tearing could be due to any of the problems that cause the discomfort.*

DOCTOR: Do you find that you need to hold reading material farther away from you than you like to see it?

PATIENT: Yes, it does help some if I hold it farther away.

DOCTOR: Do you feel that you have any eyestrain or get headaches when you read?

PATIENT: My eyes do feel tired after I read a little while, and occasionally I do get headaches with reading.

DOCTOR: Do you ever see double or two of some things when you should not?

PATIENT: I have not noticed that.

DOCTOR: Do you have any difficulty seeing at a distance, for example, while driving?

PATIENT: Sometimes when I'm driving, my vision will blur, and I have to blink several times to clear it. When my eyes water, my distance vision blurs.

DOCTOR: When was your last vision examination?

PATIENT: About 3 years ago.

DOCTOR: Have you had your present glasses since that time?

PATIENT: Yes, I got them at that time.

DOCTOR (*thinking*): *The patient certainly could need an increase in her bifocal power by this time and possibly need a change in her prescription.*

DOCTOR: When do you notice the feeling that something is in your eyes? How often does it happen?

PATIENT: If I read for some time, my eyes feel tired, and I have discomfort. It also occurs sometimes when I ride in the car. It happens every day.

DOCTOR: When do you notice the excessive tearing?

PATIENT: This usually occurs a little while after the discomfort starts. There often seems to be a sharper pain before the tearing. I will tear up and may have to wipe tears away with a tissue, and then it will reoccur if I read some more.

DOCTOR: For how long has this discomfort been occurring?

PATIENT: Probably for about 3 or 4 years, but it has gradually gotten worse.

DOCTOR: Do you have any allergies, such as hay fever or reaction to cats?

PATIENT: No, I have never had any allergies that I am aware of.

DOCTOR (*thinking*): *The problem does not appear to be due to allergies. It is probably not a foreign body or infection because it is not constant and has been occurring for so long. A foreign body or concretion under the lid also would cause pain on blinking. It may only be a need for a refractive error change; however, it could be a dry-eye problem. I need to question the patient more about possible dry-eye symptoms.*[1-3]

DOCTOR: Are you taking any medications? Even something that was not prescribed by a doctor for you, such as antihistamines for colds?

PATIENT: No.

DOCTOR: Do you notice that the discomfort is worse at any particular time of the year.

PATIENT: It seems to be worse in the winter, starting about this time (November).

DOCTOR: Do you feel you are more sensitive than many other people to smoke or smog?

PATIENT: Yes, if I am around smokers, my eyes get very irritated.

DOCTOR: Do you have any eye discomfort, irritation, or pain on awakening in the morning?

PATIENT: Yes, many mornings when I wake up, my eyes feel very uncomfortable.

DOCTOR: Do you do anything about this discomfort?

PATIENT: It feels better if I wash my face and splash water on my eyes and then hold a warm wash cloth over my eyes for a few minutes.

DOCTOR: Have you taken any trips where you have flown recently?

PATIENT: Yes, I travel by plane several times a year.

DOCTOR: Have you noticed that your symptoms are worse during or after you have flown?

PATIENT: Yes, my eyes become very irritated and red during such flights.

DOCTOR: Has anyone told you that you might have dry eyes or prescribed artificial tear drops for you?

PATIENT: No, no one has.

DOCTOR (*thinking*): *The patient has symptoms that are consistent with a dry-eye problem. I need to explore whether there is a related systemic problem.*

DOCTOR: Do you ever notice any dryness of the mouth or have difficulty eating dry foods?

PATIENT: No, I haven't noticed any such problem.

DOCTOR: Have you ever been diagnosed as having arthritis or noticed any problems with sore joints?

PATIENT: No, I haven't, but my mother does have arthritis.

DOCTOR: Have you ever received a diagnosis of any other chronic diseases?

PATIENT: No.

DOCTOR: Do you have any problems with sinus congestion, nasal congestion, or a chronic cough?

PATIENT: I occasionally have some sinus problems, but not very often.

DOCTOR (*thinking*): *The patient does not appear to have any indication of Sjögren's syndrome or related systemic problems.*[4]

DIAGNOSTIC HYPOTHESES

1. *An insufficient near add.* This may be causing at least some of her vision symptoms.

2. *A tear film deficiency.* The symptoms of grittiness or feeling of sand in the eyes are typical of dry eyes. The increased symptoms—with reading (tending not to blink, which makes the drying worse), during the winter when the heat is on and the humidity decreases, with air travel because the humidity in aircraft is very low, and symptoms on awakening, because there is a decreased tearing at night—all indicate a possible decrease in tear volume.

Unusual sensitivity to smoke is common with dry-eye patients. The increased tearing is again common with dry eyes, because the dryness irritates the ocular surface, thereby causing reflex tearing. The condition most likely is keratoconjunctivitis sicca (KCS). It does not appear that there are any signs or symptoms of a dry mouth or systemic condition suggesting Sjögren's syndrome.

3.   *Uncorrected distance refractive error.* ML may have some uncorrected astigmatism or hyperopia. However, if this is the case, it appears it is a rather small amount.

4.   *Binocular vision problem.* However, there are no indications of diplopia, and a binocular vision problem usually would not cause the grittiness and pain sensation. It could account for the tiredness and general ocular discomfort.

5.   *An allergy.* ML may have recently developed an allergy.

DIAGNOSTIC TESTING

The first diagnostic procedures were selected to test the hypotheses as to whether the refractive error was fully corrected and whether the near power was adequate. I tested uncorrected and corrected (habitual spectacle correction) visual acuities at distance and near. I performed a distance and near refraction to determine the patient's best correction. The present spectacles were neutralized for comparison to my refractive findings (given in Table CS6.1). These findings suggest that the patient's present distance correction is adequate; however, as suspected, the near add is not sufficient and should be increased. The question now is whether there are any other problems causing the symptoms or whether it is due totally to the refractive error.

To test whether there was a binocular vision problem, I performed a distance and near cover test to ensure that there was not a significant heterophoria causing the symptoms. The fusional vergences indicated that the phorias should not be a problem. From the findings, one would not expect any binocular vision problems.

To delve into the diagnostic hypothesis that the patient may have a tear film deficiency, I conducted a biomicroscopy examination,[5–7] paying particular attention to the following areas:

- Evaluating the lids for blepharitis and meibomianitis
- Examining the tear prism along the lower lid (whether it is continuous and full, any scalloping of the edge of the tear prism)
- Determining any dried mucus on the lower lid margin
- Determining injected lid margins
- Examining the cornea for fluorescein and rose bengal staining
- Everting the upper lid to look for signs of allergy, irritation, foreign bodies, or concretions

The biomicroscopic findings are presented in Table CS6.2.

From these findings, one would expect a tear film problem. The reduced tear prism and scalloping with the abnormally high debris and

Table CS6.1
Hypotheses 1 (inappropriate correction for presbyopia), 3 (uncorrected refractive error), and 4 (binocular vision problem): problem-specific testing results.

Entering visual acuities
   Uncorrected: 20/25 OD, OS at 6 m; 20/50 OD, OS at 40 cm
   With habitual correction: 20/15 OD, OS at 6 m; 20/25 OD, OS at 40 cm
Habitual correction
   OD +1.00 –0.50 × 180
   OS +0.75 –0.75 × 180
   +1.00 add OU
   D-28 flat-top segment
Subjective refraction and visual acuities
   OD +1.00 –0.50 × 180 (20/15)
   OS +1.00 –0.75 × 180 (20/15)
   +1.75 add OU (determined by plus build-up and checking the range of
      clear vision)
Cover test
   Unilateral cover test: nonstrabismic at distance and near
   Alternate cover test
      Distance: 2Δ exophoria, no vertical phoria
      Near: 5Δ exophoria, no vertical phoria
Fusional vergences, horizontal:
   Distance: negative fusional convergence, 8/6; positive fusional conver-
      gence, 10/12/7
   Near: negative fusional convergence, 16/23/15; positive fusional conver-
      gence, 16/18/10

Table CS6.2
Hypothesis 2 (tear film deficiency); biomicroscopic examination:
problem-specific testing results.

Lids
   Mild blepharitis with collarettes OU
   Mild meibomianitis
   Lid margins slightly injected, some debris caked on the margin
   Eversion: no papillae or cysts, no unusual injection, no concretions
Conjunctiva
   Grade 1 superficial injection
   Mild stipple staining (fluorescein and rose bengal) in exposed region
Tear film
   Moderate debris
   Tear prism varies in height, edges scalloped
Cornea
   Line of inferior, midperiphery fluorescein staining
   Mild stipple staining (fluorescein and rose bengal) on inferior portion
Other structures: normal

Table CS6.3
Additional database testing results.

Tonometry: 18 mm Hg OD and OS at 11:30 AM
Automated visual fields
    Equal sensitivity OD and OS at 36 dB
    No fixation losses, no false-positive or false-negative results
    No significant depression in sensitivity within central 30 degrees
Fundus examination through dilated pupils
    Cup-to-disc ratio: 0.4/0.4 OU
    ONH: healthy rim tissue 360 degrees OU
    Background: healthy retina, even pigmentation to periphery, no holes,
        tears, flat 360 degrees OU
    Vitreous: clear OU
    Vessels: healthy, no abnormal crossings OU

ONH = optic nerve head.

mucus along the lid margin strongly suggest a dry-eye problem. The inferior corneal and conjunctival staining, and the small amount of rose bengal staining, further confirm the hypothesis of a tear film problem. The mild blepharitis and meibomianitis may be at least a contributing factor to the symptoms. Because lid eversion and examination of the cul-de-sac did not indicate any signs of allergy or foreign bodies, these hypotheses can be ruled out. All the other routine testing uncovered no unusual or suspicious findings (Table CS6.3).

DIAGNOSTIC SUMMARY

This presbyopic patient was experiencing undercorrection at near, which was causing the visual symptoms at near. However, she had an additional tear film problem, causing dry-eye symptoms. The symptoms and signs were very consistent with a tear film deficiency. This deficiency may have been a decrease in the production of the aqueous component of the tears (KCS) or it could have been secondary to blepharitis and meibomianitis. Often such patients have both decreased tear production and lid hygiene problems. It is suspected that the meibomianitis and blepharitis at least contributed to the dry-eye symptoms, but a definitive diagnosis could not be made until the lid problems had been cleared with at least a 2- to 4-week intensive lid hygiene program.

TREATMENT OPTIONS

First, the patient's spectacle correction was changed to give her good near vision and relieve any eye strain due to the undercorrection, using the same straight-top bifocal design as her habitual correction. The distance prescription had not changed, and a +1.75 D add was prescribed. Second, the dry-eye symptoms had to be addressed. The first step was to place ML on warm compresses and lid scrubs three times a day for 2–4 weeks. After this treatment, she reported significant improvement in the dry-eye symptoms. The patient was informed that the lid problems are a chronic condition and that she must use the warm compresses and do the lid scrubs twice a week indefinitely. She still reported an occasional gritty and foreign-body sensation, especially with periods of reading and other concentrated visual tasks. ML was told to use nonpreserved lubricating drops when she was doing these tasks and to use them before the development of the symptoms, as a preventive measure. She reported that since doing the lid hygiene, she seldom has discomfort on awakening. Therefore, it was decided not to have her use an ointment at night, because usually this results in some blurred vision for a time after awakening. She was informed that, if the symptoms on awakening worsened, we would start the use of the ointment.

REFERENCES

1. McMonnies CW, Ho A. Patient history in screening for dry eye conditions. J Am Optom Assoc 1987;58:296–301.
2. Holly FJ. Diagnosis and treatment of dry eye syndrome. Contact Lens Spectrum 1989;4(7):37–44.
3. McMonnies CW, Ho A. Responses to a dry eye questionnaire from a normal population. J Am Optom Assoc 1987;58:588–591.
4. Semes L. Keratoconjuntivitis Sicca and Ocular Surface Disease. In JA Silbert (ed), Anterior Complications of Contact Lens Wear. New York: Churchill Livingstone, 1994;221–236.
5. Whitcher JP. Clinical diagnosis of the dry eye. Int Ophthalmol Clin 1987;27:7–24.
6. Bowman RW, Dougherty JM, McCulley JP. Chronic blepharitis and dry eyes. Int Ophthalmol Clin 1987;27(1):27–35.
7. Hom MM, Martinson JR, Knapp LL, et al. Prevalence of Meibomian gland dysfunction. Optom Vis Sci 1990;67:710–712.

Appendix: Case Scenario 6

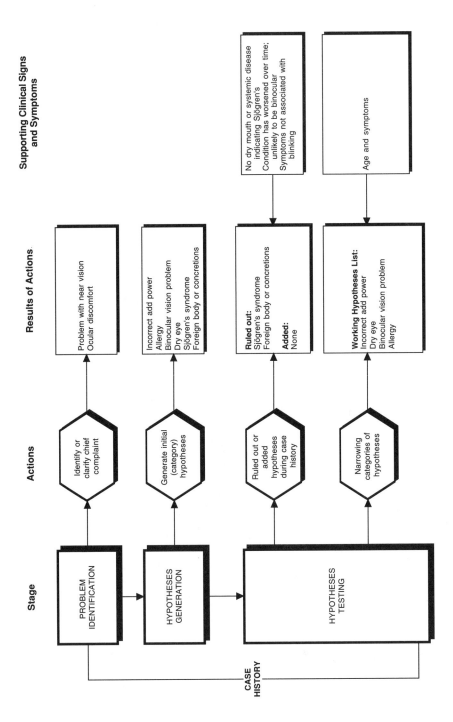

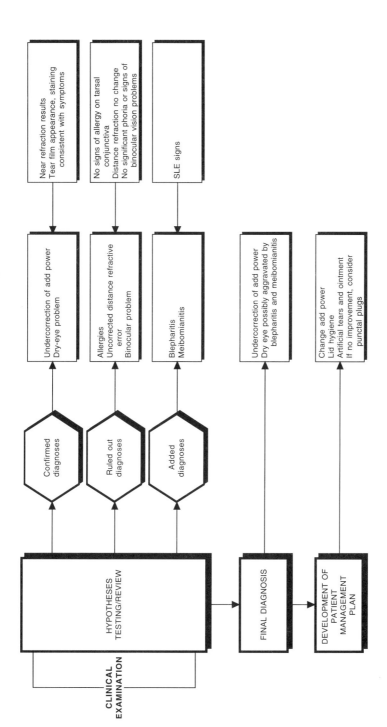

Case Scenario 6 decision-making summary. (SLE = slit-lamp examination.)

Case Scenario 7

John B. Gelvin

PATIENT BACKGROUND

MR is a 64-year-old white woman who works part-time as a greeter at a department store and as a full-time homemaker. She lives in a small Midwest town.

DOCTOR: How can I help you today?

PATIENT: I need an eye exam because I failed a screening.

DOCTOR: What type of screening was it—a vision screening or a health fair?

PATIENT: Three weeks ago, there was a Wellness Day at the hospital. I had done well on all the tests until I took the eye examination. They said that my glasses were fine but that I had failed the glaucoma test.

DOCTOR *(thinking)*: *Generally, people are screened for glaucoma by one or more of the following methods: the air-puff tonometry test (inappropriately called the* glaucoma test *at times), optic nerve evaluation by direct ophthalmoscopy, and other visual function tests (screening perimetry).*

DOCTOR: Do you remember what test you failed?

PATIENT: No, I just remember that they looked in my eyes and did some tests and said that I didn't pass.

DOCTOR: Did anyone mention high pressure in your eyes during the testing?

PATIENT: No.

DOCTOR *(thinking)*: *Screening tonometry may or may not have been performed. If tonometry was performed, the results may have been normal or may have not been emphasized. Screening patients for glaucoma by tonometry alone, with a general referral criterion set past 21 mm Hg, is useful only in detecting normal ocular hypertensive patients and will pass up to 50% of patients who will be found later to have glaucoma by complete examination.*[1] *At this point, I'll determine the patient's general ocular and health status.*

DOCTOR: How has your vision been?

PATIENT: Fine.

DOCTOR: Any blurriness in your vision while driving or when performing near-point tasks?

PATIENT: No.

DOCTOR: When was your last eye examination and who performed it?

PATIENT: Three years ago by an eye doctor in town.

DOCTOR: Do you remember the results of your examination?

PATIENT: I remember that the doctor gave me a new pair of glasses.

DOCTOR *(thinking)*: *If no complaints exist with current spectacles, the patient's refractive status should be stable. And if, on the basis of the patient's age, a cataract were found, it may be a nonprogressive or a slowly progressive cataract.*

DOCTOR: Did your doctor dilate your pupils at the time of your last examination?

PATIENT: Yes.

DOCTOR: And your eyes were found to be normal?

PATIENT: Yes.

DOCTOR *(thinking)*: *If borderline findings occur on this examination, it will be helpful to request records from the prior eye examination for comparison purposes.*

DOCTOR: Does anyone in your family have glaucoma?

PATIENT: No.

DOCTOR: Have you had any eye injuries or had eye surgery performed?

PATIENT: No.

DOCTOR: Do you suffer from migraines?

PATIENT: No.

DOCTOR *(thinking)*: *She has no real factors other than her age that might increase her risk of acquiring glaucoma.*

DOCTOR: Are you under the care of another doctor for any reason?

PATIENT: I see my family doctor about once a year. I have mild arthritis and take aspirin sometimes for the pain.

DOCTOR: So, you have been tested for high blood pressure, diabetes mellitus, and potential cholesterol problems?

PATIENT: Well, I have been told that my blood pressure should be checked regularly because it is borderline high.

DOCTOR *(thinking)*: *Patients who are regarded as suspect for essential hypertension should be suspect for vascular perfusion insufficiency to the eye (which might be evident as low-tension or normotensive glaucoma) as well as elsewhere in the body.[2] Diet, weight control, and exercise help reduce the risk of heart disease by allowing better oxygenation of tissues.*

DOCTOR: Do you exercise?

PATIENT: Oh, yes. I try to walk 5 or 6 miles a week.

DOCTOR: Does anyone in your family have high blood pressure, diabetes, heart disease, or cancer?

PATIENT: My brother had lung cancer. He's better now, but I don't know how he was treated.

DIAGNOSTIC HYPOTHESES

On the basis of MR's case history, the initial hypothesis list contains the following:

1. *Open-angle glaucoma (OAG).*[3] Health screenings assist practitioners in finding a small population of patients at risk for infirmity out of a large population in which there has not been a diagnosis of any conditions for which the patients are being screened. Because this patient has failed a glaucoma screening, glaucoma must be ruled out. The most prevalent form of glaucoma in a 64-year-old white woman is primary OAG.

2. *Secondary glaucoma.* It is not uncommon for patients in this age category to suffer from other forms of glaucoma. The potential for pseudoexfoliative glaucoma or low-tension or normotensive glaucoma does exist and must be ruled out.

3. *Other optic nerve dysfunction.*[4] Various insults to the optic nerve (varying from congenital problems and anomalies to acquired optic nerve dysfunction) can result in the failure of a screening fundus examination. Visual-field loss within Bjerrum's area on a screening test may be found.

4. *Retinal abnormalities.*[5] Various retinal entities (e.g., chorioretinal scars) will have retinal signs that may lead a practitioner to fail a screening patient. If screening fields are performed, absolute scotomas may be found within the visual field. This patient lives in the area in which patients are found on a rather regular basis to have chorioretinal scars secondary to presumed ocular histoplasmosis syndrome.

5. *Artifact with no real visual-field defect.*[6] There is a chance that a failed screening visual-field depicts an artifact and that no real visual-field defect exists.

DIAGNOSTIC TESTING

MR received a complete glaucoma evaluation. The examination consisted of two separate visits, allowing me to establish the diagnosis and to rule out other potential entities.

To rule out primary OAG and any secondary glaucoma, retinal ganglion cell function must be determined to be normal. If either of these conditions exists, the result will be both optic nerve damage by wasting of the neuroretinal rim and potential nerve fiber–layer defects. Visual function testing generally supports findings of optic

Table CS7.1
Hypotheses 1–5: problem-specific testing results.

Dilated fundus examination
   Optic nerve assessment (see Figure CS7.1)
      OD: round 0.5/0.5 cup-to-disc (C/D) ratio, neuroretinal rim intact, no
        pallor noted, peripapillary atrophy present
      OS: 0.75 vertical by 0.65 horizontal C/D ratio with temporal unfolding,
        no pallor noted, peripapillary atrophy present
   Maculae and vessels: unremarkable, no scars or defects bilaterally
   Periphery: cobblestone degeneration
Visual-field testing (see Figure CS7.2)
   OD: mild, generalized depression
   OS: generalized depression with a superior nasal step
Applanation tonometry
   OD: 24 mm Hg at 11 AM (first visit); 20 mm Hg at 9 AM (second visit)
   OS: 25 mm Hg at 11 AM (first visit); 22 mm Hg at 9 AM (second visit)
Diurnal applanation tonometry evaluation: 6–mm Hg shift OD/OS by three
   readings throughout a 12-hr period
Pupils: OD, OS: blue iris, PERRL, –APD

PERRL = pupils equal, round, reactive to light ; –APD = no afferent pupillary defect.

nerve damage; thus, the following tests were conducted to rule out hypothesis 1 (OAG):

- Stereoscopic optic nerve assessment
- Visual-field examination
- Applanation tonometry
- Pupil evaluation
- Contrast sensitivity

The results of this testing are presented in Table CS7.1.

   Cup-to-disc (C/D) asymmetry exists with the greatest C/D ratio (0.75/0.65) in the left eye. Vertical elongation toward the disc poles has occurred in the left eye as well. No split defects are found in the nerve fiber layer for either the right or left eye. Photodocumentation of the optic nerve heads also was conducted for future reference (Figure CS7.1).

   Threshold visual-field examination was performed twice. Of interest on the first field was that the right eye showed a high number of fixation losses (7 of 18). The left eye showed a wide short-term fluctuation (4.0 dB). Humphrey 30-2 visual fields were obtained at both visits. A +5.25 D lens was in place during testing of each eye. The second visual-field test showed a slight reduction in decibel sensitivity in the right eye, which heightens one's suspicion regarding a decline in optic nerve function in the right eye. The left visual field shows a supe-

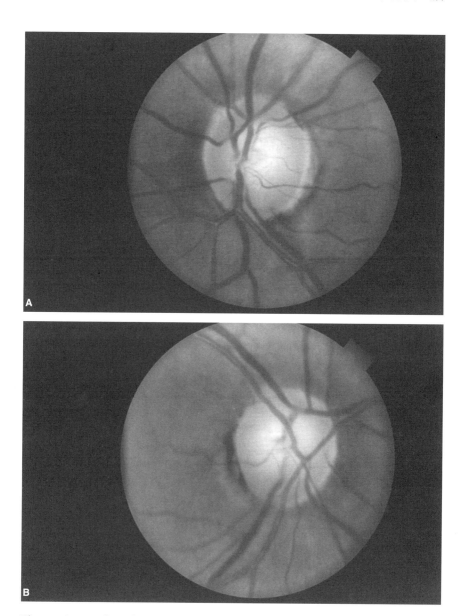

Figure CS7.1 Photodocumentation of glaucomatous optic nerve heads and those suspect for glaucoma is important in monitoring the condition. A. Right eye. B. Left eye.

rior nasal step associated with a mild depression (Figure CS7.2). Thus, the optic nerve findings correlate well with the visual-field findings, verifying optic nerve disease in the left eye. Damage to the right eye is still clinically unproven at this point. An attempt to measure the

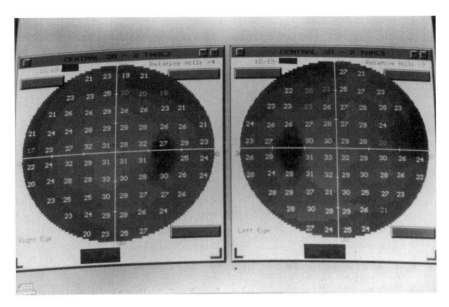

Figure CS7.2 Threshold visual-field testing to 30 degrees shows a mild general depression in the right eye and early superior arcuate defect in the left eye.

afferent system of both optic nerves by the swinging penlight test resulted in a normal finding, which suggests there is currently not a clinically detectable loss of afferent function in the left optic nerve when compared to the right. This finding, is consistent with early glaucoma disease.

Figure CS7.3 shows the results of the contrast sensitivity testing, indicating reduced central visual function in the left eye only. A reduction of contrast at 12 cycles per degree with asymmetry between the eyes lends credibility to the diagnosis of optic nerve disease in the left eye. Traditionally, contrast sensitivity is believed to be helpful only in macular dysfunction or cataracts in which overall depression throughout all cycles per degree is found.

To rule out secondary glaucoma (hypothesis 2), the testing comprised slit-lamp examination and gonioscopy (Table CS7.2). With normal lens, anterior chamber, and gonioscopic findings, no involutional secondary glaucoma was found. Applanation tonometry revealed elevated intraocular pressure (IOP) in both eyes, with a normal diurnal variation. This finding told me that the patient suffers from chronic OAG as opposed to normotensive or low-tension glaucoma.

Both optic nerve dysfunction (hypothesis 3) and retinal abnormalities (hypothesis 4) were ruled out by dilated fundus examination.

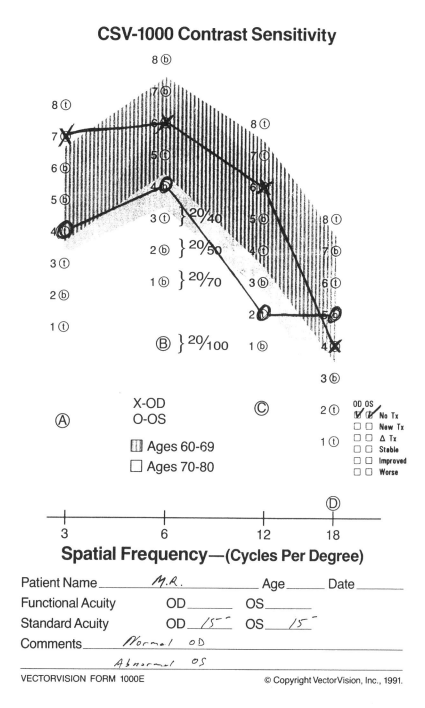

CSV-1000 Contrast Sensitivity

X-OD
O-OS

▥ Ages 60-69
☐ Ages 70-80

	OD	OS	
No Tx	☑	☑	
New Tx	☐	☐	
Δ Tx	☐	☐	
Stable	☐	☐	
Improved	☐	☐	
Worse	☐	☐	

Spatial Frequency—(Cycles Per Degree)

Patient Name _____ M.R. _____ Age _____ Date _____
Functional Acuity   OD _____ OS _____
Standard Acuity   OD _/5⁻⁻_ OS _/5⁻_
Comments _____ Normal OD _____
_____ Abnormal OS _____

VECTORVISION FORM 1000E   © Copyright VectorVision, Inc., 1991.

Figure CS7.3 Contrast sensitivity testing reveals a normal curve in the right eye and depressed overall sensitivity plus a notch at 12 cycles per degree in the left eye.

Table CS7.2
Hypothesis 2 (secondary glaucoma): problem-specific testing results.

Biomicroscopic evaluation
  Normal findings for lids, lashes, conjunctiva, anterior chambers, and
    irides OU
  Crystalline lens: clear OU
  Corneal examination: positive arcus senilis OU
Gonioscopy findings: OD/OS, iris inserted at the ciliary body with a regular
  configuration and an open 30-degree angle, no pigmentation or anomaly
  bilaterally

Congenital anomalies (e.g., optic nerve pit) and acquired anomalies
(e.g., buried drusen of the optic nerve) were ruled out by observation.
Acquired optic nerve disease (e.g., anterior ischemic optic neuropathy)
was ruled out by the lack of pallor in the optic nerve and by the
absence of a relative afferent pupillary defect. A complete evaluation
of the fundus revealed only peripheral cobblestone degeneration. Thus,
presumed ocular histoplasmosis syndrome and other retinal abnormalities were ruled out.

Artifactual visual fields (hypothesis 5) was ruled out by repeat visual-field testing. A full-field, 60-degree screening field could have been
performed to rule out a visual-field defect, yet if numerous points are
missed, a threshold visual field must be performed. The reproducibility of the visual-field defect and the associated optic nerve findings confirmed a true loss in peripheral visual function. Hence, a visual-field
artifact was ruled out.

Because it had been more than 3 years since MR's last eye examination, testing of the following was conducted as baseline:

- Visual acuities
- Refraction
- Near add determination
- Cover test at far and near
- Extraocular muscle function
- Blood pressure

The results of this testing are presented in Table CS7.3.

The patient had good entering visual acuities at far and near with
her habitual prescription. There was a small increase in hyperopia
found on the refraction, with a minor improvement in visual acuity.
There was no change in the add power. Cover test revealed the patient
was nonstrabismic at far and near, with an orthophoria at far and small

Table CS7.3
Additional database testing results.

Habitual spectacle visual acuity
    OD 20/20 at 6 m, 20/20 at 40 cm
    OS 20/20 at 6 m, 20/20 at 40 cm
Spectacle prescription
    OD +2.00 –0.50 × 110 +2.50 add
    OS +2.25 –0.50 × 120 +2.50 add
Subjective-objective refraction and visual acuities
    OD +2.50 –0.75 × 105 (20/15^{-2}) +2.50 add (20/20)
    OS +2.50 –0.25 × 120 (20/15^{-2}) +2.50 add (20/20)
Unilateral cover test: no movement at far and near
Alternate cover test: orthophoria at far, 5Δ exophoria at near
Extraocular muscle testing: normal muscle function, no limitation of gaze
Blood pressure: 140/85 mm Hg with a pulse of 62 bpm

exophoria at near. Extraocular muscle function testing was normal. Blood pressure was within normal limits for her age.

DIAGNOSTIC SUMMARY

MR suffered from primary OAG in the left eye. This has been confirmed by the wasting of neuroretinal rim at the superior and inferior optic nerve head poles in the left eye, with an associated loss of visual function found by visual-field and contrast sensitivity testing. Secondary glaucoma was ruled out by the performance of gonioscopy and a dilated fundus examination. The diagnosis for the right eye remained potential early primary OAG versus high-risk glaucoma suspect on the basis of optic nerve and IOP findings. Again, secondary glaucoma was ruled out in a fashion similar to that used for the left eye. As a result of these findings, the IOP had to be reduced in an attempt to preserve remaining visual function.

MR was found to have compound hyperopic astigmatism with presbyopia. The prescription change was not profound, yet it improved visual acuity. A new prescription was given to her to be filled at her leisure.

Other possible optic nerve dysfunction was ruled out by the observation of normal pupil function, the optic nerve findings, and the resulting visual-field defects. Neither congenital anomalies nor optic nerve disease other than glaucoma were found by dilated fundus examination.

Retinal anomalies were ruled out by dilated fundus examination. There were no retinal lesions or scars that correspond to the visual-field defects revealed by threshold visual-field testing.

An artifactual visual field was ruled out by the reproducibility of visual-field testing. With the corresponding optic nerve findings, OAG was diagnosed.

TREATMENT OPTIONS

According to MR's optic nerve, visual-field, and IOP status, a reduction of IOP to upper teens (20–23%) would be an acceptable goal.[7] Once this goal was accomplished, visual-field and optic nerve parameters had to be monitored to assess potential progression. If progression did occur, a new IOP goal had to be established. If progression did not occur, the current goal would suffice.

Management will best be achieved by topical medication. Because MR appeared to be a motivated individual, a once-daily dose of a noncardioselective beta blocker (0.25% Betagan ophthalmic solution) will be used in only the left eye at bedtime. The drug should work well in controlling her condition, because MR does not suffer from asthma, chronic obstructive pulmonary disease, bradycardia, or hypotension. It is hoped that a contralateral effect will occur as well. Glaucoma is known as a bilateral yet asymmetric condition. A lower IOP may decrease the risk of visual-field damage due to glaucoma in the right eye.[8]

MR will need to return in 6 weeks to determine the status of her IOP and at 3- to 6-month intervals thereafter to determine the status of her optic nerves and visual function. The prognosis of her condition is good in that she has mild disease, possibly bilaterally, without any significant risk factors. Her response to the medications and her longevity will be critical factors in determining the outcome.

REFERENCES

1. Leske MC. The epidemiology of open-angle glaucoma: a review. Am J Epidemiol 1983;118:116–191.
2. Flammer J. The vascular concept of glaucoma. Surv Ophthalmol 1994;38 (suppl):S3–S6.
3. Drance SM. Glaucomatous Visual Field Defects. In R Ritch, MB Shield, T Krupin (eds), The Glaucomas. St. Louis: Mosby, 1989;393–402.
4. Acers TE. Congenital Abnormalities of the Optic Nerve and Related Forebrain. Philadelphia: Lea & Febiger, 1983;27.

5. Alexander LJ. Exudative and Nonexudative Macular Disorders. In Primary Care of the Posterior Segment. Norwalk, CT: Appleton & Lange, 1994;277–344.
6. Burde RM, Savino PJ, Trobe JD. Clinical Decisions in Neuro-Ophthalmology. St. Louis: Mosby, 1985;27–34.
7. Hodapp E, Parrish RK, Anderson DR (eds). Clinical Decisions in Glaucoma. St. Louis: Mosby, 1993;67.
8. Fingeret M, Kowal D. Medical Management in Glaucoma. In TL Lewis, M Fingeret (eds), Primary Care of the Glaucomas. Norwalk, CT: Appleton & Lange, 1993;251–275.

Appendix: Case Scenario 7

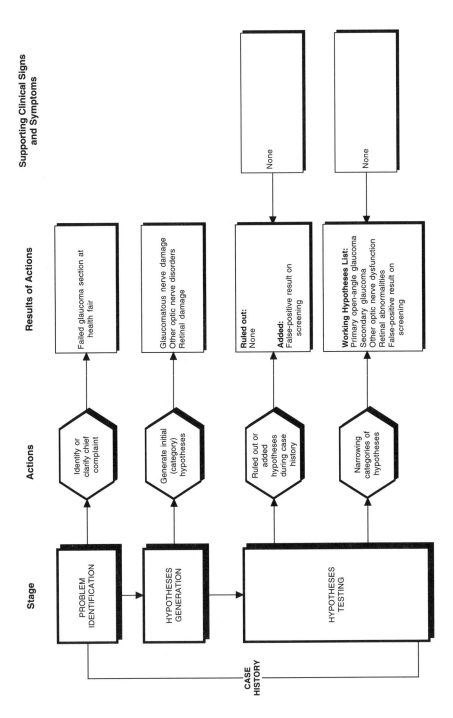

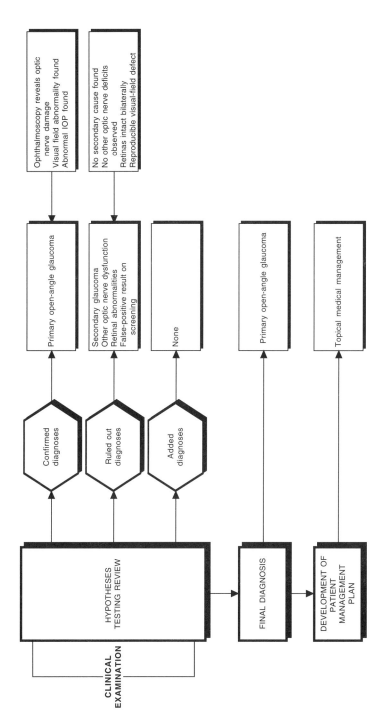

Case Scenario 7 decision-making summary. (IOP = intraocular pressure.)

Case Scenario 8

Carole A. Timpone

PATIENT BACKGROUND

GC is a 62-year-old white woman who wears bifocal spectacles.

DOCTOR: What brings you in for an eye examination today?

PATIENT: About a week ago I noticed a black spot in front of my left eye. I keep blinking to try to get it to go away.

DOCTOR *(thinking): The chief complaint of a black spot in one eye is not consistent with a refractive error problem, which would typically be reported as blurry or fuzzy vision. I'd like to determine whether the spot is a discrete black area in only part of the visual field, which might indicate a floater, or whether a large portion of the field is involved, which might indicate a more significant posterior segment condition, such as a retinal detachment or extensive vascular or optic nerve disease. I also want to verify that the problem is only in the left eye.*

DOCTOR: When you close your left eye and you're looking only with your right eye, does the black spot go away, and is the vision in your right eye clear?

PATIENT: Yes.

DOCTOR: When you close your right eye, can you still see other things clearly besides the spot, or is everything dark?

PATIENT: I can still see you and the things around the room. The spot is there too, off to the left side.

DOCTOR *(thinking): Several possible conditions could result in a noticeably darkened area in the patient's field of vision. There could be a problem in the eye's optical media, most likely in the vitreous (corneal and lenticular opacities or abnormalities usually cause more diffuse blurry or hazy vision). Considering the patient's age and the spot's relatively sudden onset, the most likely cause is a large vitreous floater secondary to a spontaneous posterior vitreal detachment (PVD).[1] By asking specific questions about the spot's appearance, its onset, behavior, and possible associated symptoms, I can determine whether it has those characteristics of a PVD-related vitreal floater.*

DOCTOR: I'd like you to describe the spot more specifically. Does it move or change its location relative to where you are looking, or does it always stay in the same place in your field of vision?

PATIENT: I always see the spot on the left side of what I'm looking at. It doesn't move.

DOCTOR: Is it there all the time?

PATIENT: Yes.

DOCTOR: You said you noticed this for the first time a week ago. Did it appear suddenly?

PATIENT: Yes, all of a sudden one morning I was aware of this dark triangular spot.

DOCTOR: Have you been experiencing any flashes of light or spots that do seem to float by?

PATIENT: I know what floaters are. I've had some for a long time. This is different. I've never had anything like this before. And no, I haven't seen any flashes.

DOCTOR: Has it changed in appearance at all over the last week; is it any larger or smaller; any darker or lighter?

PATIENT: Right when it happened, I lay back down for a while thinking it would pass, but it stayed the same. It may be a little less black now.

DOCTOR *(thinking)*: *This still could represent a relatively immobile vitreal floater secondary to a fresh PVD, although the commonly associated symptomatology, such as spots or floaters that do move and photopsia, which occurs in up to 50% of patients with acute PVD, is not present.*[1, 2] *The patient's age may suggest a cataract, but the localized, well-defined dark area that GC describes is not typical of a cataract. A cataract also is unlikely if the onset were truly rapid.*

The etiology may lie in the retinal tissue (e.g., a hemorrhage secondary to exudative age-related macular degenerative disease, vascular disease, or a retinal tear that is disrupting or blocking the sensory retina). Last, there could be an optic nerve problem (e.g., ischemia or, less likely due to the patient's age, inflammation resulting in a visual-field defect).

Because the patient confirmed the defect to be of acute onset and in only one eye, I must ask specifically about any history of trauma to that eye, which could result in damage to any of the ocular tissues as previously described. Then I'll probe for additional, routinely asked, significant symptoms and ocular and medical history, with particular attention to any vascular disease.

DOCTOR: Have you had any recent injury or surgery to your left eye?

PATIENT: No.

DOCTOR: Is there any pain or discomfort in that eye?

PATIENT: No.

DOCTOR: Are you experiencing any double vision or headaches?

PATIENT: No.

DOCTOR: And when was your last eye examination?

PATIENT: Probably a couple of years ago.

DOCTOR: Were any eye health problems, other than the need for glasses, uncovered at that examination; for example, glaucoma or cataracts?

PATIENT: No, I just got new glasses.

DOCTOR: Is there anyone in your immediate family with any eye conditions other than needing glasses, such as glaucoma, cataracts, or loss of vision?

PATIENT: No, I don't think so.

DOCTOR: I'd like to ask you some questions about your general health. Do you or does anyone in your family have high blood pressure, diabetes, or heart disease?

PATIENT: My aunt—that is, my mother's sister—has diabetes. That's all I know. I'm fine.

DOCTOR: Do you have any other medical or health problems? Are you taking any medications?

PATIENT: I have arthritis. I take Clinoril for that.

DOCTOR: When was your last medical check-up?

PATIENT: About 4 or 5 years ago.

DOCTOR *(thinking)*: *I have sufficient information to begin my examination regarding the chief complaint. New information of note is that she has not had any recent trauma. Also, she has not had a complete medical examination in at least 4 years, so she may be unaware of an existing health problem. There is some family history of diabetes. GC's eye health was reported to be normal 2 years ago. I'll inquire briefly about any more general vision and ocular problems that may be addressed during or after assessment of the chief complaint.*

DOCTOR: Are you seeing well for all your visual needs and your occupation and activities, such as driving, reading, or computer work?

PATIENT: I think I'm seeing okay. I've been reading and sewing without any problems since I got these glasses last time. I'm retired. I do some daycare in my home. Things look clear when I'm driving.

DOCTOR: Is there anything else you'd like to tell me about your eyes or your vision?

PATIENT: Maybe just that my eyes feel gritty and dry sometimes. My last doctor had me scrubbing my eyelids with baby shampoo. It helps, when I do it.

DIAGNOSTIC HYPOTHESES

GC's case history makes possible the following initial list of hypotheses:

1. *Posterior vitreous detachment.* With PVD, sudden-onset floaters, particularly those well-defined and floating in front of the optic nerve, are very common. The vitreous floaters that result can assume a number of shapes, the most classic being a ring-shaped opacity that is the remnant of the adherence of the vitreous face to the optic nerve. Such an opacity located directly anterior to the optic nerve would project into the left visual field of the patient's left eye. GC's age also supports this diagnosis.[1, 2]

2. *Subretinal hemorrhage or exudative serous detachment secondary to age-related macular degeneration.* GC's age is appropriate for this diagnosis.

3. *Preretinal or intraretinal hemorrhage.* Although the patient denies trauma, a spontaneous hemorrhage is possible: secondary to underlying diabetes or vascular disease, in conjunction with a PVD, or secondary to traction on the retina. A branch retinal vein occlusion (BRVO) causing hemorrhage as a result of vascular changes, most likely from undetected hypertension, also could produce GC's symptomatology.

4. *Localized retinal ischemia secondary to vascular occlusive disease.* Arteriolar sclerosis or an actual embolus (Hollenhorst plaque) secondary to carotid artery disease may be present. The fact that the visual-field defect has persisted rather than occurring transiently implies that a total blockage is present.[1]

It should be remembered during retinal evaluation that, if signs of vascular occlusive disease are present (and particularly if an embolus is seen), additional, more specific questions regarding GC's systemic health history should be asked (e.g., regarding symptoms of transient ischemic attacks, history of smoking, or elevated cholesterol or lipid levels). It is believed that, at this time, such inquiry that points to a more serious condition is premature until results of the examination warrant it.

5. *Visual-field defect secondary to optic nerve disease.* This disorder, which would probably be ischemic (considering GC's age), is least likely. The expected visual-field defect would be more altitudinal than temporal to fixation. However, until appropriate diagnostic testing is performed, which should include at least a screening visual field, the exact characterization of the apparent visual-field defect (including verification that it is truly unilateral, and not bilateral but asymmetric) is not yet known.

DIAGNOSTIC TESTING

The diagnostic testing is presented from a clinical decision-making approach. Any of the first four hypotheses could be confirmed or

Table CS8.1
Additional predilation database testing results.

Entering Snellen visual acuities at far and near
   20/20 OD, OS, OU at 6 m
   20/20 OD, OS at 40 cm
Pupil testing: PERRL, –APD
Biomicroscopy: anterior chamber angle estimation, grade IV (van Herick), OU
Tonometry: intraocular pressure 18 mm Hg OD, OS by Goldmann
   applanation

PERRL = pupils equal, round, reactive to light; –APD = no afferent pupillary defect.

ruled out as the definitive diagnosis by careful objective observation during a dilated fundus examination. Before performing this evaluation, it is necessary to collect the following data (presented in Table CS8.1) that would be impossible to collect or inaccurate following mydriasis:

- Entering visual acuities at far and near
- Pupillary reflexes
- Anterior chamber angle estimation by biomicroscopy
- Intraocular pressure

The normal visual acuities obtained with GC's habitual prescription allowed me to omit a pinhole or refraction to best-corrected visual acuities (BVAs). The normal and symmetric pupil reactions, with the absence of an afferent pupillary defect and good visual acuity, suggested that there was no significant optic nerve involvement.

The clinical data to determine whether age-related macular degeneration (hypothesis 2) was the diagnosis for GC's discomfort include:

- BVAs
- Amsler's grid test
- Stereoscopic, high-magnification examination of the maculae

To begin to investigate GC's perceived black spot and further to rule out my second hypothesis of age-related exudative maculopathy, Amsler's grid test was performed immediately following instillation of the mydriatic pharmaceutic agents (1% tropicamide and 2.5% phenylephrine). These data are presented in Table CS8.2. The normal Amsler's grid test results, coupled with the excellent visual acuities, continued to support the absence of macular disease. In addition, this test localizes GC's dark spot beyond 10 degrees from fixation.[1]

The posterior pole and peripheral fundus of each eye were examined with binocular indirect ophthalmoscopy, followed by fundus lens

Table CS8.2
Hypothesis 2 (age-related macular degeneration):
problem-specific testing results.

Best corrected visual acuities: 20/20 OD, OS at both far and near
Amsler's grid test: no darkened, wavy, distorted, or washed-out areas OD, OS
Stereoscopic, high-magnification examination of the macular area: both maculae clear, no evidence of edema, foveal reflexes present

---

biomicroscopy, looking particularly at the vitreous for evidence of a PVD in the left eye to confirm or reject my first hypothesis. The problem-specific clinical data to diagnose a PVD as the cause of a darkened area in the visual field include:

- Direct observation of the vitreous for evidence of a PVD
- Thorough examination of the posterior pole and peripheral fundus
- A screening visual field

Because PVDs are very common in the older population, the mere presence of a PVD-related floater did not confirm it as the etiology of the chief complaint.[2] I also had to rule out my remaining hypotheses by determining that all other findings of the fundus evaluation were normal or noncontributory to the symptomatology. Therefore, the clinical data necessary to test hypotheses 3 and 4 were being collected at the same time (Table CS8.3). The dilated retinal examination revealed a BRVO, with the accompanying vascular signs of arteriovenous nicking at vessel crossings and decreased arteriovenous ratio. The plotted visual-field defect corresponded to the location of the occlusion, GC's description of her spot, and the sectorial appearance of the hemorrhage seen on ophthalmoscopy. These results confirmed the etiology of GC's presenting chief complaint.

BRVO is believed to be the most common retinal vascular condition (after diabetic retinopathy) observed clinically.[3] The significance of a BRVO is its usual implication of underlying systemic disease and its potential for secondary retinal complications. Although BRVO has been associated with cardiovascular disease, diabetes, hyperlipidemia, and hypercholesterolemia, hypertension remains by far the single most important risk factor.[3, 4] Hypertension thus became an additional hypothesis that emerged during my diagnostic testing.

To determine whether there was undiagnosed hypertension, I measured GC's blood pressure, the results of which are presented in Table

Table CS8.3

Hypotheses 1 (posterior vitreal detachment), 3 (preretinal or intraretinal hemor-rhage), and 4 (localized retinal ischemia secondary to vascular occlusive disease): problem-specific testing results.

Dilated fundus examination
   Media: clear, no significant floaters OU
   ONH: distinct margins, healthy rim tissue OU
   Cup-to-disc ratio: 0.2 OU
   Maculae: clear, nonedematous appearance, foveal reflexes present OU
   Vessels: large, diffuse, sectorial nerve fiber–layer hemorrhage at an abnor-mal arteriovenous crossing, with adjacent dilation of associated vein in the inferior nasal quadrant OS, indicating a branch retinal vein occlu-sion; arteriovenous nicking at multiple crossings OU; A/V ratio: 1/2
   Background: clear OU
   Periphery: cystoid degeneration, temporal periphery OU
Central screening visual field: 10-dB localized relative defect, superior tem-poral quadrant OS; OD normal

---

ONH = optic nerve head; A/V = arteriovenous.

Table CS8.4

Additional hypothesis of systemic hypertension: problem-specific testing results.

Integrity of retinal vasculature: hypertensive vascular changes present; arterio-venous nicking and decreased A/V ratio, branch retinal vein occlusion
Blood pressure measurement: 165/110 mm Hg
Additional case history: new history regarding prior history of medically treated hypertension and recent discontinuation of medication

---

A/V = arteriovenous.

CS8.4 along with the other previously collected problem-specific data that support the hypothesis of hypertension. The diagnosis of hyper-tension was confirmed by a reading of 165/110 mm Hg. I explained to GC that her blood pressure was elevated and asked whether she had a history of smoking, which she denied. She then offered for the first time that she had been taking medication for high blood pressure for years but had stopped on her own in the last few years because she felt it was upsetting her stomach.

With these additional pieces of history (the retinal vascular findings and the degree of elevation of her blood pressure), I was convinced of the certainty of the diagnosis of systemic hypertension, without the

Table CS8.5
Additional database testing results.

Lensometry of habitual Rx
    OD −4.25 −3.00 × 013
    OS −4.75 −2.00 × 162
    +2.50 add OU
Cover test at near and far: orthophoric at far, 10Δ exophoria at near
Oculomotor testing: motilities smooth, full, accurate all positions of gaze
Near point of convergence: 5 cm break and 12 cm recovery
Biomicroscopy
    Lids, lashes: 2+ meibomian gland dysfunction, 1+ blepharitis OU
    Conjunctiva, cornea: trace to 1+ inferior corneal punctate staining with
        fluorescein and rose bengal
    Tear film: adequate; tear break-up time, 12 secs OU
    Lens: trace nuclear sclerosis OU

---

need to confirm the measurement on a second visit, as is the usual recommendation with initial measurement of more mild hypertension (diastolic blood pressure 90–104 mm Hg).[5]

Some eye care practitioners perform blood pressure measurements routinely as part of their baseline data collection on adult patients. In fact, because hypertensive individuals typically are asymptomatic and it is estimated that one in five patients who present to an optometrist has hypertension,[6] The Joint National Committee on Detection, Evaluation, and Treatment of High Blood Pressure (1988) recommends that optometrists, as health care providers, measure blood pressure at every patient visit.[5] Recent surveys indicate, however, that most eye care practitioners measure blood pressure in patients with risk factors, such as being overweight, having a family history of hypertension or other vascular disease, or displaying signs of hypertensive retinopathy.[7]

I collected some additional baseline clinical data (all before dilation; Table CS8.5) that were not critical to the evaluation of the chief complaint:

- Lensometry
- Cover test at near and far
- Ocular motilities to evaluate neurologic integrity
- Near point of convergence
- Biomicroscopy of the entire anterior segment. I included examination of the lids and lashes, tear film, and cornea with fluorescein and rose bengal to evaluate GC's minor complaint of gritty, dry eyes

Moderate meibomian gland dysfunction, with mild blepharitis and inferior punctate corneal staining, was observed in both eyes. All other findings were in normal range for the patient's age and lack of related symptomatology.

DIAGNOSTIC SUMMARY

The diagnosis of GC's presenting problem was BRVO, with accompanying hypertensive vascular changes, in the presence of systemic hypertension. A secondary condition of meibomian gland dysfunction with chronic blepharitis was believed to be responsible for her complaint of gritty, dry eyes. These clinical conclusions were made with a high level of diagnostic certainty and correlation to GC's symptoms.

TREATMENT OPTIONS

Treatment for BRVO consists of the following steps:

1. *Diagnosing and treating the underlying systemic disease.* Ideally, patients should have a complete physical examination with BP check, blood glucose testing, lipid profile, and complete blood cell count.[1]
2. *Careful monitoring for macular involvement.* This monitoring was accomplished with Amsler's grid and periodic retinal examination.
3. *Waiting for sufficient resolution of the retinal hemorrhages.* This delay provides time to obtain fluorescein angiograms in cases of suspected macular edema or visual acuity reduced to 20/40 or worse.
4. *Continued careful monitoring for the development of neovascularization at least every 4 months.* Laser photocoagulation is the treatment indicated for both persistent macular edema and secondary neovascularization.[8, 9]

For several reasons, the prognosis for complete resolution of the BRVO without complications was very good in GC's case. Initial visual acuity was 20/40 or better (20/20 in this case); there was no clinical evidence of macular edema; the occlusion was located inferiorly, involving a smaller-caliber vessel and far enough away from the macula to lessen the tendency for the development of macular edema, the cause of vision loss in BRVO; and cotton-wool spots were absent, which implies clinically the nonischemic variety of BRVO and, therefore, less likelihood for the development of subsequent neovascularization. GC was referred to her primary care physician for treatment of her hypertension and a complete physical examination with blood workup. She was given an Amsler's grid to self-monitor her vision and was asked to return for a follow-up examination at 1 month, at which time a complete refraction and binocular vision examination at far and near would also be performed (as it had been 2 years since her last comprehensive vision examination). She would be seen again at 3 months, 6 months, and 1 year following her occlusive episode. She also was advised to resume her lid scrubs and warm compresses for her blepharitis and meibomian glands. GC had complete resolution of her BRVO without neovascular sequelae and experienced successful medical management of her hypertension.

REFERENCES

1. Alexander LJ. Primary Care of the Posterior Segment (2nd ed). Norwalk, CT: Appleton & Lange, 1993.
2. Garston MJ. Light flashes and floaters . . . making a differential diagnosis. Contemp Optom 1988;7(1):19–30.
3. Rath EZ, Frank RN, Shin DH, et al. Risk factors for retinal vein occlusions. A case-control study. Ophthalmology 1992;99:509–514.
4. Risk factors for branch retinal vein occlusion. The Eye Disease Case-Control Study Group. Am J Ophthalmol 1993;116:286–296.
5. Good GW, Augsburger AR. Role of optometrists in combatting high blood pressure. J Am Optom Assoc 1989;60:352–355.
6. Sowka JW. What you can do to manage hypertension. Rev Optom 1994; 131(1):77–84.
7. Harris MG, Gan CM, Revelli EJ, et al. Blood pressure measurement by eye care practitioners. J Am Optom Assoc 1994;65:512–516.
8. Argon laser photocoagulation for macular edema in branch vein occlusion. The Branch Vein Occlusion Study Group. Am J Ophthalmol 1984;98:271–282.
9. Argon laser scatter photocoagulation for prevention of neovascularization and vitreous hemorrhage in branch vein occlusion. A randomized clinical trial. Branch Vein Occlusion Study Group. Arch Ophthalmol 1986;104:34–41.

Appendix: Case Scenario 8

Supporting Clinical Signs and Symptoms

No history of ocular trauma

Sudden nature and onset
Persistent in character

Results of Actions

Black spot is seen out of left eye

Posterior segment disease;
postvitreal or retinal
detachment
Media opacity
Vascular or optic nerve disease

Ruled out:
Trauma-related cause

Added:
Dry eye

Working Hypotheses List:
PVD
Subretinal hemorrhage or
exudative serous detach-
ment secondary to ARMD
Pre- or intraretinal hemorrhage
Localized retinal ischemia
Visual-field defect secondary to
optic nerve disease

Actions

Identify or
clarify chief
complaint

Generate initial
(category)
hypotheses

Ruled out or
added
hypotheses
during case
history

Narrowing
categories of
hypotheses

Stage

PROBLEM
IDENTIFICATION

HYPOTHESES
GENERATION

HYPOTHESES
TESTING

CASE
HISTORY

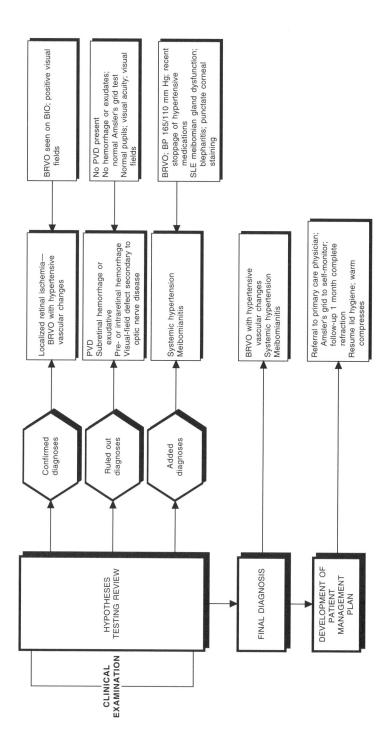

Case Scenario 8 decision-making summary. (PVD = posterior vitreous detachment; ARMD = age-related macular degeneration; BIO = binocular indirect ophthalmoscopy; BP = blood pressure; SLE = slit-lamp examination; BRVO = branch retinal vein occlusion.)

Case Scenario 9

Timothy B. Edrington

PATIENT BACKGROUND

KA is a 23-year-old male graduate student majoring in business administration.

DOCTOR: Are you having any problems with your vision or eyes?

PATIENT: Yes, my vision isn't clear. The blackboard at school is blurry, and it's becoming more difficult to see my homework clearly. I no longer see well through the glasses I received 9 months ago, and my left eye seems more blurred than my right eye.

DOCTOR *(thinking)*: *The chief complaint is blurred vision at distance and near. On the basis of the entering complaint, the patient's refractive error probably has changed over the past 9 months. If the patient is myopic and there has been an increase in refractive error, I also have to be concerned about accommodative or binocular problems because of the near complaints through his spectacle prescription. If the patient is hyperopic and testing reveals an increase in refractive error, my concerns regarding visual efficiency will be reduced, but I'll still investigate fully the accommodative and convergence systems. Another refractive error possibility is a change in astigmatism. A change in astigmatic amount or orientation could lead to symptoms of distance and near blur.*

DOCTOR: At the time your spectacles were dispensed 9 months ago, was your vision clear through your new glasses?

PATIENT: Yes, better than it is now, but I've noticed that even with new glasses, my vision seems better on some days than others. My vision has been this way for the past 5 years. I've had to have my glasses changed each year. Recently, even that doesn't seem to make my vision that much clearer.

DOCTOR *(thinking)*: *The comment about new spectacles not adequately correcting his vision diminishes the likelihood that KA's past symptoms are due simply to myopic or astigmatic refractive changes, because one would expect him to report that his vision is clear through a new spectacle prescription that simply incorporated increases in minus power or changes in cylinder correction. Hyperopia and accommodative problems still exist as possible causes of the patient's symptoms and the fluctuating quality of his vision. Another possibility for fluctuating spectacle vision is "spectacle blur" induced by rigid contact lens wear.*

DOCTOR: Have you ever worn contact lenses?

PATIENT: No.

DOCTOR *(thinking):* *To complete my understanding of the patient's case and collect database information, I'll investigate the patient's personal and family eye and medical histories.*

DOCTOR: Have you experienced any eye injuries or eye diseases?

PATIENT: No.

DOCTOR: Is there any family history of eye disease, such as glaucoma or cataracts?

PATIENT: My grandfather had cataracts when he was in his eighties. Otherwise, no.

DOCTOR: How is your general health?

PATIENT: Good, I had a physical 6 months ago. The doctor gave me a clean bill of health.

DOCTOR: Are there any health problems in your family?

PATIENT: My father has high blood pressure and takes medication for it. My blood pressure was normal at my physical.

DOCTOR *(thinking):* *This information reduces my suspicion that the patient's reduced, fluctuating vision is caused by an ocular or systemic disease, such as diabetes. I'll still perform a routine ocular health examination including a dilated fundus examination and visual-field screening.*

DIAGNOSTIC HYPOTHESES

On the basis of KA's case history, the initial hypothesis list is as follows:

1. *Uncorrected refractive error.* A spectacle prescription change probably is necessary, and testing will be performed to update the patient's refraction. However, the symptom of fluctuating vision probably is not due to refractive error change alone.

2. *Accommodative anomaly.* KA could have an accommodative anomaly contributing to the symptom of fluctuating vision.

3. *Irregular astigmatism.* Keratoconus is a possibility because of the history of several pairs of spectacles and the fluctuating vision over the past 5 years. Also, the patient reports that one eye is more affected than the other. Keratoconus generally presents as an asymmetric disease. Also, the age of the patient is consistent with the onset or initial presentation of keratoconus.[1] If keratoconus is diagnosed, his prescription probably will increase in minus. A change in the amount of astigmatism, as well as its orientation, also is likely to occur.

Table CS9.1
Hypothesis 1 (uncorrected refractive error): problem-specific testing results.

Habitual spectacle prescription
    OD −1.00 −0.50 × 090
    OS −2.75 −1.50 × 085
Distance visual acuities through habitual spectacle Rx
    OD 20/25
    OS 20/50
Near visual acuities through habitual spectacle Rx
    OD 20/20⁻
    OS 20/30
Static (retinoscopy) refraction
    OD −1.00 −1.25 × 095
    OS −3.75 −2.75 × 075
Subjective refraction and visual acuities
    OD −1.25 −0.75 × 100 (20/20⁻)
    OS −3.25 −2.50 × 073 (20/25)

DIAGNOSTIC TESTING

The diagnostic testing is presented in a decision-making format, not necessarily in the order in which the examination should be sequenced. To arrive at the definitive diagnosis, the clinical data to either confirm or deny the most likely hypotheses regarding KA's symptoms were gathered.

To explore hypothesis 1 (uncorrected refractive error), I collected problem-specific clinical data (Table CS9.1) that included:

- Habitual spectacle prescription analysis
- Entering visual acuities at distance and near through habitual spectacle prescription
- Static refraction (retinoscopy)
- Subjective refraction with visual acuities

The reduced visual acuity obtained at both distance and near through the subjective refraction were indicative of the presence of ocular disease. The cornea, crystalline lens, media, and fundus had to be examined to determine the cause of the reduction in visual acuity.

The testing presented in Table CS9.2 was performed to investigate hypothesis 2 (accommodative anomaly). Accommodative testing fell within normative clinical standards for a patient of KA's age.

To explore hypothesis 3 (keratoconus), I collected the following problem-specific clinical data:

Table CS9.2
Hypothesis 2 (accommodative anomaly): problem-specific testing results.

Accommodative amplitude
  10 D OD, OS
Accommodative accuracy (lag)
  +0.75 D OD, OS
Accommodative facility
  12 cpm OD, OS
  9 cpm OU
Negative/positive relative accommodation: +2.25 D/–2.75 D

Table CS9.3
Hypothesis 3 (irregular astigmatism–keratoconus):
problem-specific testing results.

Keratometry readings
  OD 43.75 @ 128, 45.25 @ 038 1$^+$ mire distortion
  OS 44.75 @ 057, 47.12 @ 167 2$^+$ mire distortion
Static (retinoscopy) refraction
  OD –1.00 –1.25 × 095 0$^+$ reflex distortion
  OS –3.75 –2.75 × 075 1$^+$ reflex distortion (irregular scissors motion)
Subjective refraction and visual acuities
  OD –1.25 –0.75 × 100 (20/20$^-$)
  OS –3.25 –2.50 × 073 (20/25)
Biomicroscopy
  OD subtle partial (arc) Fleischer's ring, otherwise cornea clear
  OS partial (arc) Fleischer's ring; Vogt's striae

- Keratometry readings (including mire image quality)
- Static refraction (retinoscopy) including reflex clarity
- Subjective refraction with visual acuities
- Slit-lamp biomicroscopy

The clinical data are presented in Table CS9.3.

The problem-specific testing revealed data consistent with the diagnosis of keratoconus. The change in refractive error was consistent with the progression of keratoconus. As the disease becomes more advanced, the sphere and the cylindrical component of the refraction generally increase in minus and the cylinder axis is variable. This variability in refractive error can occur from one visit to the next, and the variability tends to increase as the disease progresses. KA's left cornea exhibit-

Table CS9.4
Additional database testing results.

Pupil testing: PERRLA, –APD
Oculomotor testing
　No restrictions of gaze
　Pursuits: 3+ (SCCO rating scale)
　Saccades: 3+ (SCCO rating scale)
Phorometry
　Distance phoria: 1Δ XP
　Distance negative fusional vergence: 8/4
　Distance positive fusional vergence: 10/18/10
　Near phoria: 3Δ XP
　Near negative fusional vergence: 14/22/14
　Near positive fusional vergence: 16/20/12
Tonometry (Goldmann): 10 mm Hg OD and 8 mm Hg OS at 3:00 AM
Screening visual field: no misses OD, OS
Dilated fundus examination:
　Media: clear OU
　ONH: margins distinct OU; rim pink and healthy OU
　Cup-to-disc ratio: 0.3/0.3 OU
　Vessels: A/V ratio 4/5 with normal crossings OU
　Macula: homogeneous OU
　Retina background: homogeneous OU
　Retina periphery: no holes, tears, flat 360 degrees OU

PERRLA = pupils equal, round, reactive to light and accommodation; –APD = no afferent pupillary defect; SCCO = Southern California College of Optometry; XP = exophoria; ONH = optic nerve head; A/V = arteriovenous.

ed moderate keratoconus, whereas his right cornea would be classified as mild keratoconus, due to its lesser degree of progression at this time. Keratoconus is typically an asymmetric disease, with one cornea more affected or advanced in presentation. The Collaborative Longitudinal Evaluation in Keratoconus study group defines keratoconus in a working diagnostic context as an eye exhibiting distortion (as measured by keratometric mire, videokeratographic map, or retinoscopic or ophthalmoscopic reflex) combined with either a biomicroscopic sign of Fleischer's ring or Vogt's striae.[2] The diagnosis of keratoconus has been confirmed on the basis of clinical evidence of corneal distortion, positive biomicroscopic signs, and refractive error changes.

Additional baseline or database information collected (Table CS9.4) included:

- Pupil testing
- Oculomotor testing
- Phorometry

- Tonometry
- Visual fields
- Dilated fundus examination

This testing revealed no additional clinical problems, as all obtained values fell within normative standards for a patient of KA's age. Of interest, relative to the diagnosis of keratoconus, are the relatively low intraocular pressures, commonly seen in patients with keratoconus.

DIAGNOSTIC SUMMARY

The diagnosis of keratoconus was confirmed by the presence of corneal distortion and positive slit-lamp biomicroscopy signs. Corneal distortion can be confirmed by eliciting keratometry mire, retinoscopic reflex, or ophthalmoscopic reflex distortion. KA's keratometry mires and retinoscopic reflexes showed distortion (greater in the left eye than in the right eye). Keratometric mire distortion is more pathognomonic of keratoconus than steep or highly toric keratometry readings. Many keratoconus patients have normal keratometry values. Corneal topography changes consistent with the diagnosis of keratoconus also can be demonstrated by mapping the corneal contour with a videokeratoscope. Fleischer's rings (an iron deposition in the cornea) and striae (corneal folds) were present on biomicroscopy. These slit-lamp signs along with corneal thinning (viewed by optic section) are pathognomonic of keratoconus.[1]

Frequent refractive error changes, especially increased minus in the sphere and cylinder components, are common with keratoconus patients. KA's refractive changes occurring over a 9-month period are typical for mild presentations of the disease. Best-corrected visual acuity and contrast sensitivity measurements decrease as the disease progresses. These visual acuity changes generally are asymmetric in their presentation (i.e., one eye leads the other in terms of progression). KA's keratoconus was more advanced in his left cornea, as evidenced by keratometry values and mire quality, retinoscopy reflex distortion (irregular, scissors motion), best spectacle-corrected visual acuity, and degree of biomicroscopic signs.

TREATMENT OPTIONS

Mild presentations of keratoconus can be managed optically by spectacles or soft toric contact lenses. The patient decides, on the basis of counseling provided by the eye care practitioner, when spectacle corrected vision is unacceptable for vocational or avocational needs. When corneal distortion produces unacceptable vision, rigid gas-permeable contact lens management should be initiated. (I fit rigid lenses to provide optimal optical correction, not to retard the progression of keratoconus.) Many contact lens–fitting strategies have been proposed and are described in the literature.[3–7] I recommend that he be fitted with rigid gas-permeable contact lenses at this time.

REFERENCES

1. Zadnik K, Edrington TB. Keratoconus. In JA Silbert (ed), Anterior Segment Complications of Contact Lens Wear. New York: Churchill Livingstone, 1994;367–377.
2. Zadnik K, Barr JT, Gordon MO, et al. Biomicroscopic signs and disease severity in keratoconus. Cornea 1996;15:139–146.
3. Soper JW, Jarrett A. Results of a systematic approach to fitting keratoconus and corneal transplants. Contact Lens Med Bull 1972;5:50–59.
4. Caroline PJ, McGuire JR, Doughman DJ. Preliminary report on a new contact lens design for keratoconus. Contact Intraocul Lens Med J 1978;4(3):69–73.
5. Korb DR, Finnemore VM, Herman JP. Apical changes and scarring in keratoconus as related to contact lens fitting techniques. J Am Optom Assoc 1982;53:199–205.
6. Burger D, Barr JT. Effects of Contact Lenses in Keratoconus. In JS Silbert (ed), Anterior Segment Complications of Contact Lens Wear. New York: Churchill Livingstone, 1994;379–399.
7. Edrington TB, Barr JT, Zadnik K, et al. Standardized rigid contact lens fitting protocol for keratoconus. Optom Vis Sci 1996;73:369–375.

Appendix: Case Scenario 9

Stage

Actions

Results of Actions

Supporting Clinical Signs and Symptoms

PROBLEM IDENTIFICATION → Identify or clarify chief complaint → Vision is blurred at distance and near

HYPOTHESES GENERATION → Generate initial (category) hypotheses → Refractive error change / Accommodative anomaly

HYPOTHESES TESTING → Ruled out or added hypotheses during case history →
Ruled out: "Spectacle blur" from contact lens wear
Added: None
← No contact lens wear

→ Narrowing categories of hypotheses →
Working Hypotheses List: Uncorrected refractive error / Accommodative anomaly / Irregular astigmatism
← Blur at distance and near / Fluctuating vision / Several pairs of spectacles / One eye more affected / Age of patient

CASE HISTORY

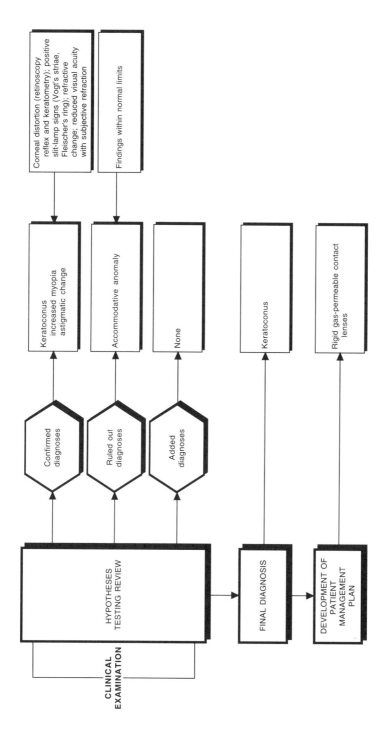

Case Scenario 9 decision-making summary.

Case Scenario 10

Kia B. Eldred

PATIENT BACKGROUND

IC is a 76-year-old white woman accompanied to the optometric examination by her daughter-in-law.

DOCTOR: What brings you in for an examination today?

PATIENT: I'm beginning to have difficulty with knitting and needlepoint and reading the patterns. I also have a slight problem seeing the television, especially the words.

DOCTOR *(thinking)*: *This patient's chief complaint is difficulty in seeing print, needlepoint, and knitting and some difficulty seeing print on the TV. Considering the visual complaint, the possible causes of difficulty with these tasks are numerous. It could be as simple as a change in refractive error, or the cause could be a pathologic condition. It would be best to determine the duration of the problem and the length of time since her previous eye examination. If it occurred suddenly, it is less likely to be a refractive problem and more likely an ocular pathology.*

DOCTOR: How long have you noticed this difficulty with reading, knitting, and needlepoint?

PATIENT: I noticed it about 2 weeks ago.

DOCTOR: Does the problem start as soon as you begin reading, or does it occur after some time?

PATIENT: The words are blurry as soon as I look at them.

DOCTOR: How long has it been since your last eye examination, and what were you told about your eyes at that time?

PATIENT: My last eye exam was about 1½ years ago, and they told me my eyes looked pretty good considering my age.

DOCTOR: Did you purchase new glasses at that time?

PATIENT: I did buy new glasses shortly after that.

DOCTOR: When the change in vision occurred, was it a slowly progressive change or a sudden change?

PATIENT: It seemed to have occurred overnight.

DOCTOR *(thinking)*: *The sudden onset of vision change would support the idea of a pathologic condition versus a refractive problem. The problem could occur in several different structures. The cornea, the lens, the optic nerve, or the retina could be affected. She could have a cataract, but a sud-*

den onset of vision loss is unlikely with a cataract. An optic nerve disorder is a possibility and so is a retinal pathology. I should determine whether she has had any type of ocular surgery and get more information about the reading problem.

DOCTOR: Have you had any type of eye surgery or injury?

PATIENT: No.

DOCTOR: Do you have any pain in your eyes? Do you have any problems with bright light indoors or outdoors?

PATIENT: I have no pain in my eyes. Bright light helps indoors but causes too much glare outdoors.

DOCTOR: When you're reading, is the whole page blurry, or do the words come and go or seem to move around?

PATIENT: The words do seem to come in and out of focus, but the whole page does not seem blurry. My eyes feel strained after reading for about 15 minutes.

DOCTOR: Does anything make it easier to read?

PATIENT: If I use a bright light next to my chair, it seems to make the print easier to see. When I sit by the window, sunlight is very helpful when I read.

DOCTOR *(thinking)*: *It now seems to be more likely an optic nerve or retinal disorder, due to the lack of any problems with pain, photophobia, or glare and the fact that there is a specific area that's blurry when she is reading.[1] I should find out more about her general health and medications she is taking to determine whether there's a link with her systemic health.*

DOCTOR: How would you say your general health is?

PATIENT: Good.

DOCTOR: Do you have any systemic disease, such as diabetes?

PATIENT: Yes, I was diagnosed with diabetes 16 years ago, and I take Glucatrol to control it.

DOCTOR: Do you have high blood pressure?

PATIENT: Yes, I was diagnosed with it at the same time they found the diabetes. I take Lopress and Dyazide to control it.

DOCTOR: Do you have any heart disease, cancer, or thyroid problems?

PATIENT: No.

DOCTOR: Are you taking any other medications?

PATIENT: Only multivitamins.

DOCTOR *(thinking)*: *Now there are several possibilities that could be considered, including wet macular degeneration, macular hole, diabetic macular edema, anterior ischemic optic neuropathy, or diabetic macular edema. I should continue to look for any other health risks based on her current health status and her family history.*

DOCTOR: When was your last visit with your physician?

PATIENT: Two months ago.

DOCTOR: What did he or she say about your high blood pressure and blood sugar level at that time?

PATIENT: He said my blood pressure and blood sugar level were very good.

DOCTOR: In your family, is there a history of cancer, heart disease, or thyroid disease?

PATIENT: No.

DOCTOR: Is there a history of cataracts, glaucoma, or retinal problems in your family?

PATIENT: Not that I know of.

DOCTOR (thinking): *It appears that IC has the diabetes and hypertension well controlled and there is no family history of ocular pathology. I'll complete my history by asking a few more questions.*

DOCTOR: Do you have any allergies?

PATIENT: No, I don't have any allergies.

DOCTOR: Do you see any flashes or small floating dots when looking at a blank wall or at the sky?

PATIENT: Well, I don't see any flashes. I do see those dots occasionally, but they don't bother me.

DIAGNOSTIC HYPOTHESES

On the basis of IC's case history, the list of initial hypotheses points to retinal involvement and includes the following disorders:

1. *Diabetic macular edema.* This is possible because of IC's 16-year history of diabetes.

2. *Macular hole.* This macular defect may be indicated because of the sudden onset of reading problems.

3. *Atrophic macular degeneration.* Though not a strong possibility because of the sudden onset, wet macular degeneration (possibly subretinal neovascularization) is a more likely possibility.

4. *Anterior ischemic optic neuropathy.* This disorder is considered because of the patient's age, sudden vision loss, the diagnosis of hypertension, and diabetes. If there were a problem involving the optic nerve, it could manifest as decreased visual acuity and impaired reading ability.

5. *Change in refractive error or inappropriate correction for presbyopia.* Though possible, it is fairly unlikely because of IC's response that there was a sudden onset of decreased vision and her observation that words came in and out of focus.

6. *Cataract.* This condition also would be an unlikely diagnosis because of the rapid onset and the comment that the whole page was not blurry.

Table CS10.1
Hypothesis 5 (change in refractive error or inappropriate correction for presbyopia): problem-specific testing results.

Entering visual acuities at distance and near
   20/60 OD, 20/30 OS, 20/30 OU at 6 m
   20/100 OD, 20/40 OS, 20/50 OU at 40 cm
Static refraction-retinoscopy
   OD +1.25 −0.25 × 110
   OS +1.25 −0.25 × 085
Subjective refraction and visual acuities
   OD +1.25 −0.25 × 110 (20/60)
   OS +1.50 −0.25 × 085 (20/30)
   +2.50 D age-appropriate bifocal power showed no improvement in near
     visual acuities
Previous prescription
   OD +1.25 DS
   OS +1.25 −0.25 × 090
   +2.25 D add OU

DS = diopter sphere.

DIAGNOSTIC TESTING

The diagnostic testing is presented in the format of a decision-making sequence, not necessarily the order of the examination. To arrive at the definitive diagnosis, I started with the tests that would yield the most information and eliminate the most possibilities. Then I continued through the examination to the tests that could confirm my diagnosis.

To rule out the less likely causes of change stated in diagnostic hypotheses 5 (uncorrected refractive error or inappropriate near add power) and 6 (cataract), I collected the following problem-specific clinical data (Table CS10.1):

- Entering visual acuities at distance and near
- Objective refraction (retinoscopy) with visual acuities
- Subjective refraction with visual acuities
- Comparison of previous prescription and subjective refraction

The reduced visual acuities confirm the patient's entering complaint of reduced vision greater at near than at distance. The patient had a compound hyperopic refractive error in both eyes. When the previous prescription and the subjective refraction are compared, there is no improvement in visual acuity and little difference in the prescriptions. This finding would rule out a refractive change as a cause of decreased

Table CS10.2
Additional baseline testing results.

Binocular vision testing
    Cover test: far, orthophoria; near (with +2.50 add), 10Δ exophoria
    Phorometry:
        von Graefe phoria at far 1Δ exophoria, at near (with
            +2.50 add) 10Δ exophoria
        Negative fusional convergence at near x/20/14
        Positive fusional convergence at near x/22/12
Assessment of bifocal power (to assist with reading)
    Plus build-up +3.00 D 0.30/0.5 M (0.5-M letter read at 30 cm or 0.3 m)
        with subjective improvement in reading
Intraocular pressure
    Goldmann pressures at 11:15 AM
    OD 16 mm Hg
    OS 17 mm Hg

M = meter letter size for Snellen notation.

visual acuity. The near add power for her age is slightly less than that expected, but no significant improvement was found with a +2.50 D add power. This result ruled out the possibility that an inappropriate correction for her presbyopia was the cause of her decreased visual acuity at near. Later, when I understood the cause of the reduced visual acuity, I attempted to see whether additional magnification at near could improve her visual acuity at near (Table CS10.2). The possibility of a cataract was less likely, as lens changes induce shifts in refractive error toward myopia in most cases.

To further rule out initial hypothesis 6 (cataract), I collected problem-specific clinical data from a biomicroscopic examination (Table CS10.3). Only mild lens changes were apparent in the examination, which would not account for the reduced acuity in either eye. The other structures were intact and would not contribute to the patient's symptoms.

To determine whether the retinal pathologies (diagnostic hypothesis 1, 2, or 3) or the anterior ischemic optic neuropathy (diagnostic hypothesis 4) are the cause of the reduced vision, I completed the following tests (Table CS10.4):

- Pupillary response
- Extraocular movements
- Amsler's grid test
- Confrontation fields
- Red cap test
- Photostress test

Table CS10.3
Hypothesis 6 (cataract): biomicroscopic examination;
problem-specific testing results.

Lids and lashes: no flakes, dermatochalasis present OU
Conjunctiva: 1+ follicles inferior palpebral conjunctiva, otherwise clear OU
Cornea: arcus senilis 360 degrees, otherwise clear OU
Anterior chamber: deep, quiet OU
Iris: blue, evenly pigmented OU
Lens: OD brunescence 2, nuclear sclerosis 1+, OS brunescence 2, nuclear
    sclerosis 1+

Table CS10.4
Hypotheses 1–4 (differentiating optic nerve or retinal disorder):
problem-specific testing results.

Pupillary testing
    PERRL, –APD
Extraocular muscles: full range of motion, no pain or diplopia
Amsler's grid test
    OD: 2-degree area of metamorphopsia 1 degree nasal to central fixation
        point
    OS: no metamorphopsia or scotoma
Confrontation fields: full in each eye
Red cap test: equal color and saturation in each eye
Photostress test
    OD: recovery time 80 secs
    OS: recovery time 60 secs

PERRL = pupils equal, round, reactive to light; –APD = no afferent pupillary defect.

No afferent pupillary defect was present, and the pupils were
responsive to direct and consensual light. This suggests that the optic
nerve was functioning normally. The extraocular muscle movements
showed no sign of restriction or pain on testing. Amsler's grid test did
reveal a 2-degree area of metamorphopsia in the right eye, 1 degree
nasal to the central fixation point. This finding of metamorphopsia
directed me more toward a macular edema hypothesis than to optic
nerve involvement.[2] Confrontation fields showed full peripheral fields
confirming the presence of only a central visual-field defect. The red
cap test was negative, indicating no difference in color perception in
each eye; therefore, the vision decrease is more likely a macular problem than an optic nerve disorder. The photostress test was positive for

Table CS10.5
Hypotheses 1–3 (retinal pathology): problem-specific testing results.

Blood pressure: 140/80 mm Hg
Computerized visual fields—Humphrey's 10-2
    OD: depression in the central 6 degrees
    OS: depression in the central 3 degrees
Dilated fundus examination with a biomicroscope and 78 D lens
    OD: macular thickening, several soft white drusen or choroidal infiltrates
        overlying the macula, appear confluent; a few calcified drusen present
    OS: soft drusen, early depigmentation of overlying pigment epithelium
    OU: vasculature of normal caliber; cup-to-disc ratios of 0.3/0.3, good disc
        color, even disc margins
Dilated fundus examination with binocular indirect ophthalmoscopy: OU
    biomicroscopic examination confirmed; normal blonde peripheral fundus,
    no holes, tears, flat 360 degrees OU
Fundus photographs: taken for baseline

a prolonged recovery time, being greater in the right eye than in the left eye. This also suggests a macular pathology.[3]

The following clinical data are the final rule-out for possible macular pathologies. These tests were completed to determine and document the type of macular pathology present and the level of involvement, so that appropriate management could be instituted.

- Blood pressure
- Computerized visual fields
- Dilated fundus examination with a 78 D lens biomicroscopic evaluation
- Dilated fundus examination with binocular indirect ophthalmoscopy
- Fundus photographs

The clinical data from these tests are presented in Table CS10.5.

Blood pressure was measured as 140/80 mm Hg. Humphrey visual fields 10-2 revealed a 10-dB relative depression in the central field of the right eye and no depression in the left field, which appears to be consistent with the Amsler's grid findings. The biomicroscopic examination of the right macula with the 78 D lens revealed an apparent macular thickening, most likely due to fluid. There were several soft white drusen or choroidal infiltrates overlying the macula, which appeared to be confluent. Among the confluent drusen were a few smaller calcified drusen. In the left eye, soft drusen were present with early depigmentation of overlying pigment epithelium. I also noted an arteriovenous ratio of 2/3 and no abnormal crossing changes. A 0.3/0.3 cup-to-disc ratio was present in each eye, with good color of the disc and even disc margins. The binocular indirect ophthalmoscopy examination confirmed these results, and no holes, tears, or degenerations were noted. Fundus photographs were taken as part of the baseline information and for further comparison.

At this point, I felt that I had sufficient problem-specific data to arrive at a tentative diagnosis to account for the patient's entering signs and symptoms. The tentative diagnosis at this time appeared to be subretinal neovascularization (wet maculopathy) in the right eye and atrophic age-related maculopathy (dry) in the left eye, based on the fundus appearance. Diabetic macular edema and macular hole were ruled out because of the absence of hard exudates, dot-blot hemorrhages, and macular hole on fundus evaluation.

I also collected some information as database and baseline information (see Table CS10.5):

- Binocular vision testing with cover test and phorometry at distance and near
- Assessment of bifocal power to assist with reading
- Intraocular pressure

This testing revealed normal binocular findings, a +3.00 D reading add gave adequate near vision, and intraocular pressures were normal in both eyes.

DIAGNOSTIC SUMMARY

IC was found to have possible subretinal neovascularization in the right eye and atrophic age-related maculopathy in the left eye. These findings correlated highly with IC's entering complaint of difficulty in reading, eye strain after 15 minutes of reading, and improvement with bright illumination.[1, 4] To refine our diagnosis, a fluorescein or indocyanine green angiogram is indicated.[2] The patient was referred to a retinal specialist's office immediately, and fluorescein angiography was completed the following day. The results indicated late venous-stage hyperfluorescence caused by intense leakage of dye from a subretinal neovascular network located outside the fovea (confirming my tentative diagnosis of subretinal neovascularization in the right eye). The results also indicated early venous-stage hypofluorescence caused by pigment clumps and hyperfluorescence caused by depigmentation and drusen in the left eye (also confirming my tentative diagnosis of atrophic age-related maculopathy).

TREATMENT OPTIONS

The patient was treated at the retinal specialist's office with argon blue-green laser photocoagulation 24 hours after the detection of the neo-vascular network.[5] The patient was referred back to our office for follow-up and for assistance with her main complaint of reading. I advised her that her vision would be reduced for 1–2 months following the laser treatment but should stabilize at that point. We discussed the use of magnifiers and spectacles. She preferred spectacles because of her knitting and needlepoint and the ease of looking at patterns and then doing the handwork. I noted that she was right-handed and suspected she also was right-eye dominant prior to her decreased vision in that eye. She agreed that was why she was having so much difficulty in reading, even though the left eye acuity was relatively good at near. Patients with a decreased level of acuity in their dominant eye and a better visual acuity in their nondominant eye can experience some difficulty in adapting to use of the nondominant eye initially. We agreed on a +3.00 D reading add for near, with occlusion of the right eye for reading until her vision stabilized and we could determine whether she could use her eyes binocularly. I also advised a high-intensity reading lamp at all times to assist her with her near work.[4] She was to return to train with the new bifocals after she received them so that I could ensure comfort and proper use of the lens regarding working distance and illumination. I suggested that she return again 1 month after dispensing to assess the progress of the vision in her right eye after the laser treatment. She also would be returning to the retinal specialist for progress visits. She was instructed to use an Amsler's grid on a daily basis to monitor her vision and to call our office immediately if she noted any change. I also discussed nutritional supplements with her and the use of the prepared over-the-counter vitamins specifically for ocular nutrition. I counseled her that a definite answer was not yet available on their efficacy and that a diet including fruits and vegetables was very important.[6] I also recommended the use of ultraviolet coatings in all her spectacles, and for outdoors she purchased a NoIR amber lens (NoIR Medical Technologies, South Lyon, Michigan) with 10% transmission.[7]

REFERENCES

1. Faye E. Clinical Low Vision. Boston: Little, Brown, 1984;171–196.
2. Alexander L. Primary Care of the Posterior Segment. Norwalk, CT: Appleton & Lange, 1989;165–174.

3. Lovie-Kitchin JE, Bowman KJ. Senile Macular Degeneration: Management and Rehabilitation. Boston: Butterworth, 1985;57–77.
4. Eldred KB. Optimal illumination for reading in patients with age-related maculopathy. Optom Vis Sci 1992;69:46–50.
5. Macular Photocoagulation Study Group. Argon laser photocoagulation for neovascular maculopathy. Three-year results from randomized clinical trials. Arch Ophthalmol 1986;104:694–701.
6. Kaminski MS, Yolton DP, Jordan WT, et al. Evaluation of dietary antioxidant levels and supplementation with ICAPS-Plus and Ocuvite. J Am Optom Assoc 1993;64:862–870.
7. Rosenberg R. Light, Glare, and Contrast in Low Vision Care. In E Faye (ed), Clinical Low Vision. Boston: Little, Brown, 1984;197–212.

Appendix: Case Scenario 10

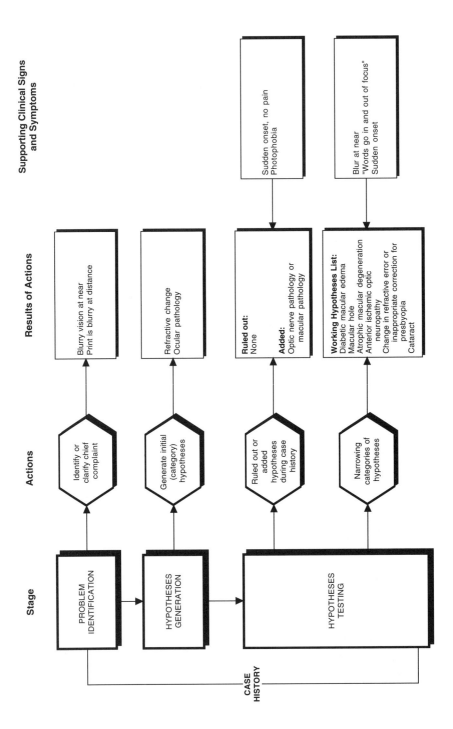

Supporting Clinical Signs and Symptoms

Results of Actions

Actions

Stage

Sudden onset, no pain
Photophobia

Blur at near
"Words go in and out of focus"
Sudden onset

Blurry vision at near
Print is blurry at distance

Refractive change
Ocular pathology

Ruled out:
None

Added:
Optic nerve pathology or macular pathology

Working Hypotheses List:
Diabetic macular edema
Macular hole
Atrophic macular degeneration
Anterior ischemic optic neuropathy
Change in refractive error or inappropriate correction for presbyopia
Cataract

Identify or clarify chief complaint

Generate initial (category) hypotheses

Ruled out or added hypotheses during case history

Narrowing categories of hypotheses

PROBLEM IDENTIFICATION

HYPOTHESES GENERATION

HYPOTHESES TESTING

CASE HISTORY

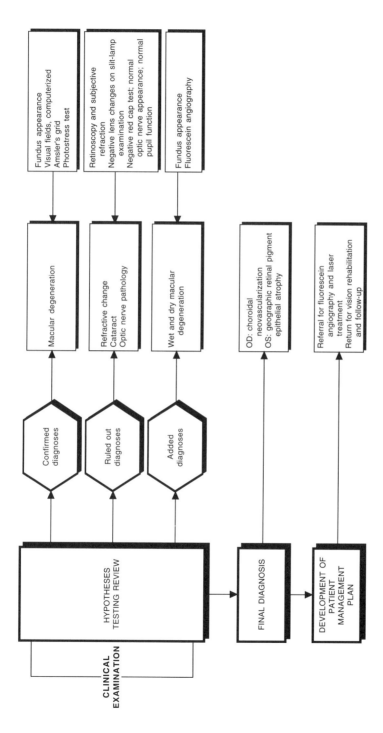

Case Scenario 10 decision-making summary.

Case Scenario 11

Cristina M. Schnider

PATIENT BACKGROUND

JN is a 32-year-old female contact lens wearer being seen for the first time in this office, having relocated from out of state 3 months ago.

DOCTOR: What brings you into the office today?

PATIENT: My friends keep telling me that my eyes are bloodshot, so I decided to have them checked out. I think it's just from wearing my contacts too long since I've been working the evening shift. I don't really think it's much of a problem.

DOCTOR (*thinking*): *Red eyes with contact lens wear can be due to a multitude of causes, including poorly fitting lenses, solution reactions, and a marginal dry-eye condition. They can occur secondary to conditions totally unrelated to the contact lenses, such as seasonal allergies and viral infections. Because this patient is new to the office, a very thorough case history with respect to contact lens wear and care is indicated, as well as a careful look at general ocular health.*

DOCTOR: Have you had any other problems with your eyes, recently or in the distant past?

PATIENT: Not really, but a doctor once told me that I had blood vessels in my eye and fit me with soft lenses. I asked him what that meant, but he never really explained it to me. I never really liked the soft lenses, though, so the last doctor finally put me back into the gas-permeable lenses. I was supposed to go back to have these checked a while ago, but I got busy with moving and changing jobs, so I never went back.

DOCTOR: Can you tell me what you didn't like about the soft lenses?

PATIENT: My eyes always seemed dry, and my vision wasn't as good. Since I switched back to the gas-permeable lenses, I haven't really had any problem.

DOCTOR: Sometimes other medications or health conditions can cause dry-eye problems. Do you take any medications, either prescribed or purchased over-the-counter?

PATIENT: No, my health is perfect, and I never take drugs of any kind.

DOCTOR: You mention your good health. Do you know whether anyone else in your family has had problems with their eyes or general health?

PATIENT: My parents have never had any problems that I know of, but I think my grandmother on my Dad's side had diabetes when she was in her late 80s, right before she died.

DOCTOR: It sounds like you have pretty healthy genes! Now, let's get back to your reason for coming in today. Tell me as much as you can about your contact lens–wearing experience: how long you have worn them, how old this pair is, and how you take care of them.

PATIENT: I've been wearing contact lenses since I was 18. I started wearing the old-fashioned hard ones and then switched to the gas-permeable kind about 3 years ago. This pair is about 6 months old. I think they're called *Boston Vision* or something, and I use the Boston solutions to take care of them. As I said, I wore those soft lenses for about a year before these lenses.

DOCTOR (*thinking*): *The lenses are reasonably new, so they should be in fairly good condition. It's unusual for a patient to be put into soft lenses because of neovascularization, so this should be investigated objectively, because JN got little information on the condition from her previous practitioner. Also, some patients have experienced mild adverse reactions to the Boston Advance conditioning solutions, so it's important to clarify which Boston solutions she is using.*

DOCTOR: Do you know which Boston care system you have been using—the original formula or the Advance formula?

PATIENT: I tried the Advance for a while but didn't like it as well, so I switched back to the original Boston. My eyes seemed to be kind of gooey with the Advance version.

DOCTOR (*thinking*): *I need to clarify the influence of lens wear on the problem. I'll use the DOFDAR questioning strategy* (description, onset, frequency, duration, associations, and relief) *to isolate possible causes more fully.*

DOCTOR: Can you tell me more about how and when the redness occurs?

PATIENT: Well, it's usually just like a red line across the middle of my eyes, and it starts a couple hours after I put my lenses on.

DOCTOR: How long have you noticed the redness? Does it happen every day, only when you wear your lenses, or just once in a while?

PATIENT: My eyes seem to get red easily, even without lenses, but it's gotten worse since I got these new lenses. The doctor made them bigger because I'd been having problems with night driving with my old rigid lenses. My eyes got red with the soft lenses, too, but it was more an all-over redness with them. This is really more like a stripe across the middle of my eyes.

DOCTOR: Is there anything that seems to make it worse, such as air conditioning or driving? And is there anything you can do to make it better?

PATIENT: It does seem to get a little worse if I have to use the computer for a long time, and using drops makes my eyes feel a little better, but the redness seems to stay about the same until I take my lenses out.

DOCTOR: Do you have any other symptoms, such as itching or watering of your eyes when they get red?

PATIENT: No, they just feel a little dry.

DOCTOR (*thinking*): *Because the condition seemed to worsen with the new lenses, it's likely that the lens design or material change has some influence on the problem. The condition also seems to be exacerbated by computer use, so there may be a dry-eye component due to the decreased blink rate often seen during periods of concentration with computer screens. The lack of other symptoms appears to rule out viral or allergic problems.*

DOCTOR: How long have you been wearing your lenses today, and what is your normal wearing time in an average day?

PATIENT: I've had them on about 8 hours today, and I usually wear them all day—probably 16 or 18 hours a day, but sometimes less on the weekends. My glasses are old and really ugly, and I hate wearing them outside the house.

DOCTOR: Here's a mirror (*handing patient a mirror*). Would you say that this is a normal amount of redness for this time of day?

PATIENT: Boy, my eyes are red! I normally never look at myself in the mirror during the day, but this is about what my friends tell me I look like! I guess maybe they're right.

DOCTOR (*thinking*): *The redness definitely seems related to the lens wear, but apparently it has been a longer-term problem than just with these lenses. My objective testing will be aimed at looking at the effect of lens performance as well as looking for ocular surface problems that also might be present.*

DIAGNOSTIC HYPOTHESES

On the basis of JN's case history, the initial hypothesis list includes the following:

1. *Marginal dry eye exacerbated by contact lens wear.* This patient reports that her eyes are often red, even without lenses, thus pointing

to the possibility of a marginal dry-eye condition. Common causes include tear film abnormalities (quality or quantity) and poor ocular surfacing due to such physical problems as impaired blinking or lid configuration. That the signs and symptoms worsen with lens wear suggests a contact lens component. Many patients who are normally asymptomatic experience a relative dry-eye condition when they wear their contact lenses. Most likely this is due to the disruption of the stability of the tear film or the influence of preservatives, surfactants and other agents in the care solutions used with the lenses.

2. *Peripheral corneal desiccation (PCD).* PCD (or 3 and 9 o'clock staining) is a common clinical sign accompanying rigid lens wear and has been reported in association with many lens-fitting problems, including excessive edge lift or thickness,[1, 2] poor blinking habits[3] and, more recently, with insufficient edge clearance.[4–6] It occurs when there is disruption to the natural flow of tears over or under a rigid lens and often is accompanied by local conjunctival hyperemia in the horizontal midline, which was described by the patient in this case.

3. *Ocular inflammation caused by poorly fitting rigid lens.* When a rigid lens is fitted improperly, irritation and inflammation can result. A lens that is too large or is fitted with insufficient peripheral edge clearance can result in desiccation and mechanical chafing, leading to an inflammatory condition of the peripheral cornea, limbus, and conjunctiva.[7] A lens that is fitted too small and flat will move excessively and also will cause irritation, but it is more likely to be generalized or restricted to the inferior cornea and conjunctiva. Local hyperemia in the horizontal midline points to the large lens problem, as the horizontal region of the cornea suffers the most from poor tear exchange over as well as under the lens. The vague history of a previous problem with "blood vessels in the eye" causing a change from rigid lenses to soft, as well as the change to a larger lens diameter, are consistent with this hypothesis as well.

4. *Damaged or poorly made contact lens.* Because the problem seemed to worsen with this particular pair of lenses, it may indicate a quality problem with the manufacture of this pair of lenses. Edge and back surface finish are of particular importance for rigid gas-permeable (RGP) lenses, and a rough edge or poorly blended posterior surface could result in disruption of tear flow, leading to PCD, staining, and inflammation. A damaged front surface or inappropriate choice of lens material also could result in poor lens wetting, leading to ocular irritation.

5. *Solution reaction.* Solution problems can be either toxic reactions or hypersensitivity reactions and result in symptoms of redness and irritation. The patient appeared to have experienced a previous solution reaction with the particular solution she was using, and the chron-

ic hyperemia is consistent with a diagnosis of solution hypersensitivity. However, it is unusual for the hyperemia to be so localized in a solution reaction.

DIAGNOSTIC TESTING

Economy of time and movement are important aspects of good patient and practice management. Therefore, because the patient presented with her lenses on, all testing related to the lenses was performed first, followed by those tests requiring lens removal. Remember, however, that the fact that the patient presented while wearing lenses may significantly influence some tests following lens removal and that confirmation of an underlying dry-eye condition might be accomplished more suitably on a visit in which the lenses were not worn. The following clinical testing was conducted and allowed testing of hypotheses 1–5 (Table CS11.1):

- Visual acuity with lenses in place
- Biomicroscopic evaluation, including lens surface on the eye, lens fitting, ocular surface integrity, lids and lashes, and other anterior structures as baseline data
- Contact lens inspection and verification

(The testing of each hypothesis can be evaluated by the observations made on the biomicroscopic evaluation in combination with baseline data on inspection of the condition and parameters of the contact lenses.)

Several findings supported the diagnosis of marginal dry eye exacerbated by contact lens wear. The noninvasive 3-second breakup time over the contact lens means that the lens would be dry before the usual interblink interval of 4–5 seconds, thus setting up conditions for a lens-induced dry-eye problem. The peripheral corneal and conjunctival fluorescein staining and conjunctival hyperemia are objective signs of the desiccation but did not reveal the cause. The marginal lower lid tear prism finding suggested a problem with either tear production or retention, and the lid margin findings pointed to a seborrheic meibomianitis as a contributing factor. Because the meibomian gland secretions are key to regulating the evaporation of the tear film, the stagnation in the production of lipid layer of the tear film observed here could play a part in the underlying mechanism for the dry-eye condition. The overly steep fit with a large-diameter lens also could have contributed to a worsening of dry-eye symptoms with contact lens wear due to impeded tear flow behind the lens. The other corneal findings of inflammation and vascularization were inconsistent with a diagnosis of a marginal dry eye, however.

Table CS11.1
Hypotheses 1–5: problem-specific testing results.

Visual acuity while wearing contact lenses: 20/15 OD, OS, OU
Lens surface on eye: noninvasive breakup time, 3 secs; mild circular scratches, grade 1 protein film
Lens fitting: central position, minimal movement, apical pooling with significant midperipheral bearing; very narrow edge in horizontal periphery; bulls-eye fluorescein pattern
Tear film: lower lid tear prism, average to low; tear breakup time, 1–3 secs; large ruptures noted, tear quantity borderline
Ocular surface integrity: grade 2+ injection, fluorescein stain of horizontal conjunctiva; 2–3+ dilation of limbal arcade at 3 and 9 o'clock; fluorescein staining in triangle shape at 3 and 9 o'clock; 2-mm superficial and deep vessels in temporal cornea with 3+ staining, infiltrates, and epithelial hyperplasia overlying; no rose bengal staining OU
Lids and lashes
　Lashes: clear
　Lids: occasional pits, capped glands on margins; meibomian glands express thick white material with difficulty
Anterior segment baseline data
　Anterior chamber: deep, clear OU
　Iris: blue, clear OU
　Lens: clear OU
Contact lens inspection
　OD 7.70 mm (BC)/9.6 mm (OAD)/−5.25 D (power) /0.12 mmct/blue
　OS 7.70 mm (BC)/9.6 mm (OAD)/−5.00 D (power)/0.12 mmct/blue
　No obvious peripheral curves visible; possibly aspheric lens design; mild scratches noted but no other defects noted on or off eye; edge thickness not verified but not noted to be excessive

BC = base curve; OAD = overall diameter.

Findings that supported the diagnosis of PCD include the poor lens-wetting characteristics, poor edge lift, corneal and conjunctival punctate staining, and conjunctival hyperemia. However, the classic description of PCD does not include the inflammatory findings of vascularization, infiltration, and epithelial hypertrophy.

The observation of ocular inflammation in this case is significant in that it included not only hyperemia of the vascular conjunctiva but new vessel growth into the normally avascular cornea, which supports hypothesis 3 (ocular inflammation due to poor lens fit). According to McMonnies,[8] the limbal vasculature of rigid lens wearers is indistinguishable from that of nonwearers, so the hypothesis of peripheral corneal vascularization is not a common one for rigid lens wearers. Efron[9] defines a *normal vascular response* to contact lens wear as vessels that encroach onto the cornea not further than 0.4 mm beyond the limbal zone. He describes as abnormal any deep vessels, vessels longer than the norm, or vessels accompanied by active inflammation or degenerative fibrous changes, such as were noted in this case. The corneal vascularization, infiltration, and hypertrophy observed in this case, in addition to peripheral corneal and conjunctival staining, indicate a more severe reaction than that due to a marginal dry eye or simple PCD staining. The mechanical component of the large-diameter lens with low edge lift combined with the poor tear exchange of the steep fit and a marginally adequate tear film certainly were sufficient to cause the inflammatory response seen in this patient.

Though contact lens damage or poor manufacturing quality can cause ocular irritation that includes staining and hyperemia, the rotational nature of a spherical lens on the eye suggests a rotationally symmetric staining pattern and a more diffuse hyperemia than was observed in this case. Further, no obvious damage or defects were noted on lens inspection, which helped to rule out hypothesis 4 (damaged or poorly made contact lens). It is possible, however, that some subtle defects can be overlooked during a routine inspection and may be virtually impossible to detect with soft contact lenses, because of the many difficulties in inspecting soft lenses.

JN's case history partially ruled out a solution reaction, and objective testing further confirmed the unlikeliness of this diagnosis. Though solution toxicity or sensitivities can cause ocular redness and symptoms of dryness as reported by this patient, neither the staining nor the injection pattern fit the classic description of solution reactions. A toxic reaction usually results in a diffuse superficial punctate staining of the entire cornea, and the sensitivity reactions are more likely to cause generalized conjunctival hyperemia than the localized pattern described in this case.

Because this was the patient's first visit to my office, I conducted additional database testing to ensure that the refractive correction was correct and that binocular vision, accommodation, and ocular health findings were normal. The results of this baseline testing are shown in Table CS11.2. The patient was found to be a myopic astigmatic, which was consistent with her previous contact lens correction, and all other findings were considered to be within normal limits.

DIAGNOSTIC SUMMARY

Because it was the patient's initial visit to the clinic and a comprehensive examination was completed, there were several diagnoses

Table CS11.2
Additional database testing results.

Refraction over contact lenses: +0.25 DS; 20/15 OD, OS, OU
Keratometry: 43.00 @ 180, 44.50 @ 090 OD, OS, mires clear, regular
Refraction
    OD −4.50 −1.00 × 180, 20/20+
    OS −4.00 −0.75 × 180, 20/20+
Binocular and accommodative function
    Unilateral cover test: no movement at far or near
    Alternate cover test: orthophoria at 6 m, 4Δ exophoria at 40 cm
    Stereopsis: 20 secs Randot Stereotest
    Negative fusional convergence at 40 cm: 12/18/16
    Positive fusional convergence at 40 cm: 15/25/16
    Negative relative accommodation: +2.25 D
    Positive relative accommodation: −2.00 D
    Accommodative amplitude: 10 D OD, OS
Fundus examination through dilated pupils
    Cup-to-disc ratio: 0.4/0.4 OU
    ONH: healthy rim tissue 360 degrees OU
    Background: healthy retina with even pigmentation to periphery; no
        holes, tears, flat 360 degrees OU; vitreous clear OU
    Vessels: healthy, no abnormal crossings OU
Tonometry (Goldmann applanation): 16 mm Hg OD and OS at 9:30 AM
Automated visual fields
    Equal sensitivity OD and OS at 36 dB
    No fixation losses, false-positive or false-negative responses
    No significant depression in sensitivity within central 30 degrees

---

DS = diopter sphere; ONH = optic nerve head.

derived for this patient at this time, not all of which relate to her chief complaint. The refractive diagnosis of regular myopic astigmatism is an obvious one but certainly not the one that caused the patient to seek attention. Another important diagnosis related to the patient's problems (but not the obvious cause of the most severe signs and symptoms) is the seborrheic meibomianitis. These diagnoses are important for long-term patient management and education, but the patient's main concern was to address the cause of the redness and dryness. In this case, the findings of inflammation and vascularization of the peripheral cornea were the key signs that ruled out the more obvious contact lens–related diagnoses of contact lens–induced dry eye, simple PCD, solution reactions, and lens damage. The presence of neovascularization expanded the list slightly.

The combination of inflammation and vascularization of the peripheral cornea in response to rigid lens wear has been termed *vascularized limbal keratitis* (VLK) by Grohe and Lebow.[7] They described the classic presentation as an elevated semi-opaque lesion bridging the limbus in the peripheral cornea, accompanied by edema, staining, and vascularization. They noted that the condition tends to occur in the following stages:

- Stage I: epithelial hyperplasia
- Stage II: inflammation (infiltration of the peripheral cornea and conjunctival hyperemia)
- Stage III: vascularization of the peripheral cornea
- Stage IV: erosion of the elevated area

The appearance of the hyperplasia, infiltration, and neovascularization places this patient in stage III and serves to differentiate this condition from conventional PCD staining. These findings, combined with the history of polymethyl methacrylate lens wear and a refit to a larger-diameter gas-permeable lens are all consistent with the description of the condition of VLK by Grohe and Lebow.[7]

It is important to note, however, that corneal vascularization, arguably the most significant complication in this condition, is the least likely to cause patient symptoms. Rather, it is the conjunctival hyperemia or the elevation and subsequent erosion that most often causes patients with this condition to seek attention.

TREATMENT OPTIONS

Grohe and Lebow[7] advocate treatment according to the state of the VLK. For stage III (neovascularization plus inflammation and hyperplasia), they recommend discontinuing lens wear for 5 days, topical corticosteroids, and lens redesign to include a reduced lens diameter and elimination of peripheral bearing.

Refitting with a smaller-diameter lens with a much improved edge clearance relationship was accomplished that day, using a dispensing inventory of RGP lenses in the clinic. The new lenses were 8.8 mm in diameter, with the base curves the same as the patient's current lenses. Because the patient's own lenses were far too steep for the diameter used, the significant reduction in diameter required no change in base curve to achieve a fit that centered well, moved smoothly, and provided a near alignment fitting relationship with a wide, deep edge reservoir that was maintained even in lateral gaze.

In addition to the refit, a nonsteroidal anti-inflammatory drug (NSAID) was prescribed for use four times a day for 2 weeks to hasten the regression of the inflammatory symptoms. The NSAIDs were not available at the time the Grohe and Lebow[7] paper was published, and I thought that this was a better first choice of treatment than are steroids. JN also was advised to limit her lens-wearing time to 8–10 hours per day and to begin a rigorous twice-daily regimen of lid hygiene to include hot compresses and lid massage to combat the seborrheic meibomianitis.

Because the patient was quite reluctant, for cosmetic reasons, to return to her old spectacles, she was encouraged to order a new pair with a contemporary frame and lenses of a high-index material and with antireflection coating. She.was scheduled to return in 2 weeks for a follow-up to assess the effectiveness of the lens design changes and the NSAID and lid treatment.

On the return visit, the patient's eyes were noticeably whiter on casual inspection, and she reported that her symptoms were much improved as well. She disliked the NSAID drops because they caused minor irritation on instillation. She reported fair compliance with her reduced lens-wearing schedule, reporting that she had been able to limit wear to approximately 12 hours per day during the week. She was very pleased with the appearance of her new spectacles and vowed to continue to reduce her contact lens–wearing time now that she had suitable glasses. She also reported that her eyes felt vastly better even without lenses since she began the lid hygiene regimen, and she agreed to continue it as part of her morning and evening routine.

Slit-lamp examination showed a marked improvement in the VLK, with no elevation noted and only a trace infiltrate remaining. The vessels were still present in the cornea but were much reduced in caliber, and the staining was now noted to be grade 1+ nasally, and 2+ temporally. The lens-fitting relationship remained adequate in each eye. The patient was instructed to replace the NSAID therapy with a lubricating drop with vitamin A supplement and to continue a reduced lens-wearing schedule of 10–12 hours per day. A 3-month contact lens follow-up was scheduled, as well as a 12-month annual comprehensive examination recall.

In cases in which refitting and therapeutic management do not result in a regression of the staining and inflammatory signs, the patient should discontinue rigid lens wear. In some cases, soft lens wear may be possible, but careful attention must be paid to the vascularized area of the cornea to ensure that vessel growth does not continue. A high water content lens is recommended, particularly with minus lens powers, so that oxygen transmission is maximized in the thicker peripheral portions of the lens.

REFERENCES

1. Bennett ES. The effect of varying axial edge lift on silicone/acrylate lens performance. Contact Lens J 1986;14(4):3–7.
2. Graham R. Persistent nasal and temporal stippling. Contacto 1968;12(1):20–23.
3. Sarver MD, Nelson JL, Polse KA. Peripheral corneal staining accompanying contact lens wear. J Am Optom Assoc 1969;40:310–313.
4. Williams CE. New design concepts for permeable rigid contact lenses. J Am Optom Assoc 1979;50:331–336.
5. Andrasko G. Peripheral corneal staining: edge lift and extended wear. Contact Lens Spectrum 1990;5(8):33–35.
6. Schnider CM. Clinical correlates of peripheral corneal desiccation. Masters thesis, University of New South Wales, Sydney, Australia, 1994;15–29.
7. Grohe RM, Lebow KA. Vascularized limbal keratitis. Int Contact Lens Clin 1989;16:197–209.
8. McMonnies CW, Chapman-Davies A, Holden BA. The vascular response to contact lens wear. Am J Optom Physiol Optics 1982;59:795–799.
9. Efron N. Vascular response of the cornea to contact lens wear. J Am Optom Assoc 1987;58:836–846.

Appendix: Case Scenario 11

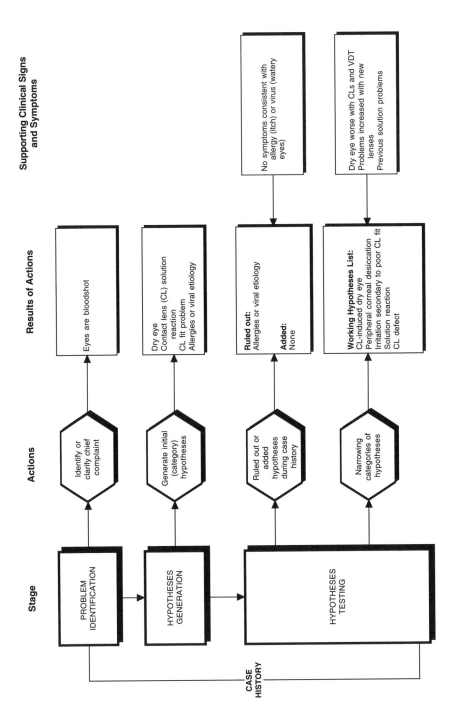

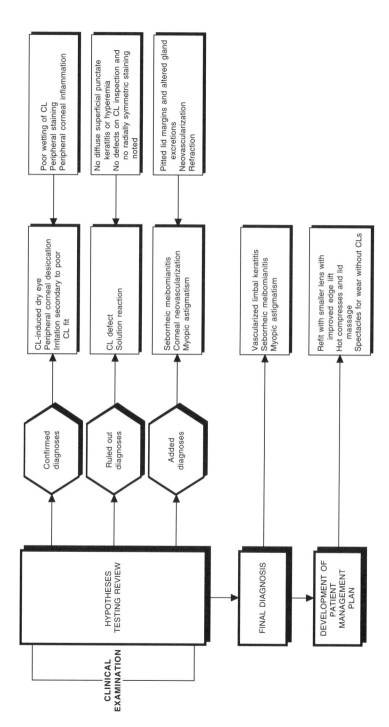

Case Scenario 11 decision-making summary. (VDT = video display terminal.)

Case Scenario 12

Michael W. Rouse

PATIENT BACKGROUND

TJ is a 9-year-old white third-grade boy, accompanied to the optometric examination by his mother.

DOCTOR: What brings you in for the examination today?

MOTHER: I'm concerned about my son's school performance. TJ has been having difficulty in school, and he's falling behind. The teacher suggested that he might have a vision problem and that he should have his eyes checked.

DOCTOR *(thinking)*: *The chief complaint for this patient is poor school performance. On the basis of the entering complaint, the possible range of vision problems that could contribute to poor school performance can be quite broad.*[1] *First, I need to identify whether there is a visual etiology or whether the problem is more likely the result of a visual information–processing deficit or a severe learning problem, such as specific dyslexia. I can obtain some insight into this question by asking about the duration of the problem. If the poor school performance has started recently, I would more likely suspect refractive or visual efficiency problems (e.g., convergence insufficiency). Visual information–processing problems and severe learning problems would probably have had an earlier effect, and the patient's school achievement probably would have been affected before the third grade.*

DOCTOR: How long has TJ had a problem in school? Is this a new problem, or has he been experiencing difficulties since he started school?

MOTHER: He was doing average work from kindergarten through second grade. It's just since the start of third grade that his performance has gotten progressively worse. The teacher has mentioned to me that he has trouble concentrating during reading tasks and that he often avoids reading and writing assignments in class. He also brings more work home than he used to because he's not able to complete his assignments in class.

DOCTOR *(thinking)*: *The recent onset (at the start of third grade) sounds more like a refractive or visual efficiency problem than a visual information–processing or learning problem. Before I totally rule out the possibility of a visual information–processing or learning problem, I'll ask a few other questions to help exclude these problems from my thinking.*

DOCTOR: Does TJ have problems in recognizing familiar words or sounding out new words while reading?

MOTHER: No, his reading skills are okay.

DOCTOR: Does TJ ever reverse letters when he writes or read letters or words backward, such as mistaking *saw* for *was*?

MOTHER: No, not at all.

DOCTOR: Is TJ's handwriting neat?

MOTHER: Yes, he writes very neatly, but often it takes him extra time to finish his work.

DOCTOR *(thinking):* It seems very unlikely at this point that a visual information–processing or severe learning problem is the cause of TJ's entering complaint. My next step is to investigate the possibility of a refractive or visual efficiency cause for the patient's entering complaint. If I find no visual basis or visual information–processing or learning problem, I will have to consider the possibility of a psychogenic etiology.[2] I'd better ask some questions now to explore whether there are any signs or symptoms that indicate a visual etiology.

DOCTOR: TJ, do your eyes ever get tired when you are studying or reading?

TJ: Yes, especially when I'm reading!

DOCTOR *(to mother):* Are you also aware that his eyes get tired?

MOTHER: Yes, he frequently complains that his eyes are tired.

DOCTOR: How often does he complain about this?

MOTHER: About three to four times a week.

DOCTOR: TJ, does your head ever hurt while you're studying or reading?

TJ: Yes, the front part of my head.

DOCTOR *(to mother):* Are you also aware that he experiences headaches?

MOTHER: Yes, he complains about headaches in the afternoons and often at night while doing his homework.

DOCTOR: When did he start reporting the eye fatigue and headaches?

MOTHER: You know, I think that it started about 1 month after the start of third grade.

DOCTOR *(thinking):* The reported symptoms strongly support a refractive or visual efficiency problem. Eye fatigue and headaches often accompany these types of problems.[3] The possibility that the headaches are associated with a systemic or pathologic cause in this case is remote, because they're associated with tasks that require visual concentration.

Why would the visual efficiency problems start to affect him as he enters the third grade? It is possible that these conditions pre-existed, but with the increased emphasis on "reading to learn" as he moved from the early grades (i.e., kindergarten, first, and second) to the higher grades, there's an increased requirement for him to sustain his visual concentration for longer periods.[1] This can stress a poor or borderline visual efficiency system, resulting in the reported signs and symptoms. Then these symptoms can lead to avoidance of near visual tasks, as was described in this patient. To complete my understanding of TJ's case and to collect database information, I'll investigate his and his family's eye and medical history.

DOCTOR: Has TJ had his eyes examined before?

MOTHER: No, but he passed the school vision screenings done in kindergarten and second grade.

DOCTOR: How is TJ's general health?

MOTHER: Good, he sees the pediatrician each year before school for a general physical, and I was told he was in good health. By the way, he passed the eye-chart test in the pediatrician's office this year.

DOCTOR: Are there any health problems in the family?

MOTHER: The only person with health problems is my husband's father. He is 60 and has high blood pressure. He takes medication that controls the problem.

DOCTOR: Are there any eye problems in the family?

MOTHER: TJ's father wears glasses for driving and watching television. I don't wear glasses. I think my mother has beginning cataracts.

DOCTOR *(thinking)*: *The only new information helpful in formulating my diagnostic hypotheses would be that the patient has passed recent school screenings. This suggests that if there is a refractive anomaly, it is more likely to be low to moderate hyperopia and low astigmatism. Myopia, significant astigmatism, or high hyperopia probably would result in a failure on the school screenings.*

DIAGNOSTIC HYPOTHESES

On the basis of the patient's case history, the initial hypothesis list emerges:

1.   *Uncorrected refractive error.* There probably is no significant myopia, astigmatism, or anisometropia because TJ has passed previous vision screenings. Most probably, TJ might have low (<1.00 D) to moderate (1.25–3.00 D) uncorrected hyperopia, which can be missed easily by vision screenings. Low amounts of hyperopia probably would have to be associated with accommodative or vergence anomalies to cause TJ's entering signs and symptoms. A moderate amount of hyperopia might cause his symptoms directly.

2.   *Vergence anomaly.* The vergence problem could be convergence insufficiency (CI), convergence excess, fusional vergence dysfunction (small phoria, but reduced or limited positive fusional convergence [PFC] and negative fusional convergence), or vertical heterophoria. There is a remote possibility that the vergence anomaly is nonconcomitant (e.g., paresis), because the patient does not report diplopia, and no one has observed a manifest eye turn. If present, the nonconcomitancy probably would be mild. The vergence anomaly could exist in isolation or in combination with uncorrected refractive error or accommodative anomalies.

3.   *Accommodative anomaly.* TJ could have accommodative insufficiency or infacility. This problem could exist in isolation, but it is more probable that the accommodative problem would be associated with an uncorrected refractive error or vergence anomaly.

4.   *Psychogenic symptomatology.* There is a remote possibility that, if TJ is having problems achieving, he might respond with a manifestation of physical signs and symptoms associated with conversion hysteria.

DIAGNOSTIC TESTING

Diagnostic testing is presented in a decision-making format, not necessarily the order in which I sequenced the examination. To arrive at the definitive diagnosis, I started with the most likely hypothesis and gathered all the clinical data to either confirm or deny its relationship to the patient's presenting problems. I then continued through the hypothesis list.

To rule out the initial hypothesis of uncorrected refractive error, I collected the following problem-specific clinical data (Table CS12.1):

- Entering visual acuities at far and near
- Static refraction (retinoscopy)
- Subjective refraction with visual acuities

The normal visual acuities and low refractive error that I found suggested that uncorrected refractive error was not responsible for the patient's entering complaints. The decision to conduct a cycloplegic refraction was delayed pending the results of additional clinical data. If I uncovered no significant data suggesting latent hyperopia or the need to prescribe maximum hyperopia (e.g., esophoria at near or high accommodative lag), cycloplegia would be performed as a baseline procedure coincident with the dilated assessment of ocular health.

To rule out the initial hypothesis of a vergence anomaly, I collected the problem-specific clinical data of unilateral and alternate cover test at near and far, and phorometry phoria and vergence ranges at near and far if any significant heterophoria were detected (Table CS12.2).

Table CS12.1
Hypothesis 1 (uncorrected refractive error): problem-specific testing results.

Entering visual acuities
   20/20 OD, OS, OU at 6 m
   20/25 OD, OS at 40 cm
Static refraction—retinoscopy
   OD +0.50 –0.25 × 180
   OS +0.50 –0.25 × 180
Subjective refraction and visual acuities
   OD +0.25 DS (20/20)
   OS +0.25 DS (20/20)

DS = diopter sphere.

Table CS12.2
Hypothesis 2 (vergence anomaly): problem-specific testing results.

Unilateral (UCT) and alternate cover test (ACT) at near and far
   UCT: at far, no movement; at near, no movement
   ACT: at far, no movement; at near ~10Δ XP; with prism neutralization,
      12Δ XP
Phorometry phoria and vergence ranges at near
   von Graefe phoria: at far, 1Δ XP; at near, 12Δ XP (no vertical phoria far or
      near)
   Negative fusional convergence at near: x/18/12
   Positive fusional convergence at near: 6/14/10

XP = exophoria.

This information (12Δ exophoria [XP] with low PFC at near) confirmed the presence of a vergence anomaly, specifically CI.[4, 5] Sheard's criterion (the blur point needs to be twice the phoria) was used to test whether there was sufficient PFC to manage the 12Δ XP demand. TJ failed to meet this criterion. Now that the diagnosis of CI had been confirmed, I collected some additional baseline information (Table CS12.3):

- Near point of convergence (NPC) checks TJ's gross convergence ability, because the NPC often is reduced as part of the CI syndrome
- Gradient AC/A
- Concomitancy testing with alternate cover test (ACT), up-down and right-left, to confirm or deny whether the deviation was concomitant

Table CS12.3
Hypothesis 2 (vergence anomaly): database testing results.

Near point of convergence: 8-cm break and a 12-cm recovery; after five
    attempts, 12 cm/15 cm
Gradient AC/A: 12Δ XP, with +1.00 14Δ XP, 2/1 gradient AC/A
Concomitancy testing
    Left, 12Δ XP; right, 12Δ XP
    Up, 8Δ XP; down, 15Δ XP
Stereopsis: 50 secs of arc, Randot Stereotest

AC/A = accommodative convergence/accommodation ratio; XP = exophoria.

- Stereopsis to check TJ's level of sensory processing and the presence of any suppression

The NPC was found to be reduced and fatigued easily on repeated attempts. The deviation was found to decrease in upgaze and increase in downgaze, suggesting an A-pattern exophoria at near. This finding is important because it requires the doctor to be careful to repeat measurements of the deviation in primary gaze. Observed variations in the deviation may be due simply to the target being placed in different positions rather than to real variations. This finding might also contribute to the symptoms the patient was experiencing, because the XP increases in downgaze, increasing the demand on the patient's already limited PFC. I went back and observed TJ attempt to compensate for the increased deviation by depressing his chin into the affected field so that he was looking in either primary or upgaze.

Some doctors might collect such additional baseline data as forced vergence fixation disparity curve, second-degree fusion, and vergence facility. I reasoned that in this case there was little clinical uncertainty regarding the diagnosis and that these tests were redundant.

To rule out associated accommodative problems, I collected the following problem-specific clinical data (Table CS12.4):

- Accommodative amplitude
- Accommodative accuracy (lag)
- Accommodative facility
- Negative and positive relative accommodation

This information confirms that the patient has an associated accommodative problem, specifically accommodative insufficiency (reduced amplitude, increased lag) and accommodative infacility (monocular and binocular).[6] The reduced binocular accommodative facility and negative relative accommodation are a result of the 12Δ XP demand and inadequate PFC at near.

Table CS12.4
Hypothesis 3 (accommodative anomaly): problem-specific testing results.

Accommodative amplitude: 10 D OD, OS
Accommodative accuracy (lag): +1.00 OD, OS
Accommodative facility: 6 cpm OD, OS; 0 cpm OU (cannot clear plus lens)
Negative/positive relative accommodation: +1.25 D/−2.00 D

Because there is a confirmed diagnosis of CI and accommodative dysfunction that correlates well with the entering complaints, the need to conduct specific testing to rule out a psychogenic etiology of the entering complaints was considered unnecessary.

At this point, I felt that I had sufficient problem-specific data to arrive at the definitive diagnosis to account for TJ's entering signs and symptoms and how these problems could be contributing to his problems in school. Then I collected additional clinical data (considered baseline or database information) consisting of color vision screening (because this was TJ's first vision examination), pupil testing to investigate TJ's general neurologic integrity, and oculomotor testing to evaluate his binocular saccades and pursuits. Although TJ did not have specific signs or symptoms of oculomotor problems, these problems can be a contributing factor in poor school performance and should be subject to screening as baseline information. I also used biomicroscopic examination to evaluate the health and integrity of anterior segment and dilated fundus examination to evaluate the health and integrity of retina. Cyclopentolate was used as the dilating agent so that a baseline cycloplegic refraction could be conducted. (The clinical results from this testing are presented in Table CS12.5.)

The testing revealed normal color vision, normal pupil responses, and normal anterior segment and fundus ocular health. Oculomotor testing revealed reduced saccadic eye movement ability, which could be secondary to the CI or an isolated additional diagnostic problem. To quantify this deficit, additional testing was conducted (the Developmental Eye Movement test). This test revealed a fifth percentile ability when compared to children of a similar age. This problem also could be contributing to TJ's school problems.

DIAGNOSTIC SUMMARY

TJ was found to have a nonconcomitant (A-pattern) CI and accommodative and oculomotor dysfunction. The CI and accommodative

Table CS12.5
Additional database testing results.

Color vision screening: passed all plates on Ishihara
Pupil testing: PERRLA, –APD
Oculomotor testing
   Pursuits: 3+ (SCCO rating scale)
   Saccades: 2+ (SCCO rating scale)
   DEM testing: ratio score, 5th percentile
Biomicroscopy
   Lids and lashes: normal
   Conjunctiva and cornea: normal
   Anterior chamber: clear, deep, quiet
   Iris: blue and normal
   Vitreous: clear
Dilated fundus examination
   Media: clear OU
   ONH margins: distinct OU
   ONH rim: pink and healthy OU
   Cup-to-disc ratio: 0.3/0.3
   Vessels: A/V ratio 4/5, normal crossings OU
   Macula: homogeneous OU, foveal reflex present OU
   Background: homogeneous OU
   Periphery: no holes, tears, flat 360 degrees OU
Cycloplegic refraction
   OD +0.75 –0.25 × 180
   OS +0.75 –0.25 × 180

PERRLA = pupils equal, round, reactive to light and accommodation; –APD = no afferent pupillary defect; SCCO = Southern California College of Optometry; DEM = Developmental Eye Movement; ONH = optic nerve head; A/V = arteriovenous.

dysfunction were correlated highly with TJ's entering complaints whereas the oculomotor deficit was considered to be a secondary problem. The level of diagnostic certainty and the relationship with the entering signs and symptoms was high. These problems were seen as having a significant correlation with the primary entering complaint of a recent onset of poor school performance.

TREATMENT OPTIONS

The best treatment approach for TJ's visual problems was optometric vision therapy.[5, 8] No optical correction was considered necessary at this time. The therapy would be directed at improving his gross convergence, PFC, accommodative amplitude, accommodative facility, accommodative accuracy, and the accuracy and speed of his saccadic eye movement skills. The estimated treatment time is approximately 10–15 office visits. Therapy would consist of one office visit per week combined with daily home vision therapy. The prognosis for resolving both TJ's objective visual problems and associated signs and symptoms was considered excellent. The prospect for improved school performance appeared good, based on the fact that the major obstacles to TJ's achieving in school related highly to his visual problems.

REFERENCES

1. Flax N. Relationship Between Vision and Learning: General Issues. In MM Scheiman, MW Rouse (eds), Optometric Management of Learning-Related Vision Problems. St. Louis: Mosby, 1994;127–152.
2. Weller M, Wiedemann P. Hysterical symptoms in ophthalmology. Doc Ophthalmol 1989;73:1–33.
3. Cooper J, Selenow A, Ciuffreda K, et al. Reduction of asthenopia in patients with convergence insufficiency after fusional vergence training. Am J Optom Physiol Opt 1983;60:982–989.
4. Cooper J, Duckman R. Convergence insufficiency: incidence, diagnosis, and treatment. J Am Optom Assoc 1978;49:673–680.
5. Scheiman M, Wick B. Clinical Management of Binocular Vision. Philadelphia: Lippincott, 1994;225–246.
6. Rouse MW. Optometric Assessment of Visual Efficiency Problems. In MM Scheiman, MW Rouse (eds), Optometric Management of Learning-Related Vision Problems. St. Louis: Mosby, 1994;267–297.
7. Garzia R. The Relationship Between Visual Efficiency Problems and Learning. In MM Scheiman, MW Rouse (eds), Optometric Management of Learning-Related Vision Problems. St. Louis: Mosby, 1994;153–178.
8. Rouse MW. Management of binocular anomalies: efficacy of vision therapy in the treatment of accommodative deficiencies. Am J Optom Physiol Opt 1987;64:415–420.

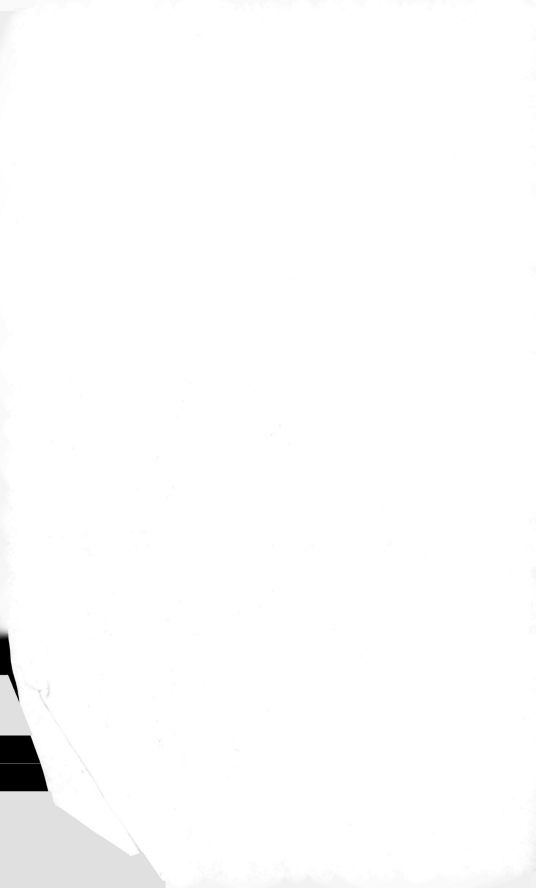

Appendix: Case Scenario 12

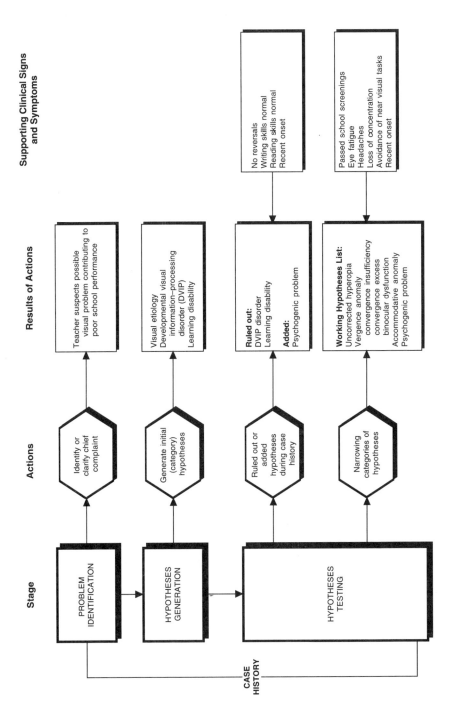

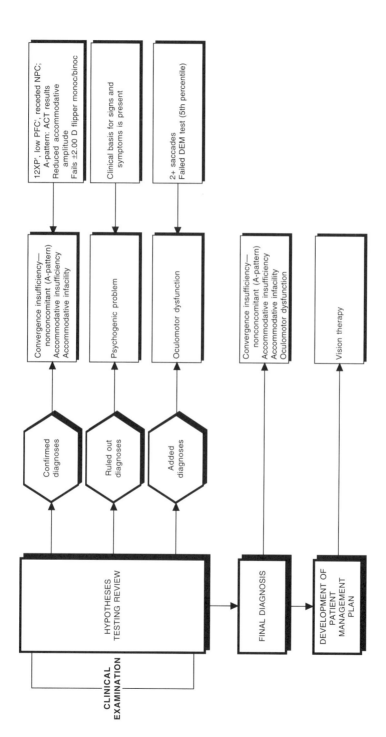

Case Scenario 12 decision-making summary. (XP' = exophoria at near; PFC' = positive fusional convergence at near; NPC = near point of convergence; ACT = alternate cover test; monoc = monocularly; binoc = binocularly; DEM = Developmental Eye Movement.)

Case Scenario 13

Michael H. Cho

PATIENT BACKGROUND

MB is a 46-year-old white woman who recently purchased her progressive-addition lenses (PALs) from another optometrist.

DOCTOR: What seems to be the problem?

PATIENT: I can't seem to get used to these progressive lenses. I've had them for a month, and I can't wear them.

DOCTOR *(thinking)*: *The patient's problems could be caused by a prescription problem, a fitting problem, or the inability to adapt to PAL optics.*

DOCTOR: What kind of problems are you having?

PATIENT: Well, I get dizzy when I wear them for too long. My eyes begin to hurt, and I get a headache.

DOCTOR: How long do you have to wear the glasses before you notice these problems?

PATIENT: Not too long. If I wear them for a few hours, I can also get a neckache.

DOCTOR: Have you tried to wear them every day?

PATIENT: Yes. I try to put them on when I get up, but I usually have to take them off after a little while and go back to my old bifocals.

DOCTOR *(thinking)*: *The presence of her symptoms indicates that either the prescription or the fit is grossly in error. Adaptation problems are not usually this severe and usually show some improvement over time.*

DOCTOR: How's your distance vision with them?

PATIENT: My distance vision is fine. Everything seems to be clearer than with my bifocals.

DOCTOR *(thinking)*: *The distance prescription may be correct; however, if the prescription is overminussed (or underplussed), she can compensate for it by looking slightly into the intermediate zone. If she has to look into the intermediate channel to see clearly, she may experience waviness or blurring in the periphery at distance, because of the narrower channel of the intermediate zone.*

DOCTOR: Do you notice blurred borders or waviness at distance?

PATIENT: No. At distance, I don't seem to have that problem.

DOCTOR *(thinking)*: *It appears likely that her distance prescription is correct because her vision is clear. Because she's not experiencing blurred borders at distance, she doesn't appear to be trapped in the intermediate channel.*

DOCTOR: How's your near vision with them?

PATIENT: Pretty good, except that I have such a small reading area. I have to keep moving my head to read one sentence. I have this blur around the edges of what I am reading.

DOCTOR *(thinking)*: *Blurred edges outlining a reading zone or being limited to a small reading area usually indicate an overplussed prescription at near. She appears to be using the intermediate zone to see clearly where the reading area is narrower, and that produces symptoms of blurred borders. It also could be caused by incorrect near IPD* (interpupillary distance).

DOCTOR: Have the PALs helped your intermediate vision?

PATIENT: Some, but I don't wear them long enough to notice. I have to keep taking them off.

DOCTOR *(thinking)*: *She seems to be having problems with her near and intermediate vision. Her problems are likely to be caused by a gross error either in the fitting of the PALs or in the power of the near prescription. Now that I understand the probable reason for her entering complaints, I need to investigate her general health for any significant factors.*

DOCTOR: How's your health?

PATIENT: Fine. I had a general physical 2 months ago, and my physician gave me a clean bill of health. I've never had problems with headaches or dizziness until I got these glasses. However, my previous optometrist gave me a complete eye exam about 6 weeks ago and told me my eyes were healthy.

DOCTOR: Does anyone in your family have any health problems?

PATIENT: My father has high blood pressure, but he exercises and watches his diet.

DOCTOR: Does anyone in your family have any eye problems?

PATIENT: Both my parents have cataracts, but they're both in their seventies.

DOCTOR *(thinking)*: *Because the patient is in good general and ocular health, it's unlikely that her headaches or dizziness could be caused by a pre-existing condition. In addition, MB correlates the onset of her symptoms with her new glasses.*

DIAGNOSTIC HYPOTHESES

On the basis of MB's history, the initial hypothesis list contains the following:

1. *Overplussed at near.* The optics of PALs are more complex than single-vision lenses, bifocals, or trifocals; consequently, proper pre-

scribing is essential for patient adaptation and good lens performance. An incorrect prescription can result in a wide variety of symptoms. The most likely cause of her problems is an overplussed near prescription. This will force her to use the intermediate channel for reading where the reading area is narrower and give her symptoms of blurred borders. In turn, this will increase her head movements to compensate for the small reading area and give her neckaches and possibly headaches.[1]

2.   *Improper fitting.* Proper fitting is imperative to the success of PALs. There are a number of potential fitting problems that can impede adaptation to the lenses.

- *IPD:* If one lens or both lenses have an incorrect IPD, the channel will not align properly to the convergence of the eyes. This effect can create the blurred borders around the reading area described by the patient. MB would have to make constant eye and head adjustments that could result in her neckaches.
- *Fitting height:* If the fitting height is fitted too low (i.e., >3 mm), the patient may complain of a small reading area. This effect could be caused by MB's failure to lower her eyes sufficiently to reach the full reading add where the reading area is largest. She would use the intermediate area to read where the channel is narrower. She may or may not notice near blur, depending on whether she adjusts her reading distance to the lens power.
- *Vertex distance:* If the vertex distance is too large, the effective channel is reduced and creates symptoms of a small reading area. As with any multifocal, a large vertex distance reduces the field of view through the reading area.
- *Pantoscopic tilt:* If the pantoscopic tilt is inadequate, the effective channel is reduced, creating symptoms of a small reading area. As with vertex distance, this would give MB symptoms of blurred borders at near with adequate near vision. If it is too severe, it may allow the frame to come into contact with the patient's cheeks. This will cause the PALs to move up and down with the patient's facial expressions and eventually slide down the patient's nose.
- *Parabolic curve (face form):* If the parabolic curve is inadequate, the effective channel is reduced, creating symptoms of a small reading area in the manner of a large vertex distance and inadequate pantoscopic tilt. Peripheral temporal blur may be more noticeable than nasal blur.

3.   *Nonadaptation.* This hypothesis operates by exclusion (i.e., only after all other possibilities have been investigated). Occasionally, a

patient cannot adapt to PALs, but this is usually the exception and not the rule.[2] This patient's adaptability can be determined only after her attempts to wear PALs, because success cannot be predicted on the basis of gender, lens history, refractive error, or age.[2] Some patients may be sensitive to the peripheral astigmatism, causing symptoms of dizziness and nausea. Typically, these symptoms are not severe unless there are contributing factors, such as incorrect power or fit. In some cases, nonadaptation may be due to incorrect lens selection. PALs are general-purpose lenses. If a patient requires special task-specific lenses, PALs may not be the appropriate lenses. Wearing an inappropriate lens is not the same as inability to adapt to the optics of PALs.

DIAGNOSTIC TESTING

Although overplussing is the most likely problem, it is important to check the fit systematically, first because there are a number of fitting factors that can contribute to poor adaptation in addition to overplussing. Once the fit has been verified, the distance and near refraction will follow. A summary of fitting factors, comparing habitual glasses to current measurements, is presented in Table CS13.1.

The first procedure was to re-mark the PALs. The engraved circles were made more visible by holding the lenses up to fluorescent ceiling lights and marking them, using a felt-tipped marker. The fitting crosses and the distance and near prescription circles were re-marked using the cut-out chart for that specific PAL. Because each PAL has a specific channel length and fitting cross location, the cut-out chart for that PAL must be used.

The second procedure was to place the glasses on MB's face and to verify the fitting height. I asked her to sit comfortably in her chair and look at a distant target that she felt was at eye level. This allowed me to fit the PALs at the center of the patient's pupil while she was in her natural head posture and her eyes were in a natural straight-ahead gaze. Many dispensers ask the patient to sit up or lean forward in the chair, hold their head straight, and look at a fixed location (e.g., penlight, dispenser's eye). This unnatural posture may be acceptable for fitting bifocal or trifocal lenses, but not for PALs. In an unnatural posture, the lenses may fit differently from the way they fit a patient who is in a natural posture. I stooped to MB's eye level and looked at the fitting crosses relative to her center pupil. In her case, the fitting heights were reasonably accurate.

The third procedure was to check monocular IPDs. The distance between fitting crosses of her PALs was measured by using the cut-out

Table CS13.1
Hypothesis 2 (improper fitting): problem-specific testing results.

	PAL (1 month old)	PAL (new)
Height (OD, OS)	29 mm, 29 mm	29 mm, 29 mm
IPD (OD, OS)	29.5 mm, 29.5 mm	30 mm, 30 mm
Vertex distance	Adequate	Adequate
Pantoscopic tilt	Adequate, no change	Adequate, no change
Parabolic curve	Adequate, no change	Adequate, no change

PAL = progressive-addition lens; IPD = interpupillary distance.

chart and was compared to her monocular IPDs measured with the corneal reflection pupillometer. Both measurements were approximately the same.

Incidentally, PALs should be ordered with reference to the patient's distance monocular IPDs. Most PALs have a 2.5 mm–segment inset for each lens. This means that the optical center of the add is positioned 2.5 mm nasally to the fitting cross. If the PALs are fitted by measuring the distance IPDs, the lenses may not be centered at near if the patient's eyes do not converge 5 mm. This discrepancy may affect the alignment of the channel. I prefer to measure the near monocular IPDs and add 2.5 mm to each eye to determine the distance monocular IPDs. This aligns the near optical centers and allows any discrepancy at distance, where there is more room for error.

The horizontal and vertical alignment of the fitting crosses was checked by having MB align her right eye with my left eye while her left eye was occluded. This allowed me to determine the location of each cross relative to the center of her pupil in primary gaze while wearing the lenses. The same was done with her left eye. The fitting cross was within 1 mm from her center pupil for each eye; therefore, I did not consider this to be a factor contributing to her problem.

The fourth procedure was to check the lens-to-eye relationship. The vertex distance, pantoscopic tilt, and parabolic curve were checked to ensure a proper lens-to-eye relationship.

The vertex distance should be approximately 14 mm; however, it is best to minimize vertex distance, being careful not to cause a fitting problem. MB's vertex distance was approximately 14 mm, but a minor adjustment was made to reduce it further. I did not believe vertex distance to be the cause of MB's problems.

The pantoscopic tilt was adequate to provide the proper lens-to-eye relationship. Enough clearance of her cheeks and eyelashes was pre-

Table CS13.2
Hypothesis 1 (overplussed at near): problem-specific testing results.

Lensometry: FT-28 bifocals (2 years old)
OD +0.75 DS, +1.75 D add
OS +1.00 DS, +1.75 D add
Progressive-addition lenses (1 month old) and visual acuities
OD +1.00 –0.50 × 180 (20/20)
OS +1.25 DS (20/20)
+2.00 D add OU with 0.37-M print (OD, OS)
Interpupillary distance (OD, OS): 29 mm, 29 mm
Pupil height (OD, OS): 29.5 mm, 29.5 mm
Distance refraction and visual acuities
OD +1.00 –0.25 × 180 (20/20)
OS +1.25 DS (20/20)
Add determination
Negative-positive relative accommodation: +2.25 D add with 0.37-M print
Cross-cylinder: +2.00 D add
Trial frame: +1.25 D add with 0.62-M print

FT = flat-top; DS = diopter sphere.

sent. The pantoscopic tilt should be between 5 and 10 degrees. It is not necessary to use a protractor to measure the exact pantoscopic tilt of the frame; it is sufficient to allow just enough clearance from the cheeks when the patient smiles. Some patients require more pantoscopic tilt than do others, owing to their facial contour.

The frame had a parabolic curve adequate to create the proper eye-to-lens relationship. The contour of the frame fit MB's face properly.

To investigate whether MB's prescription was overplussed at near (hypothesis 1), I conducted the following testing (Table CS13.2):

- Lensometry
- Visual acuity testing
- Distance refraction
- Near add determination

After the lenses were re-marked, the distance power and near add were read through the appropriate power circles. MB's PALs had the add power engraved under the temporal engraved circles. Later, the power of the lenses would be compared to her refraction. MB's 2-year-old bifocals were neutralized to determine the history of her add powers.

The distance acuities were checked monocularly, and each eye was 20/20. MB reported that her vision was clear. The distance acuities were rechecked by having MB look higher in the lens by tilting her head forward. This ensured that she was not looking through the intermediate channel. Because this did not improve her acuities, it was likely that the prescription was correct. If her acuities decreased, it would have indicated that she was using the intermediate channel to compensate for an underplussed prescription.

Her near acuities were checked monocularly, and each eye read 0.37-M print at 40 cm. This indicated that the add power was adequate but did not rule out overplussing, because she may have been using the intermediate zone to read. MB was given a magazine with print across the page and asked whether she noticed any blurred borders around her reading area. She said that when she looked at the left side of the page, the print on the right side of the page was blurry. She also said that when she looked in the middle of the page, both sides of the page were blurry. Each eye was tested with similar results. Because both sides of the page were blurry when she looked in the middle of the page with either eye or both eyes, overplussing was considered likely. Misalignment of the intermediate channel was thought unlikely because only nasal or temporal borders would have been blurry.

If the acuities were decreased, the patient would have been asked to look lower in the lens by raising her chin or by lifting the glasses higher. If this did not improve acuities, it would suggest the add power was inadequate or the distance prescription was incorrect. If acuities improved, it would imply that either the fitting height should be raised or the add power increased. Raising the height is a better option as long as it does not affect distance acuities or cause adjustment of her normal distance head posture. I noted any unusual head posture and determined whether any adjustments improved the width of her reading area.

I conducted the refraction, and there was no significant difference in the distance refraction from the prescription in MB's PALs. The refraction corresponded closely with her distance acuities.

A careful determination of the add power was important. For this, I used the cross-cylinder, negative-positive relative accommodation (NRA-PRA) balance, and trial frame to test for the add power, and I compared it to the age method. The cross-cylinder test indicated a +2.00 D add, and the NRA-PRA method indicated a +2.25 D add. However, by the age method, MB should have an add of +1.00 D or +1.25 D (Table CS13.3).[3] When there is a significant difference between the age method and other add tests, there is a risk of overplussing the prescribed add power. Overplussing is more likely to occur in early presbyopes than in absolute presbyopes, because there is a higher variation in the add powers for early presbyopes.[4] The add may range from +0.75 to +1.75 D for patients near age 45. For absolute presbyopes, the range is smaller, usually either +2.25 or +2.50 D, and error is less likely.

Table CS13.3
Add power by age.

Age (yr)	Add (D) for 13 in.[2]	Add (D) for 16 in.[2]
45	1.00	0.75
48	1.50	—
50	2.00	1.25
55	2.50	1.75
60	—	2.00
65	—	2.25
70	—	2.50
75	3.00	—

Overplussing is particularly a problem when converting a bifocal wearer to PALs, because there is a tendency to maintain or increase the add power with new prescriptions. We are trained to be cautious about reducing a presbyope's habitual add power. A patient who has habituated to a working distance using a particular bifocal lens add power may not require the same add for PALs because of the way the patient learns to use each lens. Most bifocal wearers adapt to whatever add power the optometrist prescribes because they learn to adjust their working distance to the add power. They learn to use a specific location in the lens and use a specific working distance when they read. This is aided by the segment line in the bifocals. PAL wearers do not have a segment line to guide them to any particular location in the lens. Therefore, PAL wearers learn to use the location in the lens that gives them adequate clarity for their working distance. They use the least amount of plus power in the progression that provides clear vision for that distance. In other words, they will adjust the lens power to suit their working distance. If a +2.00 D add is prescribed when a lower add (i.e., +1.50 D add) would suffice for working distance, a patient will lower the eyes only to the +1.50 D add level. However, the +1.50 D add will be located in the intermediate channel, where the channel is significantly narrower for all PALs (Figure CS13.1). This will give the wearer a small reading area outlined by blurred borders. Some patients may be able to use a slightly lower add for PALs than they use for bifocal lenses.

Trial framing is critical in determining the patient's add power. This is particularly important in MB's case because the NRA-PRA balance and cross-cylinder showed a large discrepancy from the age method. Based on the severity of her symptoms, a significantly lower add than

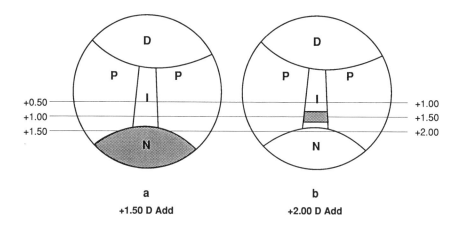

Figure CS13.1. Overplus Diagram. Shaded area represents the usable area for a patient requiring a +1.50 D add. (D = distance; P = periphery; I = intermediate; N = near.) (Reprinted with permission from MH Cho, C Spear, L Caplan. The effect of excessive add power on the acceptance of progressive addition lenses. J Am Optom Assoc 1991;62:672–674.)

her habitual +2.00 D add seemed likely. I began with a +1.25 D add and asked MB to look at 0.62- or 0.75-M print and hold it where she did most of her reading. (I use 0.37-M print to check acuities, but do not use it to determine add power unless the patient uses this size print habitually. It often causes the patient to shorten the working distance, requiring a higher add.) I was careful not to let her prop her arms up on the chair arms, as this also can shorten her working distance artificially. After placing the tentative add power in place, I asked her to adjust the reading card distance until the print was clearest. If she had to adjust the card closer than her preferred distance, the add power was too strong. If she had to adjust it farther, the tentative add was too weak. I increased and decreased the add power until the print was the clearest at her preferred reading distance. MB reported that the +1.25 D add gave her an adequate range (see Table CS13.2); however, her tendency was to shorten her working distance when I checked her acuity with the 0.37-M print.

DIAGNOSTIC SUMMARY

Two years ago MB, at age 44, was given a prescription for bifocal lenses with an add power of +1.75 D. Her most recent refraction indicated a +0.25 D change at distance and a 0.25 D increase in add power. As she had reported some difficulty with intermediate vision with her bifocals, her previous optometrist prescribed PALs with the new prescription. When she had difficulty adjusting to her new eyeglasses, she sought a second opinion.

All fitting measurements were retaken and compared to her habitual PALs. There were no problems with the fit. The PALs were verified and compared to MB's distance refraction. There were no significant changes to her distance prescription that could account for her problems. Cross-cylinder and NRA-PRA tests determined an add power of +2.00 and +2.25 D, respectively; however, the age method indicated +1.25 D. Trial frame determined an add of +1.25 D. Because she was 46 years old and already symptomatic with a +2.00 D add, the +2.25 D add was not considered. On the basis of her age and trial frame and the severity of her symptoms, I determined a +1.25 D add to be optimum for her working distance.

TREATMENT OPTIONS

It is best always to prescribe the lowest add power necessary for the patient's habitual working distance and thereby avoid overplussing. It is necessary to ensure that the patient's complaint justifies the prescription change. Any change in plus at distance will have an effect on the total plus at near. A +0.25 D change at distance and +0.50 D change of the add power will result in a +0.75 D change of total plus at near. This may be too large a change if the patient's only complaint were a little blur with fine print. One option is to consider reducing the add power for PALs if the habitual bifocals have an add power that appears slightly high for a patient's age. It is better to err on the low side. It is not routinely necessary to add plus to the near or to perform add determinations at a closer working distance.[1] The key is to position the required add power at the widest portion of the channel. This is why the patient can adapt more easily to an undercorrected add power than to an overcorrected add power. Unless the add is undercorrected grossly, the patient may complain of having to look too low in the lens with an undercorrected add. This may cause some mild neckaches in a few patients, but they will adapt to the lens periphery much more easily. If the add is overcorrected even as little as 0.50 D, the patient may have difficulty in wearing the PALs[1]; hence, the patient may experience symptoms such as headaches, neckaches, dizziness, and eye strain. This can be interpreted incorrectly as a nonadaptive patient.

I ordered the same PALs with my distance refraction and a +1.25 D add. The fitting height remained at 29 mm OD and OS. The distance monocular IPDs were ordered at 30 mm OD and OS.

When the new PALs were dispensed, MB immediately walked around the room without any symptoms of dizziness or nausea. Her response to the new lenses was that they were much improved and that she thought she could adjust to them.

On follow-up 2 weeks later, MB reported that her only complaint with the lenses was that she felt she had to look a little too low in the lenses to read. However, she was wearing the lenses full-time without any complaints of dizziness, neckaches, headaches, or nausea. Her new symptom indicated that her lenses were either fitted too low or that the add power was too low. Because her lenses were at the proper height, I increased her add to +1.50 D to alleviate her symptom of look-ing too low in the lens, and I ordered new lenses.

There were no additional charges to the patient for reordering her lenses, because the PAL lens manufacturer and wholesale laboratory have a warranty on doctor's errors. Although warranties may vary, most PAL manufacturers have a warranty for doctor's errors in addi-tion to a nonadaptation warranty. Some optical laboratories may charge an edging fee.

REFERENCES

1. Cho MH, Spear CH Jr, Caplan L. The effect of excessive add power on the accep-tance of progressive addition lenses. J Am Optom Assoc 1991;62:672–675.
2. Cho MH, Barnette CB, Aiken B, et al. A clinical study of patient acceptance and satisfaction of Varilux Plus and Varilux Infinity lenses. J Am Optom Assoc 1991;62:449–453.
3. Borish IM. Clinical Refraction (3rd ed). Chicago: Professional Press, 1970;182.
4. Hanlon SD, Nakabyashi J, Shigezawa G. A critical view of presbyopic add deter-mination. J Am Optom Assoc 1987;58:468–472.

Appendix: Case Scenario 13

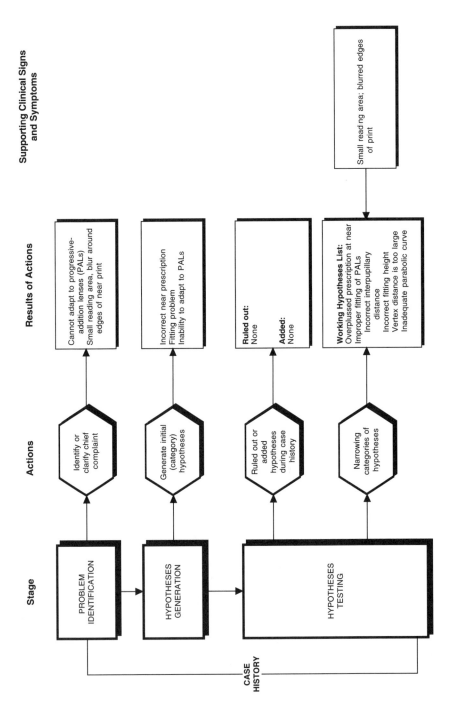

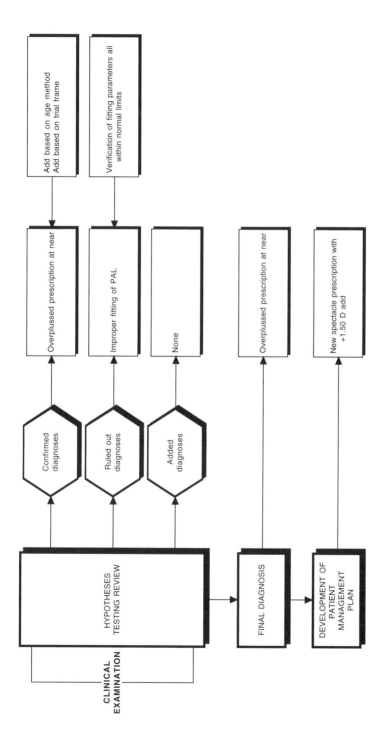

Case Scenario 13 decision-making summary.

Case Scenario 14

Dennis L. Smith

PATIENT BACKGROUND

NB is a 45-year-old female assistant vice president of the loan department of a large bank.

DOCTOR: What brings you in to see me today?

PATIENT: I'm having some difficulty with my vision, especially when I'm reading my daily reports. I've also noticed some distance blur.

DOCTOR *(thinking)*: *The principal concern of this patient is her difficulty with reading daily reports, which is a near-vision task. At 45, the patient's near complaint could be the result of incipient presbyopia[1] or the result of an uncompensated refractive error. The complaint of distance blur also needs investigation, as it could be the cause or the effect of the near concerns. The distance blur could be the result of an uncompensated refractive error, such as hyperopia or astigmatism, or a vergence anomaly.[2] She also may be experiencing the visual side effects of an undiagnosed metabolic or neurologic disorder.[2] An understanding of the duration, onset, periodicity, and associated concerns is necessary.*

DOCTOR: How long have you experienced this problem?

PATIENT: I've noticed it for about the past 2 months after I was promoted to my new position. At first I thought it was just the lighting in my new office, but I don't think so any longer, because I have the same difficulty in reading the reports at home.

DOCTOR *(thinking)*: *Another possibility may well be stress-induced accommodative dysfunction.[3] NB was recently promoted and probably is working very hard to establish her credibility in the new position. Some questions to ascertain her level of comfort and confidence in her new job might give some indication.*

DOCTOR: Tell me about the new job. How's it going?

PATIENT: I'm real happy with the position and additional responsibilities. It keeps me very busy, but I love the job. It allows me to be more focused in my area of interest, and I think it's what I do best.

DOCTOR *(thinking)*: *She seems pretty happy with her new job, so I'm going to think less of "new job" stress and more about a refractive, convergence, or presbyopia etiology.*

DOCTOR: What about the distance blur? Have you ever been examined for this in the past?

PATIENT: I've never had a problem with distance vision. I'm a pilot in the Air Force Reserve and have always tested to 20/15 without glasses.

DOCTOR: Does the distance blur come and go, or is it constant?

PATIENT: Now I seem to have problems seeing clearly when I look up from my desk—the clock on the wall is blurry for a little while.

DOCTOR: Is the blur in one or both eyes?

PATIENT: I don't know. Nothing is clear, so I guess both are blurred.

DOCTOR: How long do you have to be doing close work before you notice this blur, and if you wait a while, does the clock get clearer?

PATIENT: It starts early in the day, I think. Sometimes if I rub my eyes and take a few seconds it'll clear up. By the end of the day, though, it takes up to 5 minutes to clear my vision.

DOCTOR *(thinking)*: *This transient blurring associated with near tasks sounds like accommodative dysfunction. It also could be secondary to a small, uncompensated refractive error, vergence anomaly, or early presbyopia. Periodic headaches, asthenopia, diplopia, tearing, and fatigue are common with these conditions, so some questions in this area are warranted.*[1]

DOCTOR: What about headaches or eye pain?

PATIENT: I've noticed a few headaches in the front of my head around my eyes, and my eyes ache and throb sometimes after a busy day.

DOCTOR: How often do you have the headaches, and what do you do about them?

PATIENT: I have about two a week now. I take some ibuprofen and then rest for 30 minutes to an hour, and they go away.

DOCTOR: Do you ever wake up with a headache?

PATIENT: Never. Sleep always makes the headache and eye-aches go away.

DOCTOR: Do you have the headaches on the weekend?

PATIENT: No, not unless I take a lot of work home with me.

DOCTOR *(thinking)*: *Headaches and asthenopia that occur at the end of the day and that disappear with rest, or those that occur only during the work week, commonly are of visual etiology.*[4]

DOCTOR: How about your work stamina? Have you found yourself tiring earlier in the workday?

PATIENT: Definitely! I used to be able to read all day long. Now I'm fatigued after 20 or 30 minutes and exhausted after 4 hours, and I have a hard time concentrating.

DOCTOR: How close do you normally hold your reading material or other close work?

PATIENT *(demonstrating)*: Oh, about this far *(45 cm)*, and my computer screen is about this far *(50 cm)*.

DOCTOR: Do you experience any doubling of vision for distant or near objects? Even when you "let your eyes go"?

PATIENT: No. I've never seen double unless I consciously attempt to do so.

DOCTOR *(thinking)*: *The fatigue with reading is consistent with an accommodation or vergence problem.[5] That she denies diplopia doesn't totally rule out a vergence dysfunction, but it does decrease the likelihood. Though the complaints and symptoms are strongly suggestive of a nonpathologic visual etiology, I should rule out the possibility of an underlying medical condition (diabetes[6] or multiple sclerosis[7]), which might present with similar ocular signs and symptoms.*

DOCTOR: Are you currently on any medications?

PATIENT: None at all.

DOCTOR: When was your last physical examination, and what were the results?

PATIENT: Last month, at the military base. I had a periodic flight physical, so maybe it wasn't complete, but I was told everything was great.

DOCTOR: Did the physical include a blood workup?

PATIENT: Yes. I keep a very close watch because both my mother and brother are diabetic and take insulin.

DOCTOR: How about your physical stamina? Have you noticed any change in it, or numbness or tingling in the extremities after exercise or with heat?

PATIENT: I feel great. I've never noticed any numbness or tingling or a change in my vision after exercise or with heat.

DOCTOR *(thinking)*: *That NB has had a recent physical examination, including lab work, decreases the risk of diabetically induced refractive fluctuations.[6] Also, because there is a family history of diabetes, my patient is aware of the signs and symptoms of the disease and watches for them.*

DIAGNOSTIC HYPOTHESES

From the concerns expressed by the patient, a few diagnoses are possible. The hypotheses are listed here in order of *most* to *least* likely:

1. *Incipient presbyopia.* The patient is 45 years old, and early presbyopia can present initially as eyestrain and fatigue rather than as blur at near. The short periods of distance blur after prolonged near tasks are common with accommodative dysfunction or presbyopia.

2. *Uncompensated refractive error.* The likelihood of myopia is minimal, as the patient is an Air Force pilot and knows that she has always tested to 20/15. NB might have a low amount of hyperopia (more like-

ly), astigmatism (less likely), or both, which would not affect her visual acuity significantly. An uncompensated hyperope could experience some fatigue, asthenopia, and headache with prolonged near tasks.

3.   *Vergence anomaly.* NB could have convergence insufficiency or excess that results in visual fatigue and blur at near. The fact that the complaints are of rather recent onset in an older patient, and that she denies diplopia, reduces the possibility of convergence excess but not necessarily convergence insufficiency.

DIAGNOSTIC TESTING

To test the initial hypothesis of incipient presbyopia, I obtained the following data (presented in Table CS14.1):

- Entering visual acuities at distance and near
- Accommodative amplitude
- Near retinoscopy
- Binocular fused cross-cylinder
- Positive and negative relative accommodation (PRA/NRA)

The somewhat reduced visual acuity at near compared to distance indicates that accommodation is impaired somewhat. The reduced Donder's amplitude and the reduced PRA and high accommodative lags (seen with near retinoscopy and the binocular fused cross-cylinder) are strongly suggestive of the diagnosis of incipient presbyopia.

Additional testing was performed at NB's working distance to help determine the most effective near lens prescription for the patient. These tests included best-corrected visual acuity lenses for near working distance and range of clear vision through those lenses. These results are listed in Table CS14.2. The preferred near lens was determined to be the fused cross-cylinder value, and the patient demonstrated adequate ranges of clear vision through these lenses.

To rule out the possibility that the patient had a previously uncompensated refractive error (hypothesis 2) that is taxing her accommodation to the extent that she has difficulty in seeing well at near, I collected data (Table CS14.3) from:

- Keratometry
- Distance static retinoscopy
- Subjective refraction

The keratometric values revealed low corneal toricity, reducing the likelihood of a significant amount of astigmatism. The refractive sequence revealed a small hyperopic refractive error unlikely to reduce NB's near

Table CS14.1
Hypothesis 1 (incipient presbyopia): problem-specific testing results.

Entering visual acuities at distance and near
    20/15^{-1} OD, OS; 20/15 OU at 6 m
    20/20^{-2} OD, 20/25 OS at 40 cm
Donder's amplitude of accommodation (habitual)
    30 cm OD, 35 cm OS, 30 cm OU
Monocular Estimation Method retinoscopy at 50 cm: +1.50 D lag of
    accommodation
Binocular fused cross-cylinder: +1.50 D over subjective
Positive/negative relative accommodation: –0.50 D/+3.00 D over subjective

Table CS14.2
Hypothesis 1 (incipient presbyopia): additional database testing results.

Best visual acuity (BVA) lens at 45 cm (binocular): +1.50 D over subjective
Range of clear vision through BVA lens at near: 20–62 cm

Table CS14.3
Hypothesis 2 (uncompensated refractive error): problem-specific testing results.

Keratometry: 43.00 @ 180, 43.75 @ 090 OD, OS; clear mires
Static retinoscopy and visual acuities
    OD +0.50 – 0.25 × 090 (20/20)
    OS +0.75 DS (20/20)
Subjective refraction and visual acuities
    OD +0.25 DS (20/15)
    OS +0.50 DS (20/15)

DS = diopter sphere.

visual acuity, although it may have contributed to an increased accommodative demand that could be responsible for her symptoms.

To rule out a possible vergence anomaly, I collected data from distance and near cover tests and near point of convergence (NPC), and phorias and vergence ranges at distance and near (Table CS14.4). The distance and near cover tests revealed a moderate heterophoria at near, and the patient reported a small lateral (but no vertical) phi (or subjective) movement of the target. The NPC shows some reduction, but the patient reported that the target was hard to keep clear and backed away from the approaching target. Phorias and vergence ranges are

Table CS14.4
Hypothesis 3 (vergence anomaly): problem-specific testing results.

Cover test at distance and near
    Orthophoria at distance with no phi movement
    ~ 6Δ exophoria at near
Near point of convergence: 10-cm break after three repetitions
Phorias at distance and near (von Graefe method)
    Orthophoria at distance
    9Δ exophoria through +1.50 D add
    No vertical at distance and near
Vergence ranges at distance
    NFC: x/7/4
    PFC: 15/17/8
Vergence ranges at near (through +1.50 D add)
    NFC: 18/25/14
    PFC: 18/20/14

NFC = negative fusional convergence; PFC = positive fusional convergence.

well within the normal and expected amounts and demonstrate that NB's complaints are not secondary to a vergence anomaly.

By this point in the examination, I believed that the collected data supported the hypothesis of incipient presbyopia. I decided to collect additional baseline data to assess the patient's ocular health and to rule out any ocular pathology, using the following (Table CS14.5):

- Pupil testing
- Oculomotor testing
- Biomicroscopy
- Tonometry
- Automated visual fields
- Fundus examination through dilated pupils

The testing revealed normal pupil reactions and full, smooth oculomotor movements. The biomicroscopic and fundus evaluation revealed normal anterior segment, vitreous, and retinal health. The visual fields revealed normal retinal sensitivity with no significant depressions in the central 30 degrees.

DIAGNOSTIC SUMMARY

NB was found to be an incipient presbyope. Her chief complaint, the associated transient reduction in distance visual acuity, and her headaches, eye-

Table CS14.5
Additional database testing results.

Pupils: PERRL, −APD
Oculomotor testing
   Pursuits: smooth with no head movement
   Saccades: slight overshooting
Biomicroscopy
   Lids, lashes: clear OU
   Cornea, conjunctiva: clear OU
   Anterior chamber: deep, quiet OU
   Lens: clear OU
   Anterior vitreous: quiet OU
Tonometry: 18 mm Hg OD, OS at 11:30 AM
Automated visual fields
   Equal sensitivity OD, OS at 36 dB
   No fixation losses, false-positive or false-negative outcomes
   Gaze pattern: stable
   No significant depression in sensitivity within central 30 degrees
Fundus examination through dilated pupils
   Cup-to-disc ratio: 0.4/0.4 OU
   ONH: healthy rim tissue 360 degrees OU
   Background: healthy retina with even pigmentation to periphery, no
       holes, tears, flat 360 degrees OU, vitreous clear OU
   Vessels: healthy, no abnormal crossings OU

PERRL = pupils equal, round, reactive to light; −APD = no afferent pupillary defect;
ONH = optic nerve head.

aches, and visual fatigue supported this diagnosis. Though she also presented with a small amount of hyperopia that eventually will interfere with her distance visual acuity, it is not responsible for the age-related loss of accommodation that brought her into the office.[1]

TREATMENT OPTIONS

The best option for NB's vision problems was a prescription for spectacles. Though several possibilities were available to her, multifocal spectacles (including progressive-addition lenses), or "half-eyes" were recommended. Any of these would allow the patient to see well both at distance and near without having to remove her spectacles. NB selected a flat-top bifocal style.

I prescribed plano OD and +0.25 DS OS, with a +1.50 D near add. To address her occupational needs, I prescribed a 35-mm segment width and set the height so the segment would bisect her pupils. The wide segment provided a large area of clear near vision that would help to minimize head movement in working at the computer. The high placement of the segment allowed NB to see her near work without having to tilt her head back. She was informed that she would find the occupational glasses helpful and that she should wear them whenever she was indoors. This not only made it easy to remember when she should wear the spectacles but reassured her that the lenses were not necessary for driving or flying, allowing her to be a somewhat selective lens wearer. She also was advised that because of the placement of the segment height, she would probably have to drop her chin a small amount to see distant objects.

To address her normal daily needs outside of work, I prescribed the same-power lens with a 35-mm segment width, set at her lower lid margin. The segment line would be less noticeable in walking, driving, and doing normal tasks that might require the bifocal for clear near vision (e.g., reading a map).

REFERENCES

1. Fannin TE. Presbyopic Addition. In JB Eskridge, JF Amos, JD Bartlett (eds), Clinical Procedures in Optometry. Philadelphia: Lippincott, 1991;198–205.
2. Grosvenor TP. Primary Care Optometry: A Clinical Manual. Chicago: The Professional Press, 1982;23.
3. Grunberg NE. Stress and vision: some historical perspectives and possible future directions. J Optom Vis Dev 1986;17(4):7–9.
4. Amos JF. Patient History. In JB Eskridge, JF Amos, JD Bartlett (eds), Clinical Procedures in Optometry. Philadelphia: Lippincott, 1991;3–16.
5. Borish IM. Clinical Refraction (3rd ed). Chicago: The Professional Press, 1970;149–188.
6. Cavallerano JD. A review of non-retinal ocular complications of diabetes mellitus. J Am Optom Assoc 1990;61:533–543.
7. Frantsvog EB, Townsend JC, Selvin GJ. Localization of visual field defects in multiple sclerosis. J Am Optom Assoc 1991;62:100–108.

Appendix: Case Scenario 14

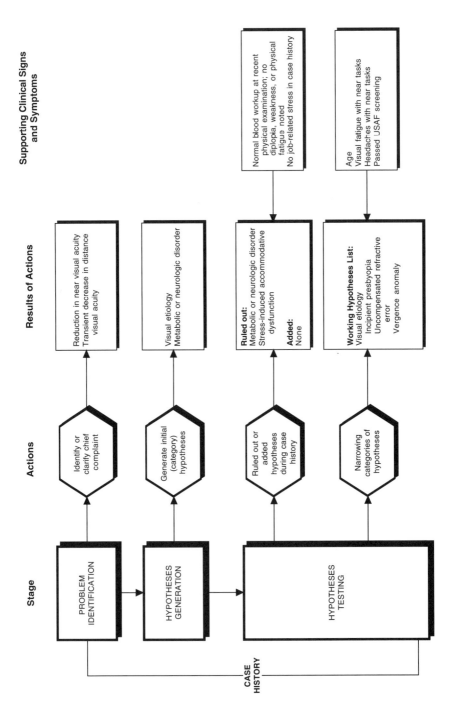

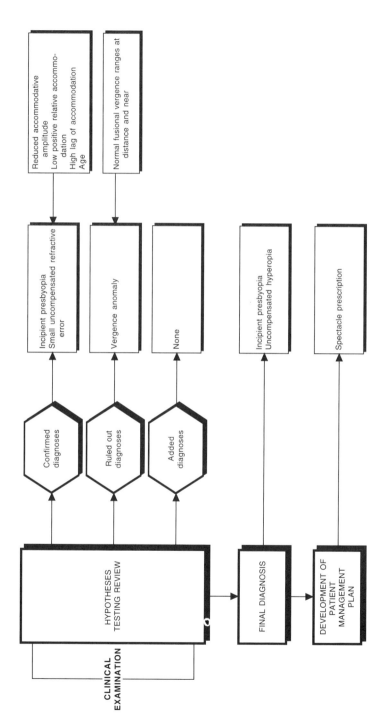

Case Scenario 14 decision-making summary. (USAF = United States Air Force.)

Case Scenario 15

Daniel Kurtz

PATIENT BACKGROUND

FF is a 26-year-old Hispanic woman.

DOCTOR: Why have you come in this morning?

PATIENT: My right eye has been bothering me for the last week.

DOCTOR *(thinking): The complaint of "bothering" is rather vague and could represent a wide variety of subjective complaints from pain to blurry vision. I'll need to clarify the complaint before I can generate any specific diagnostic hypotheses.*

DOCTOR: In what way does your eye bother you? Describe the way it feels.

PATIENT: Well, it doesn't actually hurt most of the time, but when I go outside or walk into a bright room, it feels uncomfortable for a while, as if bright lights are being shined into it.

DOCTOR: Have you noticed anything else about your eye that seems to coincide with the start of this problem?

PATIENT: No, not really.

DOCTOR: I notice that you aren't wearing glasses. Do you wear contact lenses or glasses some of the time?

PATIENT: No.

DOCTOR *(thinking): The complaint seems to fall into the general category of light sensitivity or photophobia. The first condition that comes to mind is anterior uveitis (iritis).[1] Other possible causes include optical scatter of light (irregular cornea, cataract) and keratitis. Dry eye is also a possibility if the symptom is precipitated by some peculiar circumstance that affects only her right eye; this seems remote.[2] I'll pursue iritis for now.*

DOCTOR: Has your eye been red?

PATIENT: No.

DOCTOR: Do you experience any discomfort at any time other than when you first go into the light?

PATIENT: No.

DOCTOR: Can you see well, or is your vision blurry in that eye?

PATIENT: I don't know. I've never looked with just my right eye.

DOCTOR: Have you been hit in your eye recently?

PATIENT: No!

DOCTOR *(thinking)*: *This complaint does not match well with iritis or other ocular disease. It is more likely that she's just sensitive to light. But why complain about just one eye, and why the recent, sudden onset? The cause may be psychological, related to stress on the job or at home and causing a conversion hysteria manifesting as light sensitivity. I'll ask about her occupation and general well-being and health to probe this possibility.*

DOCTOR: Tell me what you do for a living.

PATIENT: I'm a legal secretary. It's challenging and hectic at times, but I love my job.

DOCTOR: How is your general health?

PATIENT: Good, I go for a yearly physical. I went just 3 months ago, and the doctor said that I'm fine.

DOCTOR *(thinking)*: *It appears that she likes her job, and her general health is okay, so I don't see any indications suggesting a psychogenic cause for her complaint. Corneal or crystalline lens opacities can cause a complaint of photophobia because they scatter light. She has no complaints of blurred vision, but she has not had her vision tested monocularly; also, the onset might have been slow, and she may not been aware of the problem. These problems will have to be ruled out by testing. Another possibility is that she might have a mydriatic pupil that lets in too much light and can cause sensitivity to light. On general observation, it does appear that the right pupil is larger than the left. There are a number of causes of a mydriatic pupil: physiologic anisocoria, pathology in the eye, topical application of a mydriatic agent, or pathology along the sympathetic or parasympathetic pathway. I can ask for some additional problem-specific history to probe whether she may have inadvertently applied a mydriatic agent.*

DOCTOR: Have you taken any eye or other medications within the last few months?

PATIENT: No.

DOCTOR: Some plants have a potential to cause some eye irritation or discomfort. Do you garden or come into contact with any plants where you may have rubbed your eye?

PATIENT: No. I am not very good with plants. All my plants are silk plants.

DOCTOR *(thinking)*: *It doesn't appear that there was any topical application. I'll complete some baseline case history before I start the examination.*

DOCTOR: Is there any family history of eye disease, such as cataracts or glaucoma or vision problems?

PATIENT: No cataracts or glaucoma, but my father has a high amount of nearsightedness and wears contact lenses. Otherwise, I can't recall anyone else having any problems.

DOCTOR: Are there any family medical problems that I should be aware of, such as diabetes or hypertension?

PATIENT: No. All my family is pretty healthy. Although I think my grandmother, who is 72, takes some medication for high blood pressure.

DOCTOR *(thinking)*: *There isn't any additional significant information revealed from the family history.*

DIAGNOSTIC HYPOTHESES

On the basis of FF's case history, the initial hypothesis list reads as follows:

1.   *Corneal or crystalline lens opacities.* These problems might have developed to a point at which they might cause the photophobia, because they scatter light. She may have been unaware of the problems because she had not tested her vision monocularly.

2.   *Mydriatic pupil.* The increased pupil size lets in too much light and may cause the sensitivity to light. Anisocoria may be associated with four categories of problems: (1) physiologic (also called *essential* or *simple*) anisocoria (i.e., no detectable pathology), by far the most common cause of anisocoria and definitely considered, although unlikely in this case because the onset is recent; (2) pathology or a problem within the eye itself, such as topical instillation of a mydriatic agent, or ocular pathology, such as acute angle closure, iritis, or iris atrophy, also unlikely considering FF's case history; (3) pathology along the parasympathetic pathway from the oculomotor nucleus in the brain stem to the iris sphincter; or (4) pathology along the sympathetic pathway between the hypothalamus and the iris dilator.[3]

3.   *Psychogenic or idiopathic etiology.* There is a chance that there is no obvious cause for the photophobia. This diagnosis is one of exclusion and will be considered if there is no physical or neurologic reason found to account for the photophobia.

DIAGNOSTIC TESTING

Diagnostic testing is presented in a decision-making format, not necessarily the order in which I sequenced the examination. To arrive at the definitive diagnosis, I started with the most likely hypothesis and gathered all the clinical data to either confirm or deny its relationship to the patient's presenting problems. I then continued through the hypothesis list.

To rule out corneal irregularities or opacities and lenticular opacities, I conducted the following tests (Table CS15.1):

Table CS15.1
Hypothesis 1 (corneal irregularity or opacity of cornea or lens):
problem-specific testing results.

Visual acuity without correction at 6 m
OD 20/30^{-2} PH 20/20^{-2}
OS 20/15
Visual acuity without correction at 40 cm
OD 20/50
OS 20/20
Retinoscopy
OD +1.00 DS
OS +1.00 DS
Subjective refraction and visual acuities
OD +1.00 DS (20/20)
OS +1.00 DS (20/20)
Biomicroscopy
Anterior chamber: deep, quiet OU
Conjunctiva: clear OU
Cornea: clear OU
Lids, lashes: clear OU
Lens: clear OU
Tear film: normal OU
Iris: brown, normal OU

PH = pinhole visual acuity; DS = diopter sphere.

- Visual acuities at distance and near
- Retinoscopy and subjective refraction
- Biomicroscopy of the anterior segment and lens

The results of visual acuity testing revealed unequal visual acuities, with the right eye at 20/30$^-$. A pinhole visual acuity of 20/20^{-2} suggested that the decrease was either refractive or media-related. The reduced visual acuity of the right eye at near (20/50) suggested either an uncorrected anisometropic refractive error or impaired accommodative function. The results of the refraction confirmed that FF's reduced visual acuity in the right eye was secondary to an uncorrected refractive error. The pathology has left her with reduced accommodation in her right eye, so she functions like a presbyopic hyperope, without a sufficient amplitude of accommodation to neutralize her hyperopia all the time. The anterior segment evaluation was negative for lenticular opacities, and there was a normal anterior segment, except that the right pupil was greater than the left pupil (6 vs. 3 mm). There was no ptosis associated with the anisocoria; thus, the first hypothesis (corneal or lenticular opacity) was eliminated, and the second hypothesis (mydriatic pupil) was confirmed.

Table CS15.2
Hypothesis 2 (differential diagnosis of causes of mydriatic pupil):
problem-specific testing results.

Pupil testing
  –APD
  OD > OS: difference more pronounced in bright than in dim light
  OD: minimal response to light
  Both respond to near
Monocular accommodative amplitudes (minus lens to blur): OD, –1.25 D;
  OS, –6.25 D
Extraocular muscle testing: versions smooth, accurate, full in all fields of
  gaze
Near point of convergence: 5-cm break, diplopia noticed, and 10-cm
  recovery
Cover test
  Unilateral: nonstrabismic at far, near
  Alternating: orthophoria at far, 2Δ exophoria at near
Monocular color vision: 13/14 OD, OS (Ishihara plates)
Tonometry (applanation): 14 mm Hg OD, 15 mm Hg OS at 2:00 PM

–APD = no afferent pupillary defect.

To evaluate further the anisocoria and associated neurologic signs
and causes, the following tests were conducted (Table CS15.2):

- Pupil testing (under normal and dim illumination)
- Monocular accommodative amplitudes
- Extraocular muscle testing
- Cover test
- Near point of convergence
- Monocular color vision
- Tonometry

Simple anisocoria is by far the most common diagnosis for anisocoria.[4, 5] However, FF's anisocoria was more pronounced in bright light,
whereas in physiologic anisocoria, the degree of difference between
the two pupils is equal in dim and bright light. Her right pupil barely
responded to light, whereas in physiologic anisocoria, both pupils
respond briskly. Finally, patients with simple anisocoria rarely have any
symptoms, whereas FF had definite complaints.[5] Because the diagnosis of simple anisocoria is a diagnosis by exclusion, I had to consider
and rule out all possible pathologies, even if I had reason to think that
her anisocoria was physiologic.

Anisocoria due to ocular pathology is associated with acute angle closure, anterior uveitis, or atrophy or damage to the tissue of the iris.[4–6] The

results of the biomicroscopic examination allowed me to rule out all but the most unlikely of pathologies of the eye. I failed to find conjunctival injection, corneal edema, or elevated intraocular pressure, thus ruling out angle-closure glaucoma; I failed to find conjunctival injection, cells and flare in the anterior chamber, or depressed intraocular pressure, thus ruling out iritis; and the iris is intact, which ruled out iris atrophy or damage.

In pathology of the sympathetic pathway (Horner's syndrome), the affected pupil is miotic relative to the other pupil, the degree of anisocoria is greater in dim than in bright light, and the affected eye has a mild ptosis, usually involving both the upper and lower eyelid. However, none of the data suggested that FF had Horner's syndrome. Thus, her presenting complaint is sensitivity to light in the eye with the larger, not the smaller, pupil. The anisocoria is more pronounced in bright light than in dim light, and she does not have a ptosis.

Although FF has no ptosis, her entering complaint and the manner in which her right pupil reacts to light strongly suggested that her problem is located along the parasympathetic pathway. Thus, the patient's symptoms are associated with the right eye, which is the eye with the larger pupil. She has symptoms only in bright light, suggesting that the problem is more pronounced under those conditions.

The parasympathetic pathway to the iris contains three important anatomic compartments: (1) within the brain, (2) between the brain and the ciliary ganglion, and (3) between the ciliary ganglion and the iris.[6, 7] I organized my thoughts along these anatomic lines and looked for neurologic signs or symptoms associated with pathology in each of the following three locations:

1.   *Pathology located within the central nervous system (CNS).* Anisocoria due to pathology of the parasympathetic pupillary fibers within the CNS is associated with a mesencephalic (midbrain) tumor or stroke that involves either the oculomotor nuclear complex or the oculomotor axons as they traverse the midbrain.[6] Pathology in either location is almost certain to impair most or all of the muscles controlled via the oculomotor nerve; therefore, the patient would have to have some palsy of the extraocular muscles or a ptosis in addition to the anisocoria. Also, because the oculomotor axons pass through and around the red nucleus and the descending corticospinal tracts of the crus cerebri, pathology involving the axons rather than the nucleus would create serious somatic muscle weaknesses or movement disorders on the side of the body contralateral to the mydriatic pupil.[3, 6] FF revealed none of these findings, so I could rule out midbrain pathology.

2.   *Pathology located along the oculomotor nerve.* The signs and symptoms of pathology along the oculomotor nerve depend on the precise

location of the pathology. It is possible that signs and symptoms will be limited to components of the oculomotor nerve, but more than one component should be affected.[8] In FF, all of the somatic motor components of the third cranial nerve were spared; thus, pathology along the oculomotor nerve is unlikely. Nevertheless, at this point, I had to stop to consider two life-threatening conditions that strike this part of the pathway, even though they are unlikely: Hutchinson's pupil and aneurysm.

Hutchinson's pupil is an unresponsive pupil caused by herniation of the medial temporal lobe into the tentorial notch, resulting in compression of the oculomotor nerve. The herniation is caused by a space-occupying lesion inside the cranium. In addition to presenting with impairment of some of the somatic motor components of the third cranial nerve, patients usually are stuporous or even comatose.[6, 9] FF does not fit this clinical picture at all.

An expanding *aneurysm*, particularly one located at the junction of the posterior communicating artery and the internal carotid artery or elsewhere at the base of the brain, can press on the oculomotor nerve.[4, 8] Aneurysm generally is associated with headache;[6] however, a headache is not inevitable, particularly if the aneurysm has not expanded appreciably. As was the case in Hutchinson's pupil, somatic motor components of cranial nerve III should be involved.[5, 6] It is difficult to rule out this diagnosis without brain imaging, although FF presents with only a few of the signs. I kept this diagnosis in the back of my mind as I investigated further.

3.   *Pathology located in the postganglionic parasympathetic system for pupillary control.* Pathology limited to the postganglionic parasympathetic fibers making up the third compartment should produce mydriasis and cycloplegia while sparing the extraocular muscles.[5] This is precisely what is seen in FF's case. The leading diagnosis for pathology confined to this part of the system is *Adie's pupil*, also called *tonic pupil*.[4, 5] At this point, I rechecked FF's pupil reactions, observed the iris under magnification, and conducted a 0.125% pilocarpine test (Table CS15.3). I found a sluggish right pupil and the light-near dissociation characteristic of an Adie's pupil. Rechecking the pupil with the biomicroscope, I found contraction of some segments of the sphincter when I directed the beam of light into the eye. The presence of such *vermiform* contraction presumably depends on regeneration of postganglionic fibers from the ciliary ganglion to the sphincter.[5] Such regenerated fibers often serve accommodative functions as well; thus, in most cases of Adie's pupil, there is at least partial recovery from the impaired accommodation.[5] What the doctor sees depends on how much time has elapsed between the pathologic event and the presentation of the patient in the office. FF appeared to be presenting fairly

Table CS15.3
Hypothesis 2 (mydriatic pupil–Adie's pupil): problem-specific testing results.

Recheck pupil responses
OD: sluggish response to direct illumination
OD: light-near dissociation present
Re-examination of iris function under magnification: isolated segment contraction of sphincter noted
0.125% pilocarpine test
OD: brisk miotic response
OS: minimal miotic response

soon after the onset of the Adie's pupil, and regeneration had not had much time to occur; therefore, we saw only minimal contractions of the sphincter, and accommodation was still reduced significantly.

At this point, I tested both eyes with dilute (0.125%) pilocarpine, carefully comparing their relative responses.[6] FF's right eye responded much more briskly than did the left eye, which became barely smaller. A diagnosis of Adie's pupil was confirmed.[3, 6, 10]

There also was additional database testing completed to evaluate ocular health, binocular function, and near add determination (data necessary for optical management of the effects of Adie's tonic pupil on the accommodative system), and these test results are listed in Table CS15.4.

DIAGNOSTIC SUMMARY

FF was found to have pathology of the parasympathetic pathway (Adie's pupil), which is related to her entering complaint of photophobia. She also was found to have simple hyperopia. The results of the refraction confirm that the reduced visual acuity in her right eye was secondary to an uncorrected refractive error. In FF's case, although she is young, her pathology left her with an accommodative insufficiency in her right eye. In that eye, she functions like a presbyopic hyperope with insufficient amplitude of accommodation to neutralize her hyperopia at all times.

TREATMENT OPTIONS

FF needed a correction for her hyperopia to eliminate the blur resulting from the failure of the right eye to accommodate adequately. I pre-

Table CS15.4
Additional database testing results.

Dilated fundus examination
  Media: clear OU
  ONH margins: distinct OU
  ONH rim: pink and flat OU
  Cup-disc ratio: 0.1/0.1 OU
  Vessels: A/V ratio 2/3, normal crossings OU
  Maculae: clear OU
  Background: clear, no holes, tears, flat 360 degrees OU
Near refraction and visual acuity
  OD: tentative add +1.50, 20/20 at 40 cm
  OS: tentative add plano, 20/20 at 40 cm
Stereopsis: 40 secs of arc (Randot Stereotest)

ONH = optic nerve head; A/V = arteriovenous.

scribed bifocals so that she could function comfortably at near. As the fibers of her ciliary ganglion regenerate, this problem will largely correct itself.[8] She must be educated carefully to the fact that she probably will not need the glasses after some time has passed. A gradient tint was included to reduce the glare when she first goes outside; this also allows her to use the glasses for reading.

Patient education is an important consideration in Adie's pupil. First, FF needs to be reassured that she is not afflicted with a serious pathology; her condition is neither life- nor sight-threatening. Nevertheless, she is at risk that the same problem will strike her left eye at some time in the future, because the other eye acquires a tonic pupil at the rate of 4% per year,[11] and she should be aware of this possibility.[4] She also should be advised to carry some form of medical identification so that, if she should suffer a cranial injury in the future, her anisocoria will not be confused as a sign of intracranial hemorrhage (i.e., a Hutchinson's pupil).[8]

In the absence of new symptoms, she was advised to return for follow-up in 3 months. At that time, I expect to see a more typical Adie's' pupil, with some restoration of accommodation and with more pronounced and obvious vermiform contractions of the sphincter in the affected eye. I can also check for a need for any changes in her optical correction.

REFERENCES

1. Havener WH. Synopsis of Ophthalmology (6th ed). St. Louis: Mosby, 1984.
2. Semes LP. Light Sensitivity. In JF Amos (ed), Diagnosis and Management in Vision Care. Boston: Butterworth, 1987;43–82.

3. Carter JH. Diagnosis of pupillary anomalies. J Am Optom Assoc 1979;50:671–680.

4. Alexandridis E. The Pupil. New York: Springer-Verlag, 1985.

5. Slamovits TL, Glaser JS. The Pupils and Accommodation. In JS Glaser (ed), Neuro-Ophthalmology (2nd ed). Philadelphia: Lippincott, 1990;459–486.

6. Thompson HS. The Pupil. In WM Hart Jr (ed), Adler's Physiology of the Eye: Clinical Application (9th ed). St. Louis: Mosby–Year Book, 1992;412–441.

7. Netter FH. The CIBA Collection of Medical Illustrations (vol 1). The Nervous System: Part I. Anatomy and Physiology. Summit, NJ: CIBA Pharmaceutical Company, 1983.

8. Walsh TJ. Pupillary Abnormalities. In TJ Walsh (ed), Neuro-Ophthalmology: Clinical Signs and Symptoms (3rd ed). Philadelphia: Lea & Febiger, 1992;52–75.

9. Kline LB, Bajandas FJ. Neuro-Ophthalmology Review Manual (4th ed). Thorofare, NJ: Slack, 1996.

10. Beck RW, Smith CH. Neuro-Ophthalmology: A Problem-Oriented Approach. Boston: Little, Brown, 1988.

11. Thompson HS. Adie's syndrome: some new observations. Trans Am Ophthalmol Soc 1977;75:587–626.

Appendix: Case Scenario 15

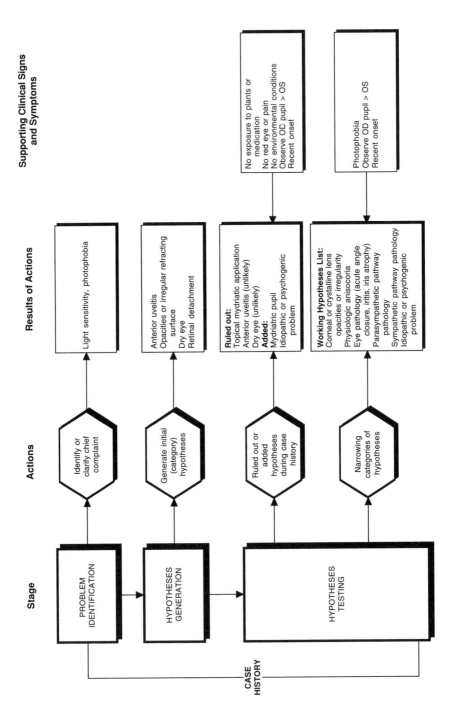

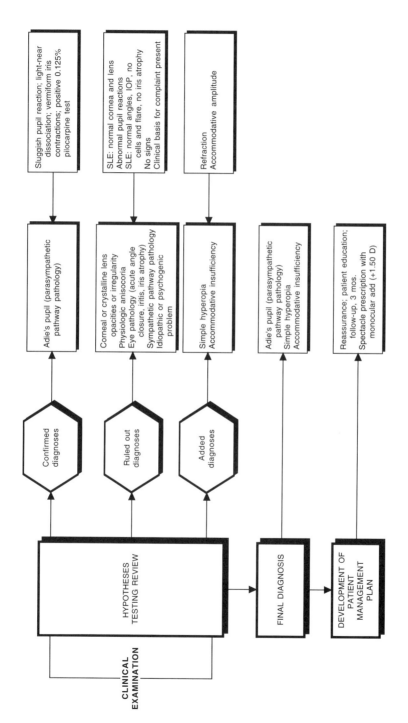

Case Scenario 15 decision-making summary. (SLE = slit-lamp examination; IOP = intraocular pressure.)

Case Scenario 16

Eric Borsting

PATIENT BACKGROUND

SK is an 8-year-old white second-grade boy.

DOCTOR: What brings you in for an examination today?

MOTHER: SK is struggling in school, and we want to know whether his eyes are causing the problem. The school recommended an eye examination as part of a psychoeducational evaluation they're performing.

DOCTOR (thinking): *A child undergoing a psychoeducational evaluation is significantly behind in school. Such an evaluation usually is recommended when the child is 2 years behind in school or has significant difficulties in the early grades. In cases of potential learning-related visual problems, the entering complaints usually are vague (such as poor school performance). I need to identify specific signs and symptoms that represent visual problems. I'm most concerned about DVIP* (developmental visual information–processing) *problems, because they often have a greater impact on learning in the primary grades.[1] Visual efficiency problems typically have a greater impact in the later grades, when the amount of near-point work increases.*

I use a standard list of questions given to the parent before the examination. The form covers behaviors that might signify one or more vision problems in school-age children (Figure CS16.1) *and the questions seek to uncover behaviors that might indicate refractive status, visual efficiency* (questions 3–19) *or DVIP problems* (questions 20–25). *The information from this form will help me focus my interview on the relevant problems.* (The responses from the patient's mother are listed in Figure CS16.1.)

DOCTOR: When did the reversal errors start, and how often do they occur?

MOTHER: The reversal errors started in kindergarten, but he still makes many errors. This occurs every week when I review his homework. My older daughter stopped making these errors at the beginning of second grade.

DOCTOR: Is handwriting also a problem?

MOTHER: It takes him a long time to write any of his assignments. He tries to avoid writing, or tries to make me do the work.

Patient: _____**SK**_____   File Number: ____**001**____

	Yes	No	
1.	✔	____	School performance not up to potential.
2.	✔	____	Attending grade level expected for age.
3.	✔	____	Skips and rereads words and/or letters.
4.	✔	____	Complains of blurred vision, during reading and writing.
5.	____	✔	Complains of headaches associated with visual tasks.
6.	____	✔	Complains of print "running together" or "jumping around."
7.	____	✔	Reports sensation of eyes "not working together."
8.	____	✔	One eye turns in or out, up or down at any time.
9.	✔	____	Experiences unusual fatigue after visual concentration.
10.	____	✔	Reports pain around or in the eye at any time.
11.	____	✔	Reddened eyes or lids.
12.	____	✔	Excessive tearing of eyes, or rubs eyes frequently.
13.	____	✔	Blinks excessively.
14.	____	✔	Frowns, scowls, or squints.
15.	____	✔	Tilts or turns head excessively.
16.	____	✔	Closes or covers one eye in bright light or during visual tasks.
17.	____	✔	Uses finger as marker when reading.
18.	✔	____	Avoids close work.
19.	____	✔	Holds books too closely.
20.	✔	____	Reversals when reading (was-saw, on-no) or writing (b for d, p for q).
21.	____	✔	Poor recall of visually presented materials.
22.	✔	____	Transposition of letters or numbers (21 for 12).
23.	✔	____	Poor handwriting.
24.	____	✔	Clumsiness.
25.	____	✔	Makes errors in copying from blackboard to paper.

Completed by _____**Mother**_____   Date ____**3/22/95**____

Figure CS16.1 History Supplement for School-Age Children.

DOCTOR: Does he skip or reread words frequently?

MOTHER: He doesn't read very often, but he tends to skip whole lines without realizing that he made a mistake.

DOCTOR: Does he report that the print appears fuzzy at times?

MOTHER: He says the print looks fuzzy, and he tells us that his eyes get tired after working on his homework for about 10 or 15 minutes.

This started at the beginning of second grade. We thought this was an attempt to get out of doing his homework.

DOCTOR (*thinking*): *Two categories of visual problems are indicated clearly in the case history. First, the reports of fuzzy or blurred vision and visual fatigue associated with near-point tasks usually are reported when the patient has uncorrected hyperopia, or an accommodation or vergence anomaly. However, such problems usually do not affect school performance until the child is reading to learn (after second or third grade) because near-point demands in the primary grades are limited.[1] Cases in which symptoms do arise usually reveal a more severe visual anomaly. The second visual problem is a possible DVIP disorder. Reversal errors, transposition of letters and words, and poor handwriting are observable behaviors that suggest a possible DVIP problem. SK also may suffer from a general learning disability. Most children with learning problems suffer from anomalies in several cognitive domains, such as auditory perception and attentional deficits. The psychoeducational evaluation will identify nonvisual factors that are causing or contributing to the learning problems.*

DOCTOR (*thinking*): *To complete the case history, I'll need information about the patient's and the family's previous eye and medical health.*

DOCTOR: Is this SK's first eye examination?

MOTHER: Yes, but he did pass the vision screening given in first grade.

DOCTOR: How is his general health?

MOTHER: Since entering school, his health is fine. When he was younger, he had several ear infections that were treated with antibiotics.

DOCTOR: Was his hearing affected?

MOTHER: No, he passed the hearing test in first grade.

DOCTOR: Are there any health problems in the family?

MOTHER: The only person with health problems is my mother, who has diabetes. She takes medications to help control the problem.

DOCTOR: Are there any eye problems in the family?

MOTHER: I wear glasses for reading, but I see fine far away. His father doesn't wear glasses.

DOCTOR (*thinking*): *He passed the school screening, which probably rules out the possibility of myopia, significant astigmatism, or high hyperopia. It appears that his mother may have hyperopia. This increases the likelihood that he may have a moderate amount of hyperopia that would be contributing to his problem.*

DIAGNOSTIC HYPOTHESES

On the basis of the case history, the initial hypothesis list includes the following:

1.   *Uncorrected refractive error.* There is a moderate probability that he has a significant amount (>1.50 D) of uncorrected hyperopia. The complaints of intermittent blurred vision at near but not distance would indicate hyperopia and not myopia. A low amount of hyperopia would not cause near-point symptoms, and very high amounts of uncorrected hyperopia (>4.00 D) usually are associated with esotropia or a bilateral reduction in visual acuity. Low amounts of astigmatism also could be present.

2.   *Vergence anomaly.* There is a moderate probability that a vergence problem could account for SK's visual fatigue at near. The vergence problem could be convergence insufficiency or convergence excess. Primary-grade children who have a mild vergence problem usually do not manifest symptoms. Because the demand on the vergence system is lower in the primary grades, symptoms usually do not arise unless the child has a marked dysfunction in the vergence system. The vergence anomaly could exist alone or in combination with an uncorrected refractive anomaly.

3.   *Accommodative anomaly.* SK could have accommodative insufficiency or accommodative infacility. These problems likely would exist in conjunction with a vergence anomaly or an uncorrected refractive error.

4.   *Visual information–processing anomaly.* There is a high probability that SK has a DVIP problem. Visual-spatial, visual-analysis, and visual-motor problems would account for many of the symptoms (reversal errors and poor handwriting) indicated in the case history.

5.   *Learning disability.* When a psychoeducational evaluation is performed, there is a high likelihood that the child has a learning disability. Such evaluations are performed when the child's school performance lags behind his or her peers by approximately 2 years. It is not my role to diagnose a learning disability directly; instead, I attempt to detect or diagnose any visual anomalies that interfere with the learning process and communicate this information to the parents and the school.[2]

DIAGNOSTIC TESTING

The diagnostic testing sequence is based in part on a hierarchy of diagnostic syndromes that may account for the patient's complaint. For example, for the complaint of intermittent blurred vision at near, the working hypothesis of hyperopia is the first problem that I would rule out. However, the sequence of the primary care examination may not match the hierarchy of diagnostic syndromes outlined previously. For

Table CS16.1
Hypotheses 1 (uncorrected refractive error) and 2 (vergence anomaly):
problem-specific testing results.

Entering visual acuities at far and near
   20/20 OD OS, OU at 6 m
   20/30 OD, OS, OU at 40 cm
Static refraction (retinoscopy)
   OD +2.50 DS
   OS +2.50 DS
Subjective refraction and visual acuities
   OD +1.50 DS (20/20)
   OS +1.50 DS (20/20)
Cover test
   Without correction: 8Δ esophoria at far, 10Δ esophoria at near
   With subjective refraction (dry): 2Δ esophoria at far, 4Δ esophoria at near
Stereopsis: Randot Stereotest
   Without correction: 50 secs of arc
   With subjective refraction (dry): 30 secs of arc
Cycloplegic examination
   OD +3.25 DS
   OS +3.25 DS

DS = diopter sphere.

example, entrance tests frequently evaluate skills in several systems to help identify the need for more comprehensive testing.

To rule out the initial hypothesis of uncorrected refractive error, I collected problem-specific clinical data (Table CS16.1) from the following:

- Entering visual acuities
- Retinoscopy
- Subjective refraction

A significant amount of hyperopia was found on dry retinoscopy (+2.50 D OD, OS) and on subjective refraction (+1.50 D OD, OS). The hyperopia probably accounts for the complaints of intermittent blurred vision and visual fatigue associated with visual tasks. The presence of a significant uncorrected refractive error also changed my diagnostic strategy. Significant refractive errors are based on the referral criteria from the Orinda study (hyperopia of >1.50 D, myopia of >0.50 D, astigmatism of >1.00 D, and anisometropia of >1.00 D).[3] An accurate measure of the binocular status may be unattainable until the refractive error is corrected. As a result, I usually perform less extensive testing of accommodative or vergence systems at the initial evaluation.

My first priority was to determine the true refractive error. A prescription determined by dry retinoscopy and subjective refraction may correct only a portion of the hyperopia, because part of the hyperopia may be latent. A cycloplegic refraction would help determine the amount of latent hyperopia present. When the dry retinoscopy is beyond 2.00 D of uncorrected hyperopia, I typically perform a cycloplegic examination.

My second priority was to address the relationship between the uncorrected refractive error and the accommodation and vergence mechanisms. Patients with significant uncorrected refractive errors frequently manifest an accommodative or vergence anomaly when testing is performed at the initial office visit.[4] However, after the corrective lenses are worn for a short period (e.g., 1 month), the visual anomaly frequently is improved or eliminated.[4] As a result, in cases with a significant uncorrected refractive error, I usually limit the testing of accommodation and vergence to the cover test and sensory fusion assessment with and without the tentative correction in place.

The results of the cover test and sensory fusion are presented in Table CS16.1. The cover test, with no correction in place, was 8Δ esophoria at distance and 10Δ esophoria at near. With the dry subjective refraction correction in place, the phoria was reduced to 2Δ esophoria at distance and 4Δ esophoria at near. Stereopsis also improved with the subjective refraction in place.

At this point, I conducted a cycloplegic examination and found an increased amount of hyperopia (+3.25 DS OD, OS). For school-age children with hyperopia greater than 2.00 D, determining the power of the initial correction is a clinical challenge. Some portion of the hyperopia usually is latent, and the major concern is whether the patient needs or will accept the full plus-lens prescription. The potential blurred vision in viewing distant targets may discourage the patient from wearing the spectacle correction. Typically, the first prescription guideline that I use is to cut the cycloplegic refraction by 1.00 D.[5] In my experience, most patients readily adjust to this initial lens prescription. In this case, a lens prescription of +2.25 OU was recommended. This is more plus than was found on the dry subjective refraction, and the patient may experience some initial distance blur, but he should adapt over a 1- to 2-week period, and the distance blur should disappear.

The second prescribing guideline I use is based on the determined or predicted effect the refractive correction will have on the accommodation and vergence system. It is difficult to determine the effect of the lenses on the accommodative or vergence systems during a cycloplegic examination. An approximate prediction of the effect of the prescription on the esophoria can be made by calculating the AC/A ratio or by using a gradient method before the cycloplegic examination. However, the true AC/A ratio may not be attainable until the refractive error is corrected fully. Before correcting the hyperopia, accommodative responses may be inaccurate and usually result in an underestimation of the AC/A ratio. For example, this patient showed 8Δ of esophoria at distance, but he may not have been accommodating the full amount of the hyperopic correction (i.e., 3.25 D). He may only have accommodated the minimum amount to identify the target. If he accommodated the full 3.25 D, a greater amount of esodeviation probably would be manifested. The use of a threshold target does minimize this effect but may not entirely remove it. Therefore, the AC/A ratio I determined from information in the initial examination is only an estimate that I use to predict the approximate change in the vergence system with the tentative spectacle correction.

In this case, I calculated the AC/A ratio to be 6.25/1 (AC/A = interpupillary distance in meters + near testing distance in meters [deviation at near – deviation at far]). The +2.25 D tentative prescription would reduce the esophoria by approximately 14Δ, but the calculated AC/A ratio usually overestimates the actual change in the vergence system. It has been recommended that multiplying the calculated AC/A by 0.8 produces a more accurate predictor of the actual change in vergence per diopter of added lens power.[6] This would result in an AC/A ratio of 5/1. A more accurate method is the gradient method. In this case, a +1.50 lens resulted in a 6Δ change in the phoria and yields an AC/A ratio of 4/1. This is less than the calculated AC/A (6.25/1) or the adjusted calculated AC/A (5/1). The actual change in the phoria following full-time wear of the spectacle correction probably would fall between the 4/1 and 6/1 values. Even using the lower value for the AC/A (4/1), I can predict that a +2.25 D spectacle correction would reduce the esophoria by 9Δ, which would leave the patient with a slight exophoria at distance and a small esophoria at near.

At this point, I had sufficient information to arrive at the primary diagnosis (hyperopia) to account for the complaints of occasional blurred vision and headaches associated with visual tasks. SK manifested a vergence anomaly when her refractive error was uncorrected, but the spectacle correction (+2.25 D OU) should result in a significant improvement or elimination of the vergence anomaly. The effect of the corrective lenses on the DVIP-related complaints is difficult to predict. Children with significant hyperopia are at a greater risk for developing certain DVIP problems.[7] However, in my experience, correcting the refractive error does not always result in improved DVIP skills. As a result, the follow-up office visit should include a screening for DVIP problems.

Table CS16.2
Additional database testing results.

Color vision screening: passed all plates on Ishihara color test
Pupil testing: PERRLA, –APD
Biomicroscopy
  Lids, lashes: clear OU
  Conjunctiva, cornea: clear OU
  Anterior chamber: clear, deep, quiet OU
  Iris: blue, clear OU
  Vitreous: clear OU
Dilated fundus examination
  Media: clear OU
  ONH margins: distinct OU
  ONH rim: pink, healthy OU
  Cup-to-disc ratio: 0.3/0.3 OU
  Vessels: A/V ratio 2/3 OU
  Macula: homogeneous OU
  Periphery: no holes, tears, flat 360 degrees OU

PERRLA = pupils equal, round, reactive to light and accommodation; –APD = no afferent pupillary defect; ONH = optic nerve head; A/V = arteriovenous.

At this point, I collected additional clinical data considered baseline or database information (Table CS16.2). I also have included clinical findings obtained before the cycloplegic examination. I recommended that SK wear the spectacle lens prescription full-time for 1 month and return for a follow-up examination. At the follow-up examination, I reviewed the initial signs and symptoms with the mother.

DOCTOR: Has SK been wearing his glasses?

MOTHER: Yes, he wears the glasses about 90% of the time. Occasionally he plays outside without the glasses.

DOCTOR: What has he told you about the glasses?

MOTHER: He told me that he no longer experiences fuzzy vision when doing schoolwork. He's also working for longer periods of time without complaining or taking breaks.

DOCTOR: Is he still making reversal errors?

MOTHER: Yes, but they occur less frequently.

DOCTOR: Is his handwriting still poor?

MOTHER: Yes, but he seems willing to write more.

DOCTOR: Does he still make errors on his spelling words?

MOTHER: Yes, this hasn't changed with wearing the glasses.

DOCTOR: Does he still skip lines of text when reading?

MOTHER: Yes, but this occurs less frequently with the glasses

DOCTOR: What were the results of the psychoeducational evaluation?

Table CS16.3
Hypotheses 2 (vergence anomaly) and 3 (accommodative anomaly):
problem-specific testing results. Follow-up examination after
wearing +2.25 DS OU for 1 month.

Entering visual acuities at far and near
   20/20 OD OS, OU at 6 m
   20/20 OD, OS, OU at 40 cm
Static refraction (retinoscopy)
   OD +3.00 DS
   OS +3.00 DS
Subjective refraction and visual acuities
   OD +2.50 DS (20/20)
   OS +2.50 DS (20/20)
Cover test (with correction): orthophoria at far and near
Stereopsis: 20 secs of arc
Comprehensive evaluation of accommodation and vergence
   von Graefe phoria: at far, 1Δ exophoria; at near, 1Δ esophoria (no vertical
     far or near)
   Negative fusional convergence at near: x/20/14
   Positive fusional convergence at near: x/24/12
   Accommodative amplitude: 13 D OD, OS
   Accommodative accuracy: +0.75 D OD, OS
   Accommodative facility (±2.00 D flippers): 8 cpm OU
   Negative/positive relative accommodation: +3.00 D/–2.25 D

DS = diopter sphere.

MOTHER: The school recommended that SK be placed in a resource
    room for one period during the day.
DOCTOR (*thinking*): *The spectacle correction for hyperopia improved the asso-*
    ciated signs and symptoms of blurred vision and visual fatigue associated
    with near-point tasks. At this point, I should perform a thorough evalu-
    ation of accommodation and vergence, because he has adapted to the cor-
    rection. However, I would suspect that a significant problem in this area
    is not present because of the positive responses in the case history. Despite
    my expectations, a thorough evaluation is indicated following the specta-
    cle correction to confirm that the accommodation and vergence systems
    have normalized. A screening for a possible DVIP anomaly also is indi-
    cated, because the behaviors of reversal errors, poor handwriting, and
    transposition errors persisted after the patient had worn the correction.
    Finally, I would evaluate saccadic skills, because the mother reported that
    SK skipped whole lines of text when reading.

The results of the evaluation for refractive status and accommodative
and vergence testing are shown in Table CS16.3. SK readily adapted to

Table CS16.4

Hypothesis 4 (developmental visual information processing [DVIP]) and additional hypothesis of oculomotor anomaly: problem-specific testing results.

Oculomotor testing
  Pursuits: 2+ (SCCO rating scale)
  Saccades: 2+ (SCCO rating scale)
DVIP screening
  Gardner Reversal Frequency Test: execution, 1st percentile; recognition,
    16th percentile
  Visual sequential memory: 37th percentile
  Developmental Test of Visual Motor Integration: 16th percentile

SCCO = Southern California College of Optometry.

the spectacle correction and now has accepted almost the full amount of the hyperopia. A small residual esophoria (1Δ) at near was compensated for readily by adequate negative fusional convergence. The accommodative findings were all normal.

At this point, I performed a screening for saccades, pursuits, and DVIP skills (Table CS16.4). Confrontational testing of pursuits and saccades revealed deficiencies in both skills. This corresponded to the complaint of skipping lines when reading. The results of the DVIP screener indicated an abnormally high frequency of reversal errors, poor visual-motor integration, and normal visual-sequential memory. This corresponds to complaints of reversal errors and poor handwriting. An inconsistency in the symptoms and test findings were found for the complaint of transposition of letters within words (e.g., thier for their). Children who make transposition errors often have difficulty remembering a sequence of items. In this case the lack of agreement between the symptom (transposition errors) and the test result (adequate sequential memory) indicates that the problem probably does not have a visual etiology.

DIAGNOSTIC SUMMARY

SK was found initially to have hyperopia with a secondary basic esophoria. The hyperopia and esophoria correspond to his symptoms of intermittent blurred vision and visual fatigue associated with near-point visual tasks. The relationship between the diagnosis and the signs and symptoms were confirmed by the improvement in symptoms after correcting the hyperopia with lenses. After the refractive error was corrected, the follow-up examination indicated that the secondary vergence anomaly was resolved. However, further testing revealed oculomotor and DVIP dysfunctions. The oculomotor problem corresponds to complaints of skipping lines and words in reading. Finally, the DVIP dysfunction corresponds to complaints of reversal errors and poor handwriting. These problems were seen as having a significant correlation with the entering complaint of poor school performance.

TREATMENT OPTIONS

Full-time wear of the spectacle lenses corrected the hyperopia and improved binocular function. The refractive correction will be monitored in subsequent primary care vision examinations. The oculomotor and the DVIP problems could be handled by two approaches. First would be to continue to monitor the effect of the lenses on the oculomotor and DVIP skills. This approach is based on the theory that abnormalities in oculomotor and DVIP resulted from lack of use. Children with uncorrected hyperopia may avoid near-point activities because of the demands on the accommodative and vergence mechanisms. As a result, the development of oculomotor and DVIP skills would be disrupted. The correction of the hyperopia could promote more near-point activity by the patient, and a normal developmental pattern could be re-established. On the basis of this approach, 6 months to 1 year would probably be needed before significant changes occur in these skills.

The second approach would be an active vision therapy program to remedy the deficient visual skills. The vision therapy program is designed to teach the patient appropriate visual strategies for improving visual processing skills. At this time, we do not know exactly which cases will improve with a spectacle correction alone and which individuals need an active vision therapy program. My decision in this type of case is based on two factors. First is the depth of the DVIP problem. When the developmental delay is equal to or greater than one standard deviation below the mean, there is an increased likelihood that the problem is affecting performance significantly.[8] A delay in treatment could result in an exacerbation of the child's learning problems. In this case, scores for the reversal frequency test and the developmental test of visual-motor integration are more than one standard deviation below the mean. Second is the presence of other learning problems. SK probably had information-processing problems in other cognitive domains besides vision, because he is enrolled in a resource room. Children with learning problems are probably less likely to make rapid gains in developmental visual skills. As a result of these factors,

I recommended that he be enrolled in a vision therapy program at this time, rather than waiting.

REFERENCES

1. Flax N. The Relationship Between Vision and Learning: General Issues. In MM Scheiman, MW Rouse (eds), Optometric Management of Learning-Related Vision Problems. St. Louis: Mosby, 1994;127–153.
2. Hoffman LG. The Role of the Optometrist in Diagnosis and Management of Learning-Related Vision Problems. In MM Scheiman, MW Rouse (eds), Optometric Management of Learning-Related Vision Problems. St. Louis: Mosby, 1994;217–225.
3. Blum HL, Peters HB, Bettman JW. Vision screening for elementary schools; the Orinda study. Berkeley: University of California, 1959.
4. Dwyer P, Wick B. The influence of refractive correction upon disorders of vergence and accommodation. Optom Vis Sci 1995;72:224–232.
5. Caloroso EE, Rouse MW. Clinical Management of Strabismus. Boston: Butterworth-Heinemann, 1993.
6. Flom MC, Wick B. A Model for Treating Binocular Anomalies. In AA Rosenbloom, MW Morgan (eds), Principles and Practice of Pediatric Optometry. Philadelphia: Lippincott, 1990;245–273.
7. Rosner J, Gruber J. Differences in the perceptual skills of young myopes and hyperopes. Am J Optom Physiol Opt 1985;62:501–504.
8. Scheiman MM, Gallaway M. Visual Information Processing: Assessment and Diagnosis. In MM Scheiman, MW Rouse (eds), Optometric Management of Learning-Related Vision Problems. St. Louis: Mosby, 1994;127–153.

Appendix: Case Scenario 16

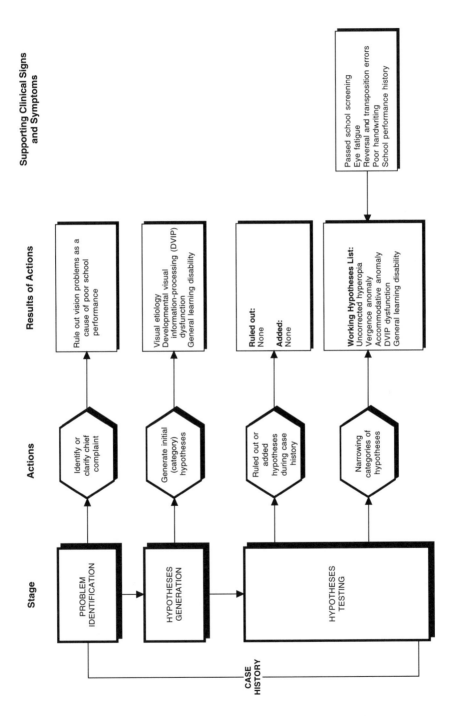

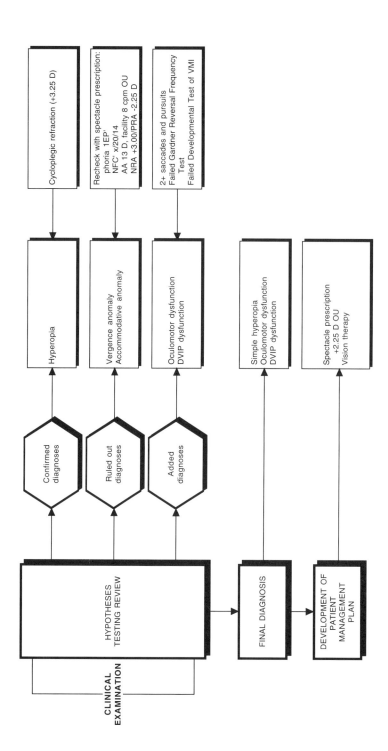

Case Scenario 16 decision-making summary. (EP' = esophoria at near; NFC' = negative fusional convergence at near; AA = accommodative amplitude; NRA = negative relative accommodation; PRA = positive relative accommodation; VMI = visual-motor integration.)

Case Scenario 17

Mitchell M. Scheiman

PATIENT BACKGROUND

DS is a 4-year-old white boy, accompanied to the optometric examination by his mother.

Doctor: Why did you bring your son in to see me today?

Mother: I am worried because lately I've noticed that his right eye has been crossing in.

Doctor *(thinking)*: *With a chief complaint of a crossed eye, my first priority is to try to differentiate whether this is an acquired or congenital strabismus. In this case, it seems likely that it is acquired (on the basis of the mother's description of the problem). If it is acquired, the question I need to answer is whether there is a functional etiology or a more serious neurologic or organic basis. I can gain some insight into these issues by asking a series of questions about the characteristics of the strabismus, such as the time and mode of onset and what makes the problem better or worse. Indications of a serious etiology would be a sudden, constant onset and a strabismus that is worse in one position of gaze. A gradual onset with an intermittent deviation that worsens when the child concentrates on an object held closely suggests an accommodative or a refractive etiology.*

Doctor: How long have you noticed that his right eye turns in? Does it cross in at all times?

Mother: I've noticed the eye turning in for the past 6 months. His eyes look straight most of the time. They just cross on occasion.

Doctor: Is there something in particular that your son is doing when his eye turns in?

Mother: Yes, it happens when he looks at and concentrates on something he is playing with, something that is close to him.

Doctor *(thinking)*: *An onset at approximately age 3–4 is considered to be a late onset and is characteristic of accommodative esotropia.[1] The fact that the strabismus is more likely to occur when he concentrates on a near task also suggests an accommodative etiology. I still want to rule out a non-concomitant strabismus, which also could have a late onset. Insights into this matter can be gained from questions about a health problem or injury associated with the onset or variability in the strabismus during the day.*

I also can determine whether the strabismus seems to be associated with a certain position of gaze.

DOCTOR: You said that you first began noticing his eye crossing approximately 6 months ago. Did he have any significant illness or injury around that time? In particular, any head injury?

MOTHER: No, he has been very healthy this past year, and he's never had any head injury.

DOCTOR: Does the eye seem to turn in more when he is tired or at the end of the day?

MOTHER: No, not really. I think it seems to occur more when he's looking at close things.

DOCTOR: Does his right eye seem to turn when he looks in one position or another? For example, is the eye-turn more likely to occur if he looks to his right, to his left, up, or down?

MOTHER: No, I never noticed anything like that. It just seems to occur when he really looks carefully at something he is holding or if he is concentrating on something.

DOCTOR *(thinking)*: *This sounds like an accommodative esotropia. Let me find out whether he is showing any signs of double vision or complaining of double or blurred vision. Blurred vision might suggest a moderate to high degree of hyperopia as the etiologic factor. If he complains of double vision or tends to cover or close an eye, it suggests that the onset of the eye-turn is recent, rather than long-standing.*

DOCTOR: Does your son ever complain of blurry vision, or does he have a hard time seeing anything?

MOTHER: No, he never complains about his eyes, and he seems to be able to see everything he needs to see.

DOCTOR: Does he ever cover an eye, close an eye, or complain of seeing double?

MOTHER: He never complains of anything, but now that you ask, I have seen him occasionally close his right eye when he is looking carefully at something.

DOCTOR *(thinking)*: *This combination of the right eye turning in when he looks at and concentrates on something up close and his closing an eye suggests a recent onset; a likely hypothesis at this time is accommodative esotropia. I'll need to differentiate the exact type of accommodative esotropia during the evaluation. Is it secondary to high hyperopia, a high AC/A ratio, or a combination of both hyperopia and a high AC/A? To complete the patient history and collect database information, I'll investigate the patient's and family's eye and medical histories.*

DOCTOR: Has your son had an eye examination before?

MOTHER: Only from his pediatrician. He never said anything was wrong.

DOCTOR: How is his general health?

MOTHER: He's always been a very healthy child. He has an occasional ear infection or fever. Other than that, there has been no other problem.

DOCTOR: So he is not taking any medication?

MOTHER: That's right.

DOCTOR: Are there any health problems in the family?

MOTHER: My father had bypass surgery at the age of 62. There are no other problems.

DOCTOR: Does anyone in the family have any vision problems?

MOTHER: His father is nearsighted.

DOCTOR: Any history of a lazy eye, a crossed eye, wearing a patch, or eye surgery?

MOTHER: No, there's no history of any eye problems.

DIAGNOSTIC HYPOTHESES

On the basis of the case history, the initial hypothesis list consists of the following:

1.   *Refractive accommodative esotropia.* The usual onset of accommodative esotropia is between 6 months and 7 years, with an average onset at approximately 3 years old.[1-3] A common form of accommodative esotropia is esotropia secondary to uncorrected moderate to high hyperopia.[4, 5] Studies have shown that approximately 50% of accommodative esotropes have a normal AC/A ratio.[1, 6] This certainly could account for the onset, frequency of the deviation, and worsening of the condition when DS looked at a close object.

2.   *Nonrefractive accommodative esotropia.* This form of accommodative esotropia is caused by a high AC/A ratio and also is a possible etiology, because the condition seemed to occur only when DS concentrated and tried to identify an object held up close. A high degree of hyperopia might lead to an occasional eye-turn even in trying to concentrate on an object held at a distance.

3.   *Combination refractive and nonrefractive accommodative esotropia.* This form of accommodative esotropia is secondary to both high hyperopia and a high AC/A ratio. There certainly could be a combination of both conditions.

4.   *Partially accommodative esotropia.* There may be only a partially accommodative esotropia that will not be eliminated completely after correction of the hyperopia and treatment of the high AC/A ratio. It is possible that the child has had a long standing small-angle esotropia

that is partially accommodative. Because of the increase in accommodative demand that occurs at this age, a variable accommodative component of the deviation now may be present and may be large enough to be observable.

5. *Strabismic amblyopia.* This is unlikely, because the strabismus is intermittent and onset is late. It still must be ruled out during the evaluation.

6. *A nonconcomitance.* There still is a possibility that there could be a condition such as Duane's retraction syndrome, Brown's superior oblique tendon sheath syndrome, or a neurologically based etiology (a unilateral or bilateral sixth nerve palsy). Although esotropia is not associated generally with Brown's superior oblique tendon sheath syndrome, parents are not always accurate when describing their observations. A parent may report that a child's eye is crossing when the eyes look abnormal in one position of gaze. In Brown's syndrome, a vertical deviation will be present when the child adducts and elevates his eyes. Parents may report this unusual appearance as a crossed eye.

DIAGNOSTIC TESTING

To arrive at the definitive diagnosis, I started with the most likely hypothesis and gathered all the clinical data either to confirm or deny its relationship to the patient's presenting problems. I then continued through the hypothesis list. Some of the diagnostic testing (the cycloplegic refraction and dilated fundus examination) are presented in a decision-making format, rather than the order in which I sequenced the examination.

To investigate the initial hypothesis of accommodative esotropia secondary to high hyperopia, I collected the following problem-specific clinical data (Table CS17.1):

- Entering visual acuities at distance and near
- Unilateral and alternate cover test at distance and near (habitual)
- Static refraction
- Subjective refraction with acuities
- Cycloplegic refraction
- Unilateral and alternate cover test at distance and near (with correction)

The normal acuities at distance and near are consistent with the possibility of moderate hyperopia. The acuity data also ruled out hypothesis 5 (strabismic amblyopia). The data from the static and subjective refraction confirmed that DS exhibited a moderate degree of hyperopia.

Table CS17.1
Hypothesis 1 (accommodative esotropia secondary to high hyperopia): problem-specific testing results.

Entering visual acuities at distance and near
  20/20 OD, OS, OU at 6 m
  20/20 OD, OS at 40 cm
Unilateral and alternate cover test
  At distance: intermittent 25Δ, right esotropia (deviates 10% of the time)
  At near: intermittent 45Δ, right esotropia (deviates 75% of the time)
Static refraction (retinoscopy)
  OD +2.00 DS
  OS +2.00 DS
Subjective refraction and visual acuities
  OD +2.00 DS (20/20)
  OS +2.00 DS (20/20)
Cycloplegic refraction
  OD +3.00 DS
  OS +3.00 DS
Cover test
  At distance (with +2.00 DS OD, OS): orthophoria
  At near (with +2.00 DS OD, OS): intermittent 20Δ, right esotropia
    (deviates 10% of the time)

DS = diopter sphere.

The cycloplegic refraction was reserved until the very end of the examination to allow completion of all other accommodative and binocular vision testing. (The results are included here as part of the analysis, however.) The cycloplegic refraction revealed only a mild amount of latent hyperopia. Generally, with hyperopia we expect to find 0.50–0.75 D more hyperopia under cycloplegic conditions.[8] Therefore, the cycloplegic refraction actually revealed only 0.25–0.50 more plus than the static and subjective refraction. The cover test results with the subjective refraction indicated that correction of the hyperopia would eliminate the esotropia at far. The cover test at near, however, suggested that, even with the subjective refraction, an intermittent esotropia was still present. This indicates that the condition is not accommodative esotropia secondary to moderate to high hyperopia alone.

To rule out the hypothesis of accommodative esotropia secondary to high AC/A ratio, I collected the following specific clinical data (Table CS17.2):

- Gradient AC/A ratio (alternate cover test at near with subjective and alternate cover test at near with +2.00 D lenses)
- Stereopsis testing (with +2.00 D add)

Table CS17.2
Hypothesis 2 (accommodative esotropia secondary to high AC/A ratio):
problem-specific testing results.

Alternate cover test
At near with subjective: intermittent 20Δ, right esotropia (deviates 10% of the time)
At near with +2.00 D lenses in addition to subjective: 4Δ esophoria
Stereopsis testing with +2.00 D add: 20 secs of arc (Randot Stereotest)
Worth's four-dot test (with +2.00 D add): four-dot response
Prism bar vergence at distance and at near
Negative fusional vergence at 6 m: x/3/1
Positive fusional vergence at 6 m: x/22/14
Negative fusional vergence at 40 cm: x/10/4
Positive fusional vergence at 40 cm: x/30/20

- Worth's four-dot test (with +2.00 D add)
- Vergence at distance and at near

An AC/A ratio between 4/1 and 6/1 is considered normal.[9] This information, indicating an 8/1 gradient AC/A ratio, confirmed the presence of a high AC/A ratio. Through a +2.00 D add, the deviation at near was a 4Δ esophoria. Thus, the esotropia was associated partially with the high AC/A ratio. The sensory and vergence testing indicated normal stereopsis and positive fusional vergence and only slightly reduced negative fusional vergence. Because the sensory and vergence testing were essentially normal, the strabismus is most likely of recent onset and is compatible with a diagnosis of accommodative esotropia. Generally, long-standing esotropia is associated with secondary sensory anomalies, such as reduced acuity, poor stereopsis, and reduced fusional vergence ranges.

The information in Tables CS17.1 and CS17.2 does tend to suggest strongly a diagnosis of accommodative esotropia secondary to both hyperopia and a high AC/A ratio. Because the distance deviation was eliminated entirely with the hyperopic correction and the near deviation is eliminated with an additional +2.50 D, the hypothesis of partially accommodative esotropia can be eliminated.

To rule out a neurologic etiology, nonconcomitant strabismus, or a congenital syndrome, I performed the following testing (Table CS17.3):

- Pupillary evaluation
- Versions in diagnostic positions of gaze
- Alternate cover test at near in diagnostic positions of gaze
- Color vision testing
- Dilated fundus examination

Table CS17.3
Hypothesis 6 (neurologic etiology, nonconcomitant strabismus, congenital syndrome): problem-specific testing results.

Pupillary evaluation: PERRLA, −APD
Ductions: full movement in all positions of gaze
Versions: full movement in all positions of gaze, no apparent restrictions
Alternate cover test at near in diagnostic positions of gaze
    Upgaze: 20Δ esophoria
    Downgaze: 22Δ esophoria
    Left gaze: 20Δ esophoria
    Right gaze: 20Δ esophoria
    Up and right: 20Δ esophoria
    Up and left: 20Δ esophoria
    Down and right: 22Δ esophoria
    Down and left: 22Δ esophoria
Color vision testing: OD and OS, passed all plates on Ishihara color test
Dilated fundus examination
    Media: clear OU
    ONH margins: distinct OU
    ONH rim: pink, healthy OU
    Cup-to-disc ratio: 0.1/0.1 OU
    Vessels: A/V ratio 2/3, normal crossings OU
    Macula: homogeneous OU
    Background: homogeneous OU
    Periphery: no holes, tears, flat 360 degrees OU

PERRLA = pupils equal, round, reactive to light and accommodation; −APD = no afferent pupillary defect; ONH = optic nerve head; A/V = arteriovenous.

All neurologic testing was normal. There was no sign of a nonconcomitant strabismus, and concomitance testing ruled out Duane's syndrome and Brown's syndrome.

At this point, I thought that I had sufficient problem-specific data to arrive at a definitive diagnosis of accommodative esotropia secondary to a combination of high AC/A ratio and hyperopia. I collected additional data from amplitude of accommodation and biomicroscopic examination, both considered baseline or database information (Table CS17.4). This testing revealed a normal amplitude of accommodation and normal anterior segment health.

DIAGNOSTIC SUMMARY

DS was found to have an accommodative esotropia secondary to both moderate hyperopia and a high AC/A ratio. This diagnosis is very com-

Table CS17.4
Additional database testing results.

Amplitude of accommodation (push-away method): can identify the picture
   at 5 cm (20 D), OD and OS
Biomicroscopy
   Lids, lashes: clear OU
   Conjunctiva, cornea: clear OU
   Anterior chamber: clear, deep, quiet OU
   Iris: brown, normal OU
   Vitreous: clear OU

---

patible with the patient's history. Accommodative esotropia has an average onset at approximately age 3 and almost always begins as an intermittent esotropia associated with near work. The normal, sensory binocular vision findings were also typical of a late-onset, accommodative esotropia. Because accommodative esotropia has a late onset and tends to be intermittent, binocular vision generally is well-developed and is essentially normal.

TREATMENT OPTIONS

The most appropriate treatment approach for the patient's problem was to prescribe spectacles (to correct the hyperopia) and a near add to manage the high AC/A ratio.[5] In this case, I recommended a prescription of:

OD +2.00 DS +2.50 add
OS +2.00 DS +2.50 add

The cycloplegic refraction indicated that another +0.50 D could be prescribed. Because +2.00 D lenses completely eliminated the distance esotropia, I chose not to prescribe more than the subjective refraction, to avoid the possibility of creating any blur that could interfere with DS's initial adaptation to the glasses. The +2.50 D add was selected because it eliminated the near deviation.

It is critical in such cases to specify the appropriate size and placement of the segment. The segment should be large and must be set considerably higher than traditional bifocals to ensure that it is used properly by the child. In this case, an FT-35 segment should be used, and it should be set high enough to split the pupil.[5] The glasses were prescribed for full-time wear, and the child should be re-examined in approximately 4 weeks. The follow-up visit is designed to ensure that the esotropia has been completely eliminated with the eyeglasses. Such a follow-up visit is critical because the initial measurements are not always accurate. Fluctuations in angle size may occur when accommodative responses are inaccurate (often the case in accommodative esotropia).[5] If the follow-up examination reveals a residual strabismus or high esophoria, a program of vision therapy should be considered.[7] The prognosis in this case for achieving normal binocular vision is excellent with spectacles alone.

REFERENCES

1. Parks MM. Abnormal accommodative convergence in squint. AMA Arch Ophthalmol 1958;59:364–380.
2. Baker JD, Parks MM. Early-onset accommodative esotropia. Am J Ophthalmol 1980;90:11–18.
3. Hiatt RL. Medical management of accommodative esotropia. J Pediatr Ophthalmol Strabismus 1983;20:199–201.
4. Helveston EM. Accommodative Esotropia. In JS Crawford (ed), Pediatric Ophthalmology and Strabismus. (Trans New Orleans Acad Opthalmol:34th:1985) New York: Raven Press, 1996;111–118.
5. Caloroso EE, Rouse MW. Clinical Management of Strabismus. Boston: Butterworth-Heinemann, 1993.
6. Raab EL. Etiologic factors in accommodative esodeviation. Trans Am Ophthalmol Soc 1982;80:657–694.
7. Wick B. Accommodative esotropia: efficacy of therapy. J Am Optom Assoc 1987;58:562–566.
8. Scheiman M, Wick B. Clinical Management of Binocular Vision: Heterophoric, Accommodative, and Eye Movement Disorders. Philadelphia: Lippincott, 1993;85–86.
9. Griffin JR. Binocular Anomalies: Procedures for Vision Therapy (2nd ed). Boston: Butterworth, 1982;36–37.

Appendix: Case Scenario 17

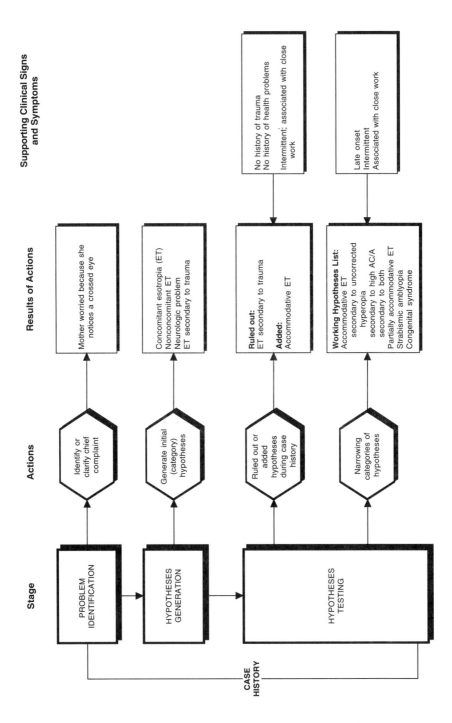

Supporting Clinical Signs and Symptoms

No history of trauma
No history of health problems

Intermittent; associated with close work

Late onset
Intermittent
Associated with close work

Results of Actions

Mother worried because she notices a crossed eye

Concomitant esotropia (ET)
Nonconcomitant ET
Neurologic problem
ET secondary to trauma

Ruled out:
ET secondary to trauma

Added:
Accommodative ET

Working Hypotheses List:
Accommodative ET
  secondary to uncorrected
  hyperopia
  secondary to high AC/A
  secondary to both
Partially accommodative ET
Strabismic amblyopia
Congenital syndrome

Actions

Identify or clarify chief complaint

Generate initial (category) hypotheses

Ruled out or added hypotheses during case history

Narrowing categories of hypotheses

Stage

PROBLEM IDENTIFICATION

HYPOTHESES GENERATION

HYPOTHESES TESTING

CASE HISTORY

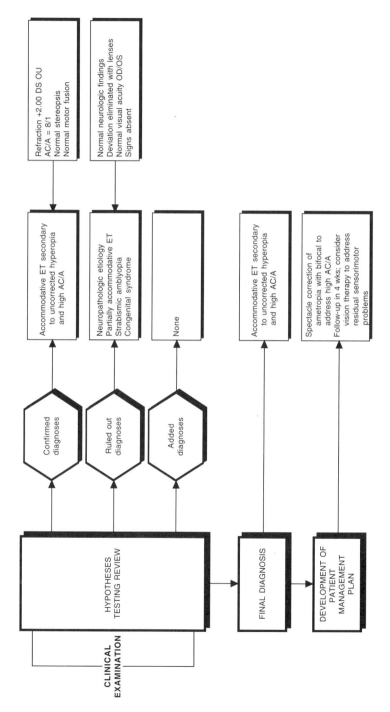

Case Scenario 17 decision-making summary. (AC/A = accommodative convergence/accommodation ratio.)

Case Scenario 18

Joseph W. Sowka and Alan G. Kabat

PATIENT BACKGROUND

JP is a 62-year-old white male executive who presents for a comprehensive eye examination.

DOCTOR: Why are you here today? What can I do for you?

PATIENT: Well, its been about 4 years since I last had an eye exam, and I wanted to have a good, comprehensive evaluation done today. I'm particularly troubled by a recent increase in the number of floating spots in my left eye.

DOCTOR *(thinking)*: *This patient's chief complaint involves a sudden increase in the amount of floaters in the left eye. On the basis of the fact that the patient volunteers this information early in the examination, I must assume that this is a significant medical event insofar as the patient is concerned. However, I must examine all the possible causes of floaters. At this point, I must consider any and all of the possible etiologies: anterior segment and tear film, vitreal disorders, retinal disorders, and neurologic events. Because the patient has reported a change in the status of the floaters, I also must consider this a new event and must explore the patient's history and experience with floaters.*

DOCTOR: When did you first notice this problem?

PATIENT: I first noticed some floaters about 4 years ago, in both eyes. At that time, I was examined by an optometrist in Chicago, where I used to live, and she said that everything was fine, not to worry. Frankly, I don't recall the term that she used to describe this condition. Those initial floaters have not really changed since then, but about 4 days ago, I noticed the floaters had gotten much worse in my left eye. I noticed one big floater almost in the center of my vision but a little to the left. It has me a little concerned because it's so different from the others, and the other optometrist told me that if I ever noticed a change in the floaters I should be checked right away.

DOCTOR *(thinking)*: *Due to the duration and stability of this new event, this is most likely not an ocular surface abnormality, such as mucus tear debris or dry eye syndrome. Most likely the previous instance of floaters was attributable to benign vitreous syneresis or asteroid hyalosis. I must elab-*

orate further on the symptoms to establish the tentative diagnostic hypothesis. However, on the basis of the information provided, the most likely etiology would seem to be a posterior vitreous detachment (PVD). However, I also must rule out retinal detachment because of recent onset of floaters, so I will ask about any recent observations of flashes of light.

DOCTOR: Have there been any other unusual occurrences associated with this problem? In particular, have you noticed any flashes of light or a loss of vision?

PATIENT: Actually, I did notice some flashes during the first 2 days, but they don't seem to be occurring anymore. I don't feel as if my vision has decreased, but the floater sometimes does get in the way. It's very annoying, but nothing else.

DOCTOR: Is there any pain in either eye?

PATIENT: No.

DOCTOR *(thinking)***:** *The flashes of light most likely are indicative of a posterior segment event, specifically vitreoretinal traction[1]; however, at this point I cannot rule out a neurologic event, such as the aura of migraine, vertebrobasilar insufficiency, or a transient ischemic attack, although they seem unlikely.*

DOCTOR: Do these floaters seem to be worse at any specific time?

PATIENT: The floaters are noticeable most of the time, but especially when the light is bright.

DOCTOR: Does the large floater in your left eye seem to move when you move your eyes, or is it stationary?

PATIENT: The big floater does seem to move about when I look in different directions, but it always seems to settle in the same place.

DOCTOR: Have you had any unusual sensations in other parts of your body associated with this condition, such as headache, nausea, vomiting, or numbness or weakness on the right side of your body?

PATIENT: No.

DOCTOR *(thinking)***:** *Because no associated symptoms have been noticed, I can be reasonably sure that this is not neurologic in nature. I still need to ensure a complete history by delving into the patient's medical background.*

DOCTOR: Has there been any recent injury to your eye, or have you ever had any eye injuries?

PATIENT: I haven't had any recent injuries that would coincide with this problem. I did have a fingernail scratch on my left cornea about 5 years ago. My optometrist in Chicago treated me for that and said I had fully recovered. Other than that, my eyes have been fine. I only need glasses for reading and my current glasses are fine.

DOCTOR *(thinking)***:** *The chief complaint is now fully elicited and established. I am reasonably certain that the floaters are organic in nature, and the* *etiology lies in the posterior segment. Now, I must investigate the patient's ocular and medical history.*

DOCTOR: How is your general health—do you have any problems with high blood pressure, diabetes, heart disease, or any other disorders?

PATIENT: Yes, I've had high blood pressure for the past 7 years, and I've had diabetes since I was about 40 years old. I've just recently had a physical, about 2 months ago, and my doctor says I'm fine otherwise.

DOCTOR *(thinking)***:** *The fact that the patient has a positive medical history of systemic vascular disease raises the very real possibility that he may have retinal neovascularization and associated vitreal hemorrhage, or even a tractional retinal detachment.*

DOCTOR: Are you taking any medications currently?

PATIENT: Yes, I'm using Lopressor for my blood pressure and Diabeta for the diabetes.

DOCTOR: Do you recall the results of your last physical, specifically your blood pressure and sugar readings?

PATIENT: My blood pressure was 130/88, and my sugar was 120. I monitor these numbers at home, and they're generally in this range.

DOCTOR *(thinking)***:** *As these values are considered within the normal and expected ranges, it is apparent that the patient is well-controlled and compliant with medical therapy. This may reduce the likelihood of retinal vasculopathy; however, even the best-controlled diabetics will develop vasculopathy given ample time.[2]*

DOCTOR: Is there anything else significant about your health or your family's health?

PATIENT: My father died at a young age from cancer; my mother was healthy her whole life. My children are all healthy.

DOCTOR: Do you have any allergies, particularly to any medications?

PATIENT: No, not as far as I am aware.

DOCTOR *(thinking)***:** *This medical history opens up an entire array of potential problems. Particularly with a long-standing history of hypertension and diabetes, this patient is at risk for significant retinal vasculopathies, such as vascular occlusions and diabetic retinopathy,[3, 4] which certainly might result in neovascular membrane formation and subsequent vitreal hemorrhage. Also, if the patient has suffered a vein occlusion, his symptoms could be directly attributable to the blood in the retina. The most likely possibility to consider, however, remains PVD, especially in light of the patient's age and history of floaters. If indeed this is a PVD, I must rule out associated retinal complications, such as tractional tears and detachment. This is a major concern because the patient did complain of flashing lights. Fortunately, as the flashes have ceased, the likelihood of a high-risk break is diminished. Finally, I must consider as a possible eti-*

ology vitreal inflammatory conditions, such as posterior uveitis or inflammatory chorioretinitis.

DOCTOR: Is there anything else you feel is important to tell me about your eyes or your vision before I begin the examination?

PATIENT: No.

DIAGNOSTIC HYPOTHESES

On the basis of the case history and patient profile, the initial list includes the following hypotheses:

1. *Posterior vitreous detachment.* On the basis of the patient's age, combined with a large, motile floater and associated flashes of light, PVD seems the most likely etiology. PVD is a common finding in patients over 60.[2] This condition has the tendency to be motile, as a result of its suspension in the vitreous cavity, although it tends to settle in the same position when the eye is stationary. If vitreoretinal traction exists, photopsia will occur on ocular movement. Thus, the patient will report flashes of light associated with the floater. If the traction is strong enough, a retinal break and subsequent detachment may occur as the most serious complication.

2. *Retinal detachment.* The patient experienced a significant increase in floaters in the left eye and also has experienced some flashes of light. Therefore, it is important to consider the possibility of retinal detachment.

3. *Vitreous hemorrhage.* Patients experiencing vitreal hemorrhage often complain of myriad floating spots that may appear to be dark or may be clear. Of course, a patient would need to have a predisposing condition to induce vitreal hemorrhage, such as a pre-existing neovascular membrane that ruptures and bleeds into the vitreous cavity. Retinal tears, whether traumatic or nontraumatic, also may cause hemorrhage into the vitreous cavity. Certainly, with a long-standing history of hypertension and diabetes, this patient has the necessary predisposing conditions to retinal neovascularization. The patient either may have had proliferative diabetic retinopathy or a long-standing, ischemic retinal vein occlusion. However, he did not report reduced acuity, whereas patients with vitreous hemorrhage often will have some degree of vision loss.[2]

4. *Posterior uveitis.* Posterior uveitis or any chorioretinal inflammatory condition associated with vitreal inflammatory cells (including intraocular tumors) can present with symptoms in much the same way as that seen in JP's case.[2, 5] Because many of these conditions are idiopathic, he is a prime candidate for such a disorder.

5.   *Asteroid hyalosis and vitreal syneresis.* These two common, yet benign, clinical entities can result in vitreal opacities. Asteroid hyalosis, despite its striking ophthalmoscopic presentation, is curiously asymptomatic in most cases. On the other hand, vitreal syneresis, a normal age-related degeneration of the vitreous, is a common cause of floaters in many patients. It certainly is possible that the degree of syneresis had progressed for JP. Vitreous syneresis is not easily observable ophthalmoscopically and often becomes a diagnosis of exclusion. This seems somewhat unlikely in this case, however, because of the reported large size of the new floater.

6.   *Retinal hemorrhages.* Retinal hemorrhages, such as those associated with a venous occlusion, can induce photopsia due to mechanical disruption of the photoreceptors by extravasated blood. The somewhat spotty nature of this hemorrhage may be interpreted as visual-field floaters reported by these patients, although there will be no mobility of these scotomata on eye movement. Also, because no retinal traction is present with this condition, the likelihood of associated flashes of light is very small.

DIAGNOSTIC TESTING

Because it is presumed that the most likely etiology of this condition lies in the posterior segment of the eye, confirmatory diagnosis was made by funduscopic examination through dilated pupils. However, I needed to complete a primary vision examination, because the patient had not had a full, comprehensive ocular evaluation for approximately 4 years. It is important to remember that a patient may have more than one disease or condition.

The following clinical database testing was performed initially: entering visual acuity at both distance and near and manifest refraction with associated visual acuity (Table CS18.1). Uncorrected visual acuity demonstrated minimal refractive error; manifest refraction showed mild hyperopic astigmatism and presbyopia, which are noncontributory to the patient's chief complaint. However, the fact that a final acuity of 20/20 in each eye was obtainable may help to rule out significant vitreal hemorrhage.

Additionally, I performed a neuro-ophthalmic screening, the clinical results of which are presented in Table CS18.2, which included:

- Pupillary reflexes
- Ocular posture and motilities
- Confrontation visual-field testing

Table CS18.1
Database testing results.

Entering visual acuity
    20/20 OD, 20/25 OS at 6 m
    20/20 OD, OS at 40 cm with +2.25 DS OU reading prescription
Manifest refraction and visual acuities
    OD +0.25 –0.25 × 120 (20/20)
    OS +0.25 –0.75 × 069 (20/20)
    OU +2.25 D (age-appropriate) add; 20/20 at 40 cm

DS = diopter sphere.

Table CS18.2
Database testing results of neuro-ophthalmic screening.

Pupils
    PERRL, –APD
    No anisocoria noted in bright or dim illumination
Cover test: orthophoria at distance; 6Δ exophoria at 40 cm
Extraocular motilities: full range of motion OU, without pain or diplopia
Confrontation visual fields: full in all quadrants OD, OS

PERRL = pupils equal, round, reactive to light; –APD = no afferent pupillary defect.

This testing revealed normal findings. The fact that no relative afferent pupillary defect was discovered in the left eye indicated that profound retinal hemorrhage with ischemia was unlikely, as was extensive retinal detachment. The likelihood of extensive vitreal hemorrhage was further refuted by normal confrontation fields.

The results of biomicroscopy and applanation tonometry are presented in Table CS18.3. Biomicroscopy demonstrated normal and consistent senescent changes. Intraocular tensions were unexpectedly elevated, but this was not especially diagnostic with regard to the chief complaint. However, further investigation into the possibility of glaucoma was warranted.

Dilated fundus examination (Table CS18.4) revealed a large annular membrane within the vitreous cavity of the left eye, confirming my diagnostic hypothesis of PVD. In addition, the absence of any vitreal hemorrhage or retinal break indicated that this was, at least initially, an uncomplicated PVD. All other diagnostic possibilities, including posterior uveitis, asteroid hyalosis, and retinal hemorrhage were ruled out by ophthalmoscopic observation. When considered along with the elevated intraocular pressure in both eyes, the moderate optic nerve head

Table CS18.3
Database testing results of biomicroscopy and applanation tonometry.

Biomicroscopy
   Lids, lashes: unremarkable OU
   Conjunctiva: unremarkable OU
   Cornea: mild arcus OU
   Tear break-up time: 12 secs OD, 13 secs OS
   Anterior chamber: deep, quiet OU
   Iris: flat, mild stromal atrophy OU
   Lens: early nuclear sclerosis with mild cortical spoking OD > OS
   Anterior vitreous: free of cells and pigment OU
Applanation tonometry: 29 mm Hg OD, 27 mm Hg OS at 9:15 AM

Table CS18.4
Hypotheses 1–6: problem-specific testing results via dilated fundus examination.

Posterior vitreous: free of cells and hemorrhage OU; large annular membrane noted inferior temporal to the optic disc OS
Optic nerve
   Distinct margins without pallor OU
   Cup-to-disc ratio: 0.4/0.5 OD, 0.5/0.5 OS
   No neovascular membranes noted OU
Macula: flat, dim foveal reflex present OU
Vasculature: mild arteriolosclerosis with focal A/V constriction OU
Background: mild presence of dot and blot hemorrhages with rare nerve fiber–layer hemorrhage, paramacular exudate without retinal thickening OU
Periphery: focal chorioretinal atrophy inferiorly OD > OS; no neovascular membranes noted OU; no retinal breaks or elevations seen OU

A/V = arteriovenous.

cupping may be indicative of glaucoma, which is an additional diagnostic hypothesis uncovered during testing.

DIAGNOSTIC SUMMARY

JP was found to have an uncomplicated PVD of the left eye. It was deemed uncomplicated because there was no evidence of vitreal hemorrhage or retinal breaks. However, this is not to say that complications may not arise at a later time. Most commonly, sequelae such as tractional retinal breaks or vitreal hemorrhages may occur within the 6 weeks immediately following the PVD. Beyond 6 weeks, the risk of complications is greatly diminished, and the condition generally is considered an ocular annoyance, as noted by this patient.

In some cases of PVD, the clinician may observe a small area of hemorrhage settled in the inferior fundus. This finding may be particularly ominous, as it strongly suggests a ruptured blood vessel due to a tractional retinal tear. In cases of small preretinal hemorrhage, however, the etiology may be merely an area of retinal capillary rupture, secondary to the detached posterior hyaloid face. In this situation, the retina itself remains intact. The clinician must still consider the worst possible scenario and examine closely for retinal breaks; scleral indentation and Goldmann contact lens funduscopy are indicated. Even if no retinal break is discovered, the possibility of an occult tear still does exist, and the patient should be re-examined every 2 weeks for the ensuing 6-week period. After 6 weeks, should the hemorrhage remain stable or resolve and no break be discovered, the patient is considered out of danger. Though retinal breaks secondary to PVD may exist without rhegmatogenous retinal detachment ensuing, the fresh break possesses no proved record for remaining stable.[6] In those cases in which the PVD leads to a tractional retinal break, popular thinking indicates that prophylactic retinal sealing be initiated. Referral to a qualified retinal surgeon for consultation and laser photocoagulation or cryopexy is indicated in these circumstances.

TREATMENT OPTIONS

The patient was rescheduled for a follow-up visit in 6 weeks, at which time the fundus would be re-examined with dilation and indirect ophthalmoscopy to rule out late complications. In the interim, the patient was instructed to self-monitor for any change in the status of the floaters or related photopsia. Should this occur, the patient was directed to return immediately. It is important to note, incidentally, that JP also manifests significantly elevated intraocular pressures and moderate optic nerve head cupping. Though unrelated to the chief complaint or to the final diagnosis of PVD, this finding underscores the need for obtaining a comprehensive database in all cases, rather than simply a problem-oriented examination. Ultimately, JP also will require a full workup with respect to glaucoma. At the follow-up visit, tonometry must be performed to establish a diurnal pressure curve. Gonioscopy as well as automated threshold perimetry also must be conducted at that time.

REFERENCES

1. Byer NE. The natural history of asymptomatic retinal breaks. Ophthalmology 1982;89:1033–1039.
2. Alexander LJ. Primary Care of the Posterior Segment (2nd ed). Norwalk, CT: Appleton & Lange, 1994.
3. Cohen RJ, Sowka JW. Hemi-central retinal vein occlusion. Clin Eye Vision Care 1993;5:154–157.
4. Sowka JW. How to identify retinal vessel occlusions. Rev Optom 1993;130:53–60.
5. Kabat AG. Primary ocular tumors: a threat to eyes and lives. Rev Optom 1994;131(4):98–107.
6. Sowka JW. How to manage retinal breaks. Rev Optom 1991;128(10):70–79.

Appendix: Case Scenario 18

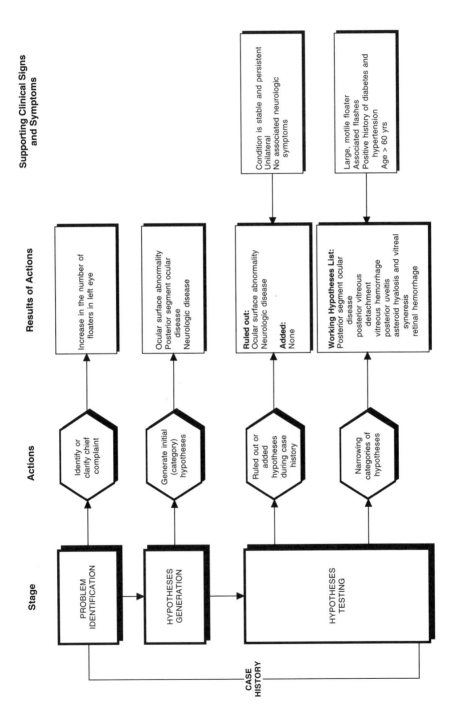

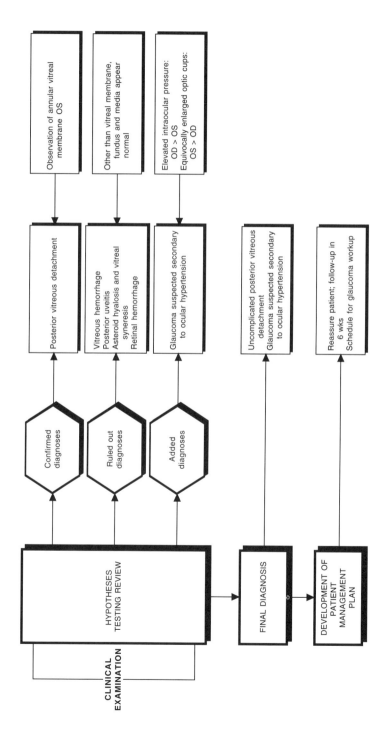

Case Scenario 18 decision-making summary.

Appendix

Key to Diagnosis of Case Scenarios

Case Scenario	Primary	Secondary
	Diagnosis/Topic	
1	Anisometropic amblyopia	Hyperopic astigmatism
2	Blepharitis (chronic staphyococcal)	None
3	Cataract	Hyperopic astigmatism
4	Conjunctivitis (bacterial)	Presbyopia; convergence insufficiency
5	Diabetes mellitus	Hyperopia; presbyopia; mild non-proliferative diabetic retinopathy; possible systemic hypertension
6	Dry eye (keratocon-junctivitis sicca)	Presbyopia; hyperopic astigmatism; blepharitis; meibomianitis
7	Glaucoma (open-angle)	Presbyopia; hyperopic astigmatism
8	Hypertension	Branch retinal vein occlusion; meibomianitis; presbyopia; myopic astigmatism
9	Keratoconus	Myopic astigmatism
10	Macular degeneration	Subretinal neovascularization; presbyopia; hyperopic astigmatism
11	Neovascularization (corneal)	Seborrheic meibomianitis; myopic astigmatism
12	Convergence insufficiency	Accommodative insufficiency and facility; oculomotor dysfunction; hyperopic astigmatism
13	Presbyopia (ophthalmic optics problem)	Hyperopia
14	Presbyopia (incipient)	Hyperopia
15	Anisocoria (Adie's pupil)	Hyperopia; accommodative insufficiency
16	Hyperopia	Developmental vision information–processing dysfunction; oculomotor dysfunction
17	Accommodative esotropia	Hyperopia
18	Posterior vitreous detachment	Presbyopia; hyperopic astigmatism; possible glaucoma

Index

Accommodative anomaly, 262, 306, 309, 362
   diagnostic testing for, 264
Accommodative esotropia, 381–382
   diagnostic testing for, 378–380
   nonrefractive, 377
   partially, 377–378
   refractive, 377
Acne rosacea, 157–158
Acquired immunodeficiency syndrome (AIDS), 118
Acute angle-closure glaucoma, 7
Acute iritis, 7
Adie's pupil, 351, 352
   treatment options, 352–353
Albinism, 5–6
Algorithmic reasoning model, 4
   for red eye, 5
Allergic conjunctivitis, 7, 10, 13, 191
   diagnostic testing for, 192
Allergic disorders, incidence of, 72
Allergies, 222
Amblyopia
   anisometropic, 142–143, 145–146
      diagnostic testing for, 146, 148
   deprivation, 142
   disease rates for, 74
   functional, 142
   isoametropic, 142–143, 145
   strabismic, 142–143, 145–146
      diagnostic testing for, 146, 378
America Online (AOL), 123
American Academy of Ophthalmology, 108, 112, 121, 123
American Optometric Association, 27, 108, 112, 121, 123
   code of ethics, 127

Amsler's grid test, 76, 175, 278
Anchoring, 16, 17
Angiography, fluorescein, 76
Angle-closure glaucoma, acute, 7
Anisocoria, 347, 349–350
Anisometropic amblyopia, 142–143, 145–146, 148
   diagnostic testing for, 146
   treatment, 149
Anterior ischemic optic neuropathy, 275
Anterior segment pathology, 143–144
Arteriolar sclerosis, 250
Artificial intelligence (AI), 53
Asteroid hyalosis, 393
Astigmatism
   disease rates for, 73
   irregular, 262
      diagnostic testing for, 264
Atrophic macular degeneration, 275

Bacterial conjunctivitis, 7, 10, 13, 191, 195
   diagnostic testing for, 192
   treatment for, 195–196
Bayes' theorem, 85–89
Biomedical literature, 101–124
   categories,
      primary, 102
      secondary, 103
      tertiary, 103
   information management skills, 116–117
   interpersonal sources, 104
   managing reprint collections, 115–116
   online services, 103
   organization of, 102–105

Online services, 103
America Online (AOL), 123
CompuServe, 123
Internet, 112–114
MEDLINE, 102, 109–111, 122
Prodigy, 123
VISIONET, 110, 122
World Wide Web (WWW),
113–114
Open-angle glaucoma (OAG), 206,
233, 239–240
treatment for, 240
Optic nerve dysfunction, 233, 250
diagnostic testing for, 238, 277
Orinda study, 363

PALs. *See* Progressive-addition lenses
(PALs)
Papyrus, 124
Parallel testing, 90
Parsimony, law of, 33
Partially accommodative esotropia,
377–378
Patients
avoiding prejudice toward,
131–132
biomedical information for,
111–112, 123
confidentiality and, 131
giving compassionate care to,
128–129
individuality of, 132
keeping their best interests,
127–128
medical ethics and. *See* Ethics
providing appropriate information
to, 130–131
referring to other doctors, 129–130
understanding, 128
unfamiliarity with, 16, 21–22
Pattern recognition, for red eye, 5–6
Pattern recognition model, 4–6
Period prevalence, 69

Peripheral corneal desiccation (PCD),
290
diagnostic testing for, 292
Photophobia, 347
Photostress test, 278
Point prevalence, 69
Positive fusional convergence (PFC), 306
Posterior segment pathology, 143–144
Posterior subcapsular cataracts, risk
factors for, 76
Posterior uveitis, 392
Posterior vitreous detachment (PVD),
250, 252–253, 392, 395–396
diagnostic testing for, 252–253
treatment for, 396
Postoperative endophthalmitis, risk
factors for, 76
Preretinal hemorrhage, 250
diagnostic testing for, 253
Presbyopia, 191, 205, 210, 275
diagnostic testing for, 193,
206–207, 223, 336, 337
incipient, 335, 338–340
Prevalence
definition, 67
period, 69
point, 69
positive predictive value vs., 82
Prevalence rates, 69–70. *See also*
Disease rates
durations of disease and, 69
examples of studies, 70
Progressive-addition lenses (PALs)
case scenario involving, 317–331
diagnostic testing for, 320–325
improper fitting of, 319
overplussing of, 318–319, 324, 325
patient having adaptation problems, 319–320
treatment for wearers of, 326–327
Pseudodiagnosticity, 16, 17–18
Psychogenic etiology, 347
Psychogenic symptomatology, 306